1

What Are Minerals?

WHEN it comes to human nutrition, the vitamins seem to hog the headlines, leaving the minerals to play catch-up. But, as important as vitamins are, we could not live very long without minerals and trace minerals. Some of the obvious health conditions involving minerals include calcium, magnesium and boron in preventing osteoporosis; iron in preventing life-threatening iron-deficiency anemia; iodine in deterring goiter; magnesium and selenium in keeping our hearts healthy.

Minerals, which are naturally formed homogeneous solids with a definite chemical composition, were among the first substances that people used and described. Egyptian paintings of 5,000 years ago reveal that minerals were used in weapons and jewelry, as well as in religious ceremonies. Theophrastus, the Greek natural scientist, wrote a short work on minerals about 300 B.C. Pliny the Elder of Rome wrote about metals, ores, stones and gems around A.D. 77. Other early studies of minerals, such as those by German scientists, included *De Mineralibus* (1262), by Albertus Magnus, and *De Re Metallica* (1556), by Georgius Agricola.

The scientific study of mineral crystals began about 1665, when Robert Hooke, an English scientist, reported that metal balls piled in different ways duplicated the shapes of alum crystals. And in 1669, Nicolaus Steno, a Danish physician, found that the angles between the faces of quartz crystals were always the same, even though the crystals had different shapes. By the late 1700s, scientists had studied many minerals, but they had yet to determine the makeup of crystals and the reasons for their shape. In 1772, Romé de l'Isle, a French scientist, postulated that Steno's discovery could be explained only if the crystals were composed of identical units stacked together in a regular way. During the 1780s, René J. Haüy, another Frenchman, made further investigations into mineral units, calling them integral molecules. About this time chemists began to develop a clearer understanding of the nature of chemical elements. Although mineralogists found that minerals were made up of chemicals, they still did not understand their structure. It would be some time before the major classes of minerals, based on their composition and structure, e.g., sulfides, halides, carbonates, sulfates, oxides, phosphates, silicates, etc., were fully understood.

With the invention of the X-ray scientists found the key to the internal structure of minerals. Scientists later learned how atoms are arranged into unit cells and, in turn, into crystals. By the 1930s, scientists had used X-rays to study and describe many different minerals. Today, new laboratory instruments are changing the study of minerals. The electron probe microanalyzer, linked to a computer, can measure changes in the chemical composition of a single crystal. A scanning electron microscope magnifies crystals many thousands of times beyond normal size. Scientists can photograph the shadows or reflections of atoms and molecules with an electron microscope to observe the internal structure of a mineral crystal.

CLASSES OF MINERALS

Several schemes have been devised for classifying minerals. The most accepted method is based on chemical composition, therefore, the following classes can be identified:

- Native elements
- Sulfides
- Oxides and hydroxides
- Halides
- Carbonates, nitrates, borates and iodates
- Sulfates, chromates, molybdates and tungstates
- Phosphates, arsenates and vandates
- Silicates

Of these classes, silicates are the most common, since silica is the most abundant component of the earth's crust, representing about 60 percent.

Since the names of some minerals are so old, their origins are unknown. However, with the development of mineralogical science at the end of the 18th century, the use of a single name for each species was established. The name of a mineral species is often given by its discoverer and the name often ends in "ite." Some of the names are derived from Greek or Latin words that help to describe the mineral, such as color (albite, from the Latin word for white, *albus*); crystal shape (sphene, from the Greek *sphen,* wedge); or density (barite, from Greek *barys,* heavy). Some of the names indicate chemical composition (calcite, zincite). As might be expected, minerals were named after mineralogists, mineral collectors, mine owners or public figures. Anglesite was named from the island of Anglesey, which is off the coast of Wales; aragonite is named after Aragon in Spain; and franklinite gets its name from Franklin, New Jersey, where it occurs as the dominant zinc mineral. Chromite gets its name because of the presence of a large amount of chromium in the mineral; magnetite because of its magnetic properties; and sillimanite is named after Professor Benjamin Silliman of Yale University.

When referring to human nutrition, the word mineral refers to certain chemical elements which are found in the ash after a food or body tissue has been burned and inspected. Some of the elements in the residue are essential to the proper functioning of the body and must be regularly supplied by the diet. Other elements, although essential, enter the body by various means. The essential minerals are referred to as "inorganic" nutrients, to distinguish them from the "organic" or carbon-containing nutrients, such as carbohydrates, fats, proteins and vitamins.

Essential elements are considered macrominerals or microminerals, depending upon the quantity which is required in the diet. Macrominerals include calcium, phosphorus, sodium, chlorine, magnesium, potassium and sulfur. Required daily amounts range from a few tenths of a gram to one or more grams. Microminerals are also known as trace elements, because they are required in minute quantities, ranging from millionths of a gram (micrograms) to thousandths of a gram (milligrams) per day. The trace elements known to be essential for humans are chromium, cobalt, copper, fluorine, iodine, iron, manganese, molybdenum, selenium, silicon and zinc. Arsenic, vanadium, tin and nickel may be added to the list.[1] Mineral deficiencies have been recognized and treated for thousands of years even though people did not fully understand the bases of these treatments. As an example, a Chinese document dated around 3000 B.C. described goiter and recommended that these patients eat seaweed and burnt sponge, which are reliable sources of iodine. Around the time of Hippocrates, or about 4th century

B.C., the Greeks gave those with anemia iron-containing water in which heated swords had been dipped.[1]

The breakthroughs in understanding the functions of minerals in the body did not come for many centuries, because research laboratories were not developed until the Renaissance. However, there is evidence that medieval alchemists may have invented some of the techniques and tools of chemistry as they attempted to change base metals into gold. In addition, all of the elements that are essential for human life are so highly reactive that they are usually found in chemical combinations with other elements, except when they are found in small amounts as charged particles (ions) in the blood. A breakthrough came in 1669, when the German alchemist Hennig Brand identified the highly combustible and toxic phosphorus as a constituent of a compound in human urine.

French chemist Antoine L. Lavoisier (1743–1794), who is credited as being the founder of the science of nutrition, predicted that such elements as sodium and potassium would soon be discovered, because he believed that they were present in mineral compounds then known as "earths." Lavoisier also discovered that oxygen, which he named, had a function in combustion and that a strict analogy occurred between combustion and human respiration. He was guillotined by the French revolutionists. British chemist Sir Humphry Davy (1778–1829) discovered sodium, potassium and other elements a few years later. He was so highly regarded by the French Academy that, in 1806, they awarded him their Volta medal, even though France and England were at war at the time the award was presented. Davy discovered the anesthetic properties of nitrous oxide by experimenting on himself and recognized its possibilities as an anesthetic during surgical operations. In addition to separating sodium and potassium from their salts, he did the same for barium, calcium and strontium. He also invented a safety lamp for coal miners.[2]

Progress in mineral research then began to accelerate. Baron Jons Berzelius, a Swedish chemist (1779–1848) added to our knowledge by: reporting his analysis of the calcium and phosphorus content of bone in 1801; and concluding in 1838 that the iron in hemoglobin made it possible for the blood to absorb oxygen. In 1822, French chemist Boussingault reported that South American villagers who used salt containing iodine were protected from goiter. Through animal feeding trials, Boussingault discovered the necessity of providing calcium and iron in the diet. Chossat, a Swiss physician, won a prize in 1840 for demonstrating that the addition of calcium carbonate to a diet of wheat and water improved bone growth in pigeons.

From the mid-19th century to the present, most of the great advances in mineral knowledge involved the trace minerals. From 1850 to 1876, French chemist Chatin analyzed the iodine content in soil and water from various regions where cretinism and goiter were prevalent. He tried, without success, to convince his contemporaries that these diseases were due to a lack of iodine. It would be almost another half century before the value of iodine became widely accepted. That accomplishment was attributed to the German biochemist Baumann who, in 1895, discovered that the thyroid gland contained iodine. Between 1907 and 1918, American medical scientist Marine and his colleagues found that a small amount of iodine prevented goiter in animals and in schoolchildren.[1]

Various minerals were found to be required by animals and man, as indicated by the dates of the discoveries: phosphorus, 1918; copper, 1925; magnesium, manganese and molybdenum, 1931; zinc, 1934; and cobalt, 1935. Even though they were known to be essential, there was often uncertainty as to the metabolic roles of minerals. It was not until 1948 that it was determined that cobalt functions as a component of vitamin B12. Between the 1930s and the 1950s, much was learned about the function of these essential elements in the body.[2]

Throughout the rest of this book, we will explore the merits of each mineral individually, examining those that are essential to our health as well as those that may cause us undue agony.

REFERENCES

1. Ensminger, Audrey H., et al. *Foods and Nutrition Encyclopedia*. Clovis, Calif.: Pegus Press, 1983, pp. 1508ff.
2. *Stedman's Medical Dictionary*. Baltimore: The Williams and Wilkins Company, 1976, pp. 361, 762.

2

Why Do We Need Minerals?

MANY people in the United States consume plenty of food, but it is not necessarily the right kind of food. Statistically, studies have concluded that almost two-thirds of an average American's diet is made up of fats and refined sugars having low to no nutrient density. This contributes to nutrient deficiencies that can rob the body of its natural resistance to disease and premature aging, while also weakening its overall physiological and psychological performance. The remaining one-third of the average diet is counted on for the essential nutrients needed to maintain health, which may or may not be from high nutrient dense food.

The U.S. Department of Agriculture has found that a significant number of Americans receive well under 70 percent of the Recommended Dietary Allowance (RDA) for vitamin A, vitamin C, the B-complex vitamins, calcium, magnesium and iron. Another study reported that many typical diets contained less than 80 percent of the RDA for calcium, magnesium, iron, zinc, copper and manganese.[1]

Historically, doctors and nutritional scientists only recognized nutritional deficiencies if they actually manifested as diseases such as beriberi, pellagra or rickets. If a patient had no overt symptoms or disease, he or she was regarded as healthy and adequately nourished. Today, doctors and scientists are beginning to recognize mild and moderate nutritional deficiencies, the symptoms of which may often be subtle, overlapping and varied, according to D. Lindsey Berkson, M.A., D.C., a nutritionist in Santa Fe, New Mexico. "Many times these symptoms are taken for granted as being part of the aging process. [Nutrionally oriented] doctors and scientists are learning, however, that these symptoms are actually subtle deficiency signs that can be responsive to nutrient supplementation and dietary improvement. Greater understanding and better testing methods are leading to the diagnosis of more and more subtle nutrient imbalances."[1]

Paul Dudley White, M.D., the eminent cardiologist, spoke in 1971 about the epidemic nature of coronary thrombosis. "I want to emphasize," White said, "that heart disease truly is an epidemic today, a fact that many people seem to refuse to accept. . . . Your generation has become so used to the specter of heart attacks, you don't even conceive of life free from this danger. But remember, when I was an intern at Massachusetts General Hospital in 1911 there was no Department of Cardiology."[2]

Coronary thrombosis was initially reported by Dr. George Dock, who wrote about his discovery in the *Journal of the American Medical Association* in 1939. But the disease was an obscure medical curiosity in 1912, when Dr. J. B. Herrick, a Chicago physician, discussed six cases in *JAMA*.[2]

When White set up the first cardiology laboratory in 1920, coronary thrombosis was so uncommon that most medical students did not know of the disease until after their formal training. Although White brought a crude electrocardiograph back from a European trip in 1914, the modern electrocardiograph did not appear until 1944. And it was not until the 1950s that physicians began routinely monitoring blood levels of cholesterol due to the steadily increasing death rate from heart disease.[2]

PROGRESS BRINGS GROSS DEFICIENCIES

The grains that compose our processed white flour and breads are more of the malignant calories Americans eat that contribute to malnutrition and ill health, according to R. O. Brennan, D.O., in *Nutrigenetics*. The industrial age of the late 18th century changed the milling process of grains, he said. Grains were once prepared for cooking by being ground in a stone mill, and as much as 85 percent of the whole grain remained in the flour with this method. Brennan added:

> The advent of the industrial age and a growing population with an increased demand for bread and mercantile pressures brought the rolling mill. The new mill could produce much more flour than the stone mill, but unfortunately it generated enough heat to destroy most of the grain's protein along with wheat germ and its oil. It removed the outer coating of the grain as well as its hull and, in so doing, removed most of the nutrients and bulk we need. The flour was bleached, aged and preserved, usually with chlorine dioxide. The chemical further destroyed many essential oils and amino acids. What was left was the grain's starch. The new process made grain much like sugar, full of quick, short-lived energy, but lacking constructive, long-term power.[3]

Brennan added that 75 percent of the value of the natural whole grain was extracted, and, while producing flour for white bread, the following nutrients were removed during the milling process:

TABLE 2.1

DEFICIENCY

NUTRIENT	% REMOVED	CAUSES	IS LINKED TO
Vitamin A	90%	Poor vision	Arthritis and reproductive failure
Vitamin B1	77%	Appetite control; beriberi	Mental illness, heart damage and mental retardation
Vitamin B2	80%		Congenital defects, rheumatoid arthritis and mucous membrane difficulties
Vitamin B3	81%	Pellagra	Mental illness and rheumatoid arthritis
Vitamin B6	72%	Insufficiency in using amino acids	Convulsive seizures, arthritis and mental illness
Vitamin B12	77%		Genetic damage
Pantothenic acid	50%	Inability to produce steroid hormones	Infertility, congenital defects and mental disease
Vitamin D	90%	Difficulty in using calcium, phosphorus	
Vitamin E	86%	Weakness in cell membranes	Heart disease and aging
Folic Acid	67%		Genetic damage, congenital defects, infertility, mental illness, some cancers and heart disease

NUTRIENT	% REMOVED	CAUSES	IS LINKED TO
Calcium	60%	Poor bone formation	Infertility
Chromium	40%		Heart disease and diabetes
Cobalt	89%	Poor red blood cell development	Sterility
Iron	76%	Anemia	Obstetrical complications
Magnesium	85%	Improper energy exchange within cells	Alcoholism, mental illness and heart disease
Manganese	86%		Sterility and mental illness
Phosphorus	71%	Improper energy exchange throughout the body	Congenital defects and infertility
Potassium	77%	Imbalance in cellular fluid regulation	Mental illness
Selenium	16%		Liver deterioration
Sodium	78%	Imbalance of body fluids	Infertility
Choline (related to B-complex)	30%	Instability of cell membrane	Some cancers and heart disease
Zinc	78%		Congenital deficiencies and infertility[3]

"The flour industry did nothing to improve its product until it was pressured to do [so] in 1941," Brennan continued. "The resulting 'enrichment', however, meant replacement of thiamine (B1), riboflavin (B2), niacin (B3) and iron. That was all. Processing took out parts of 22 elements. The industry put back parts of four. The flour industry has not bothered to add another nutrient in over 30 years, in spite of continued research that revealed many additional bodily needs from grain's natural ingredients. In fact, 60 percent less vitamin fortification is added to flour today than it was 20 years ago. The food is still deficient. Yet the bakers of white bread are allowed to print the word 'enriched' on their labels. Nutritionist Roger J. Williams notes that rats given a diet of this 'enriched' bread either died or became stunted."[3]

Mineral insufficiency and trace-element insufficiency states are actually more likely to occur than are vitamin-insufficient states, according to Sheldon Saul Hendler, M.D., Ph.D., in *The Doctors' Vitamin and Mineral Encyclopedia.* Those at increased risk of such insufficiencies include people who eat low-calorie diets, the elderly, pregnant women, people on certain drugs (such as diuretics), vegetarians and those living where the soil is deficient in certain minerals. Vitamins are usually present in foods in similar amounts throughout the world, but this is not true of the minerals, Hendler added. Because of differing geological conditions, minerals and trace elements may be scarce in the soils of certain regions and rich in those of other regions. As an example, the soil of South Dakota is very rich in selenium, while the soil in certain parts of China and New Zealand is very poor in this element. Thus, you can live in some areas, eat a perfectly "balanced" diet and still develop mineral deficiencies or trace-element deficiencies that can only be averted through dietary change or supplementation, he said.[4]

There is increasing evidence, Hendler continued, that those whose nutritional status is suboptimal in certain trace elements, such as selenium, may be at greater risk for certain forms of cancer and heart disease. But suboptimal intake can be due to factors other than soil depletion. These factors are as diverse as the effects of acid rain and the overrefining, overprocessing of foods. Hendler added:

> Our vulnerability to even minute dietary imbalances in minerals can be appreciated by comparing our daily mineral intake (about 1.5 grams) with our total intake of carbohydrates, proteins and lipids (about 500 grams). Thus our mineral intake represents only about 0.3 percent of our total intake of nutrients, yet they are so potent and so important that without them we wouldn't be able to utilize the other 99.7 percent of foodstuffs and would quickly perish. Our total daily intake of zinc accounts for only 0.003 percent of our total nutrient intake. So it becomes easier to see how even what would seem to be a tiny decrease in zinc intake can have an enormous negative impact on health, especially if that decrease persists.[4]

In his book *Natural Prescriptions*, Robert M. Giller, M.D., recommends that everyone should take a good-quality multiple-vitamin-mineral supplement and/ or supplements daily. For those who are confused about which supplements to buy, and who have to spend a lot of time reading labels, he said that the daily supplement should have approximately 50 mg of the most important B vitamins B1, B2 and B6. He has found that a multiple that contains at least this amount of the Bs will be balanced and will also contain a good range of other vitamins, minerals and trace minerals. Be sure to check the dosage instructions on the label, since some products must be taken two or three times daily.[5]

Giller does not believe that many of the vitamin-mineral supplements contain enough of the antioxidant vitamins and minerals that are needed for optimum health. He thinks these amounts are important: vitamin C, 1,000 mg; vitamin E (400 to 600 IU); beta-carotene (10,000 to 25,000 IU); and selenium (100 to 200 mcg). If your supplement does not fall within these ranges, he recommends that, in addition to your daily vitamin/mineral supplement, you take the following: vitamin C (500 mg); vitamin E (200 IU); beta-carotene (10,000 IU); and selenium (50 mcg).[5]

REFERENCES

1. Goldberg Group, The Burton. *Alternative Medicine:* The Definitive Guide. Puyallup, Wash.: Future Medicine Publishing, Inc., 1993, pp. 386ff.
2. Passwater, Richard, Ph.D. *Supernutrition for Healthy Hearts.* New York: The Dial Press, 1977, pp. 11, 14–15.
3. Brennan, R. O., D.O. *Nutrigenetics.* New York: M. Evans and Co., Inc., 1975, pp. 43ff.
4. Hendler, Sheldon Saul, M.D., Ph.D. *The Doctors' Vitamin and Mineral Encyclopedia.* New York: Simon and Schuster, 1990, pp. 112ff.
5. Giller, Robert M., M.D., and Matthews, Kathy. *Natural Prescriptions.* New York: Carol Southern Books, 1994, pp. XXIV, XXV.

High-Fiber Diets and Minerals

ONE of the controversies among nutritionists and scientific researchers is whether or not a high-fiber diet, especially one that includes whole grain cereals, binds to minerals and takes them out of the body before they are fully utilized. Since whole grains are a reliable source of many minerals, there doesn't seem to be much logic to the controversy.

However, in the January 1, 1976 issue of *The New England Journal of Medicine,* Shela W. Bordin and Gerald M. Bordin, M.D., of the University of New Mexico at Albuquerque, said that "bran enthusiasts should be advised that daily consumption of large amounts of the sawdust-like flakes may adversely affect iron absorption. However, bran buffs have no need to despair. Happily, ascorbic acid (vitamin C), among others, has been demonstrated to enhance iron absorption."

The Bordins added that, in addition to its fiber content, greater levels of iron and calcium are found in the bran layer than in other parts of the wheat kernel. As with the seeds of corn, rice, soybeans and peanuts, bran contains a large amount of phytic acid and that this compound reduces the degree of absorption of iron, as well as calcium, zinc and manganese from the small intestine.

"Phytate in the diet appears to exert its greatest influence upon iron absorption," the Bordins continued. "Experimentally, sodium phytate introduced into the diet resulted in a 'significant' reduction of iron absorption. Whether the amounts of phytates normally ingested in the diet are of practical importance for iron absorption is questioned."[1]

An article in the January 15, 1992 issue of *Family Practice News* reported that iron containing foods include fortified cereals, enriched grains, dried beans and fruit, peas and spinach, but that "iron from these foods is difficult to absorb. Inhibitors of iron absorption include calcium, fiber, bran, tannic acid in tea, phosphates and phytates. Iron absorption is autoregulated to a certain extent. Children who are iron deficient will absorb more dietary iron than those who have adequate iron stores."[2]

The concern that dietary fiber may inhibit mineral absorption, thus contributing to mineral deficiencies and such conditions as osteoporosis and anemia, may be unfounded, reported K. Behall, et al., in the *American Journal of Clinical Nutrition* in 1987. The researchers, from the USDA Beltsville Human Nutrition Research Center and the University of Maryland, gave volunteers one of three diets. They were given either a basic diet or one supplemented with an insoluble fiber cellulose or one with two added soluble fibers, locust bean gum or karaya gum. The fiber content was 7.5 grams per 1,000 calories. During the final eight days of the one-month trial, the researchers collected urine and fecal samples from the volunteers, analyzing the collections for weight and mineral content.[3]

Final results of the study showed that the insoluble fiber, cellulose, had an adverse effect on manganese absorption, but did not affect the absorption of calcium, magnesium, iron, copper or zinc. In addition, the soluble gum fibers had no effect on mineral absorption, while karaya gum improved the absorption of all minerals that were tested. The research team concluded that soluble fibers, such as the gums, which have a hypocholesterolemic effect in the treatment and prevention of cardiovascular disease, do not adversely affect mineral status. In fact, these fibers might improve the absorption of minerals in those persons consuming the Recommended Dietary Allowances for these nutrients.[3]

Some studies show that high-fiber foods may decrease the availability of calcium, magnesium, zinc and iron, but there is a problem with the research, according to *The Natural Healing and Nutrition Annual* of 1989. It seems that it is difficult to sort out the effects of fiber from the effects of other components in high-fiber foods.[4]

Wheat bran, for example contains phytate. There is reason to believe that phytate is responsible for tying up minerals, or that a combination of fiber and phytate is responsible. In spinach, for example, oxalic acid may be the culprit, but scientists believe that the responsible substances combine with minerals to make complexes that your body can't absorb.

"There *is* some effect," said Eugene Morris, Ph.D., a research biochemist at the USDA facility in Beltsville, Maryland. "We're just not sure yet how great it is or exactly what is causing it."[4]

June Kelsay, Ph.D., a research nutritionist at the Maryland research center, indicated that too much fiber and too little minerals might cause a problem. However, over a period of time, the body may adjust to this decreased availability. "So there is probably no adverse effect even when eating 30 to 35 grams of total dietary fiber a day. It would be hard to eat any more than that because of the volume of food you'd have to consume," said Kelsay.

Morris agreed, adding that, "It's my opinion that if you're eating a lot of fiber, you should make sure you're also consuming at least the RDA of minerals. If you're getting enough minerals to start with, you're probably safe."[4]

Speaking at the annual meeting of the Federation of American Societies for Experimental Biology in Anaheim, California, in 1980, Morris added whole wheat to the list of foods that provide iron and several other minerals in digestible form.

"Whole wheat contains important amounts of minerals," Morris said. "But until now it was reported they were unavailable nutritionally because they were linked to phytate. Phytate is present in cereal bran or husks at higher levels than in most other foods. Some texts have suggested that the phytate in wheat bran not only makes iron in wheat unavailable, but it also interferes with absorption of iron in meat and other foods. But," he added, "when men participating in our research ate whole wheat in normal amounts, the whole wheat actually contributed to the body's absorption of minerals, rather than subtracting from it."[5]

During the study, 10 men consumed 36 grams a day of wheat bran in muffins for 30 days. Five of the men ate phytate-free muffins with their meals for 15 days and then ate muffins with bran containing phytate for 15 days. It was easy to remove the phytate from the bran through a simple soaking process. Another group of men ate the muffins in reverse sequence. All other foods used in the Beltsville study were low in fiber and phytate. The researchers studied iron, zinc, magnesium, manganese, copper and calcium, and nutritional availability was ascertained by determining the difference between minerals in the food eaten and minerals excreted in the volunteers' urine and feces. All of the minerals were in positive balance, meaning that intake was greater than excretion.

"This indicates," Morris said, "that the men were absorbing the minerals. The sequence in which they ate the two types of bran influenced the balance, but average balances were not greatly affected by the two levels of phytate consumed."[5]

Morris admitted that the findings, although adding to nutrition knowledge, leave some questions unanswered. One of these, he said, is the threshold level of whole-grain cereals that can be consumed without causing mineral deficiencies.

"Our experimental diets included 36 grams a day of bran, an intake we considered to be in the high-normal range," Morris said. "There are documented cases of severe mineral deficiencies in people who eat exceptionally large amounts of whole grains. So our findings should not be interpreted to mean there is no limit to the amount of these foods you should consume."[5]

Another unanswered question has to do with the poor absorption of magnesium by the participants in the study. The positive balance of this mineral was very narrow, and something in the diets may have interfered with optimum availability of magnesium. Since Morris and his colleagues were concerned that people get sufficient magnesium, further studies were planned.[5]

All aspects of dietary fiber intake were chronicled by Susan M. Pilch, Ph.D., in a report, "Physiological Effects and Health Consequences of Dietary Fiber," which was prepared for the Center for Food Safety and Applied Nutrition, Food and Drug Administration, Washington, D.C., in June 1987. Pilch was with the Life Sciences Research Office, Federation of American Societies for Experimental Biology in Bethesda, Maryland. Pilch did a thorough review of the literature concerning the potential undesirable effects of dietary fiber, especially the effects on mineral bioavailability.[6] Several studies indicated that fiber intakes of vegetarians were higher than those of omnivores. Menopausal lacto-ovo vegetarian women ranging in age from 50 to 89, were compared with omnivorous women of the same age range.[15] The vegetarian women had less bone loss. However, no differences were reported between bone mineral mass in lacto-ovo vegetarian men and omnivorous men in any decade of life.[16]

Pilch reported that one study compared zinc status of adolescent lacto-ovo vegetarians with a control group. Dietary fiber intake was higher for the vegetarians, and dietary zinc intake was similar, but zinc intake was significantly higher per 1,000 kcal for the vegetarians. Hair zinc levels of both groups were within ranges obtained by other workers, but levels were significantly lower for the vegetarians (218 vs 249 mcg/g).[6]

Diets of Punjabi lacto-ovo vegetarians living in the United States showed that males and females were in positive iron balance.[17]

Better utilization of zinc from vegetarian diets than by omnivores consuming vegetarian diets was also noted in the review.[18]

"From the information available, it appears that the mineral status of vegetarians is essentially equivalent to that of omnivores, and that if vegetarians do have decreased bioavailability of minerals due to higher fiber intakes, they are able to adjust," Pilch said. "Alternately, fiber intakes of vegetarians may not be as elevated as has been assumed, which is likely to be true for lacto-ovo vegetarians."

Pilch also reviewed dietary studies of Third World populations where intakes of fiber are high.[19] There was little evidence that these populations suffer from mineral deficiencies resulting from high fiber intakes. Blood serum levels of minerals would not likely be altered by fiber unless a deficiency is well advanced, due primarily to the homeostatic maintenance of blood mineral levels. Any decreases are likely to remain within the normal ranges. However, serum mineral levels have been used to assess the effect of dietary fiber on mineral nutriture.[6]

In one study, serum levels of calcium, iron and magnesium were normal in 15 diabetics fed high-fiber diets for an average of 21 months.[20] Another study reported that serum levels of iron, total iron-binding capacity, calcium, phosphorus, zinc and magnesium were within the normal ranges for 68 adults taking two tablespoons of bran for six months, and for 20 adult vegetarians, of whom eight were taking bran supplements.[21]

When insulin-dependent diabetics in Norway supplemented their ordinary diet with low-fiber bread (15 to 20 g/day of fiber) for three months or with guar gum (29 g/day) or bran (33 g/day) for the same period, blood concentrations of calcium, inorganic phosphate, magnesium, iron, zinc and selenium did not change.[22] Urinary calcium excretion was slightly lowered during treatment with wheat bran, but inorganic phosphorus, magnesium and zinc were unchanged.

However, when 21 grams of cellulose was fed to nine adolescent girls for 21 days and results compared with those seen on a control low-fiber diet, blood calcium, inorganic phosphorus and iron levels decreased significantly.[23]

Absorption of iron as measured by changes in serum iron or in total iron content was less in human volunteers given breads made with wholemeal flour in place of white flour,[24-26] and when bran was added to rolls.[27] Whole wheat bread added to a meal also resulted in a decrease in absorption of nonheme iron which could not be explained by the presence of phytate.[28] When bran, pectin or cellulose were added to muffins prepared with wheat flour, only bran significantly lowered the absorption of iron in a meal.[29] A further study with a low-fiber versus a high-fiber meal demonstrated that the iron absorption in the low-fiber meal was about double that in the high-fiber meal. The authors suggested that this decrease from six to three percent absorption was not a major problem in iron availability in humans.[6]

Pilch reviewed another study that reported that when white and wholemeal breads contained equal amounts of zinc, the absorption of zinc from a test meal was greater from white than from wholemeal bread.[30] The addition of protein to the wholemeal bread resulted in improved iron absorption. In another study, when defatted soy flour was substituted for 25 percent of the protein in chicken in a test meal, zinc absorption was not influenced.[31] Feeding a soybean meal or an animal protein meal with the same zinc content resulted in similar absorptions of zinc.[6]

"Test meals may give information about the effects of fiber on the absorption of minerals from a particular meal, but will not necessarily indicate the overall absorption of minerals in the whole diet," Pilch continued. "Other constituents in the meal and in the diet will also affect mineral availability."[6]

Concerning the fecal excretion of minerals, Pilch described a study in which four groups of subjects ate one of the following diets: a low-fiber diet (18 grams of dietary fiber), a diet containing fruits and vegetables (43 grams of dietary fiber), a diet containing citrus pectin (28 grams of dietary fiber), or a diet containing wheat bran (37 grams of dietary fiber). The results were compared with those obtained when a low-fiber control diet was consumed for two and a half weeks. Those fed the bran diet had increased magnesium excretion, but there were no significant changes in either calcium or magnesium excretions on any of the other diets.[6]

For diets containing 2.8 grams of crude fiber or 25 grams of soy polysaccharide (60 percent total dietary fiber) fecal excretions of calcium, phosphorus, iron, magnesium, zinc and copper were not significantly different.[33]

The effects of alpha-cellulose and phytate on zinc absorption revealed that cellulose had no effect, whereas phytate decreased the absorption of zinc.[34]

Copper, iron, zinc and calcium concentrations were measured in dry-milled corn bran, wheat bran and soybean hulls before they were baked into bread and after passage through the human gastrointestinal tract. The concentrations of all four elements increased in corn bran; calcium increased in wheat bran; and zinc increased and iron decreased in soy hulls as these fiber sources passed through the gut.[6]

"If minerals are bound by fiber and are rendered unavailable to the body, increased fecal mineral excretion should result," Pilch said. "The assumption is made that urinary excretion would not be affected. However, more complete information can be obtained when minerals are determined in both urine and feces so that balances can be calculated."[6]

Pilch recapped the results of several mineral balance studies in which supplements were added to self-selected diets. Wheat bran (14 grams/day) added to the diets of four females for four weeks, did not affect zinc balances.[36] When the normal diets of two men and four women were supplemented with 21 grams of dietary fiber from a nonpurified soya pulp or a purified soya fiber for three weeks each, fecal calcium, magnesium and iron, but not zinc, were significantly increased. However, mineral intakes were also increased when the fiber was added. In another study, volunteers added 30 grams of wheat bran supplement to their diets, increasing fiber intake from 8.5 grams to 20.9 grams/day. Dietary calcium intakes were calculated, and all feces were analyzed for calcium content. Apparent calcium absorption decreased during the last eight days of the study.[38]

"Adding a fiber supplement to the usual diets of human subjects is probably the most practical way to conduct studies of this type, but results are more uncertain because of greater possibilities of inaccuracy in reporting food intakes or in making food collections," Pilch added.[6]

In a table in the publication, Pilch revealed the results of human studies in which mineral balances were determined when fiber was increased in the diet. The diets given the volunteers were controlled by the researchers. Some of the observations from the studies were:

- Decreased absorption of minerals due to binding by fiber is not so important if mineral intakes are high. When intakes are marginally adequate, negative balances of minerals are more likely to result if minerals are bound to fiber. The level of mineral intake needed to maintain balance also depends on the level of intake to which the subject is accustomed.
- Unrefined cereals are high in phytate which may be partially responsible for negative mineral balances observed on brown bread intakes. Removal of phytate in one study resulted in improved mineral balances.
- The presence of oxalic acid in the spinach fed in the diets containing fiber from fruits and vegetables was partially responsible for negative balances originally attributed to fiber. Negative balances resulted only when spinach was fed with a diet containing higher levels of fiber.
- High levels of protein intake have been shown to decrease calcium balance due to increased excretion of calcium in the urine. Detrimental effects of fiber on calcium balance may be more pronounced on high-protein diets.
- In laboratory glassware, some fibers have been shown to bind minerals more readily than others, but the *in vivo* and *in vitro* findings are sometimes contradictory. Wheat fiber, hemicellulose and cellulose resulted in negative balances in some studies. Pectin, which is a soluble fiber, did not affect mineral balances.
- Most of the negative mineral balances reported in the studies in the table resulted when more than 25 grams/day of insoluble fiber was fed.
- Most of the study periods were from two to four weeks. In two of the studies in which experimental periods were extended to eight to 18 weeks, negative mineral balance improved. Therefore, if sufficient time is allowed, the body may adjust to any decreased mineral availability.[6]

Some of the trials involved only a few people, which makes it difficult to assume that results apply to the population in general and to interpret statistical analyses. In some of the earlier studies, statistical analyses were not performed on the data; however, individual data were reported and the decreased mineral balances due to fiber in the diet appear to be real. In addition, some of the studies did not employ a crossover design, therefore, any effects of feeding one diet before another were not eliminated.

"Evidence that fiber has an adverse effect on mineral bioavailability is conflicting," Pilch said. "Although some test meals containing fiber result in decreased absorption of iron and zinc, the actual amount of decrease is probably small in relation to the total daily intake of these minerals. Some reports indicate that minerals in feces were increased due to fiber in the diet, but others report no effect. Results of balance studies showed that with high intakes of wheat fiber, mineral balances were decreased or negative."[6]

In two studies, she continued, the addition of cellulose resulted in negative balances; in two others, there was no effect. However, there are many kinds of cellulose, which might be expected to elicit different responses. For example, hemicellulose decreased zinc balance in two studies.

"Consumption of diets containing about 25 grams/day of insoluble fiber in fruits and vegetables did not affect mineral balances unless oxalic acid in spinach was included," Pilch concluded. "Locust bean gum, karaya, carboxymethylcellulose and pectin did not affect mineral balances. Given the possibility that there is likely to be an adaptation to any alteration in mineral availability resulting from an increased fiber intake, a moderate level of fiber intake of 20 to 25 grams/day of insoluble fiber does not appear to pose a problem."[6]

The problem is obviously complicated, involving a person's ability to properly absorb nutrients, the health of the gastrointestinal tract and the interplay between various minerals. The relationship between copper-zinc, sodium-potassium, calcium-phosphorus and other minerals and vitamins will be explored in more detail in later chapters.

REFERENCES

1. Bordin, Shela W., and Bordin, Gerald M., M.D. "Bran: Roughage That's Rough on Iron," *The New England Journal of Medicine* 294(1):57, January 1, 1976.
2. "Low-Normal Iron Levels in Children Said to Warrant Supplementation," *Family Practice News* 22(2):41, January 15, 1992.
3. Behall, K., et al. "Mineral Balance in Adult Men: Effect of Four Refined Fibers," *American Journal of Clinical Nutrition* 46:307–314, 1987.
4. "Minerals in Whole Wheat Are Digestible, USDA Study Shows," *USDA News*, April 16, 1980.
5. Bricklin, Mark, editor. *The Natural Healing and Nutrition Annual.* Emmaus, Pa.: Rodale Press, 1989, pp. 71ff.

6. Pilch, Susan M., Ph.D. "Physiological Effects and Health Consequences of Dietary Fiber." Prepared for Food Safety and Applied Nutrition, Food and Drug Administration, Department of Health and Human Services, Washington, D.C., June 1987, pp. 136ff.

7. Hardinge, M. G., et al. "Nutritional Studies of Vegetarians. III. Dietary Levels of Fiber," *American Journal of Clinical Nutrition* 6:523–525, 1958.

8. Anderson, B. M., et al. "The Iron and Zinc Status of Long-Term Vegetarian Women," *American Journal of Clinical Nutrition* 34:1042–1048, 1981.

9. King, J. C., et al. "Effect of Vegetarianism on the Zinc Status of Pregnant Women," *American Journal of Clinical Nutrition* 34:1049–1055, 1981.

10. Treuherz, J. "Possible Inter-Relationship Between Zinc and Dietary Fibre in a Group of Lacto-Ovo Vegetarian Adolescents," *Journal of Plant Foods* 4:89–93, 1982.

11. Gibson, R. S., et al. "The Trace Metal Status of a Group of Post-Menopausal Vegetarians," *Journal of the American Dietetic Association* 82:246–250, 1983.

12. Davies, G. J., et al. "Dietary Fibre Intakes of Individuals with Different Eating Patterns," *Hum. Nutr. Appl. Nutr.* 39A:139–148, 1985.

13. Howie, B. J., et al. "Dietary and Hormonal Interrelationships Among Vegetarian Seventh-Day Adventists and Nonvegetarian Men," *American Journal of Clinical Nutrition* 42:127–134, 1985.

14. Schultz, T. D., and Leklem, J. E. "Selenium Status of Vegetarians, Nonvegetarians and Hormone-Dependent Cancer Subjects," *American Journal of Clinical Nutrition* 37:114–118, 1983.

15. Marsh, A. G., et al. "Cortical Bone Density of Adult Lacto-Ovo-Vegetarian and Omnivorous Women," *Journal of the American Dietetic Association* 76:148–151, 1980.

16. Marsh, A. G., et al. "Bone Mineral Mass in Adult Lacto-Ovo-Vegetarian and Omnivorous Males," *American Journal of Clinical Nutrition* 37:453–456, 1983.

17. Ganapathy, S., and Dhanda, R. "Protein and Iron Nutrition in Lacto-Ovo-Vegetarian Indo-Aryan United States Residents." *Indian J. Nutr. Diet.* 17:45–52, 1980.

18. Kies, C., et al. "Zinc Bioavailability from Vegetarian Diets: Influence of Dietary Fiber, Ascorbic Acid and Past Dietary Practices." In: Inglett, G. E., editor. Nutritional Bioavailability of Zinc. ACS Series No. 210. Washington, D.C.: American Chemical Society, 1983, pp. 115–126.

19. Walker, A. "Mineral Metabolism." In: Trowell, H.; Burkitt, D.; Heaton, K., editors. "Dietary Fibre, Fibre-Depleted Foods and Disease." New York: Academic Press, 1985, pp. 361–375.

20. Anderson, J. W., et al. "Mineral and Vitamin Status on High-Fiber Diets: Long-Term Studies of Diabetic Patients," *Diabetes Care* 3:38–40, 1980.

21. Rattan, J., et al. "A High-Fiber Diet Does Not Cause Mineral and Nutrient Deficiencies," *J. Clin. Gastroenterol.* 3:389–393, 1981.

22. Vaaler, S., et al. "Trace Elements in Serum and Urine of Diabetic Patients Given Bread Enriched with Wheat Bran or Guar Gum." In: International Symposium on

Trace Element Metabolism in Man and Animals," TEMA-5. Edinburgh: Churchill Livingstone, 1985, pp. 446–449.

23. Godara, R., et al. "Effect of Cellulose Incorporation in a Low-Fiber Diet on Fecal Excretion and Serum Levels of Calcium, Phosphorus and Iron in Adolescent Girls," *American Journal of Clinical Nutrition* 34:1083–1086, 1981.

24. Dobbs, R. J., and Baird, I. M. "Effect of Wholemeal and White Bread on Iron Absorption in Normal People," *British Medical Journal* 2:1641–1642, 1977.

25. Elwood, P. C., et al. "Absorption of Iron From Chapatti Made from Wheat Flour," *American Journal of Clinical Nutrition* 23:1267–1271, 1970.

26. Vellar, O. D., et al. "Iron-Fortified Bread: Absorption and Utilization Studies," *Acta Med. Scand.* 183:251–256, 1968.

27. Bjorn-Rasmussen, E. "Iron Absorption from Wheat Bread: Influence of Various Amounts of Bran," *Nutr. Metab.* 16:101–110, 1974.

28. Simpson, K.M., et al. "The Inhibitory Effect of Bran on Iron Absorption in Man," *American Journal of Clinical Nutrition* 34:1469–1478, 1981.

29. Cook, J. D., et al. "Effect of Fiber on Nonheme Iron Absorption," *Gastroenterology* 85:1354–1358, 1983.

30. Sandstrom, B., et al. "Zinc Absorption from Composite Meals. I. The Significance of Wheat Extraction Rate, Zinc, Calcium and Protein Content in Meals Based on Bread," *American Journal of Clinical Nutrition* 33:739–745, 1980.

31. Sandstrom, B., and Cederblad, A. "Zinc Absorption from Composite Meals. II. Influence of the Main Protein Source," *American Journal of Clinical Nutrition* 33:1778–1783, 1980.

32. Stasse-Wolthuis, M., et al. "Influence of Dietary Fiber from Vegetables and Fruits, Bran or Citrus Pectin on Serum Lipids, Fecal Lipids and Colonic Function," *American Journal of Clinical Nutrition* 33:1745–1756, 1980.

33. Tsai, A. C., et al. "Effects of Soy Polysaccharide on Gastrointestinal Functions, Nutrient Balance, Steroid Excretions, Glucose Tolerance, Serum Lipids and Other Parameters in Humans," *American Journal of Clinical Nutrition* 38:504–511, 1983.

34. Turnlund, J. R., et al. "A Stable Isotope Study of Zinc Absorption in Young Men: Effects of Phytate and Alpha-Cellulose," *American Journal of Clinical Nutrition* 40:1071–1077, 1984.

35. Dintzis, F. R., et al. "Mineral Contents of Brans Passed Through the Human GI Tract," *American Journal of Clinical Nutrition* 41:901–908, 1985.

36. Guthrie, B. E., and Robinson, M. F. "Zinc Balance Studies During Wheat Bran Supplementation," *Fed, Proc. Fed. Am. Soc. Exp. Biol.* 37:254, 1978. (Abstract).

37. Schweizer, T. F., et al. "Metabolic Effects of Dietary Fiber from Dehulled Soybeans in Humans," *American Journal of Clinical Nutrition* 38:1–11, 1983.

38. Balasubramanian, R., et al. "Effect of Wheat Bran on Bowel Function and Fecal Calcium in Older Adults," *Journal of the American College of Nutrition* 6:199–208, 1987.

4

Deficiency Diseases Related to Minerals

DEFICIENCY diseases are often related to dietary shortages of one or more essential nutrients, and they may be prevented or cured by replacing the missing nutrients, unless there is irreparable damage to vital tissues of the body. Even when a variety of foods are available at a reasonable cost, some people will eat an unbalanced diet, which can lead to illness.

It is difficult to detect deficiencies in people who subsist on only a few foods. As an example, one would expect to find deficiencies of vitamins A and C in the Eskimos who still follow their primitive diet of meat and fish and little else. However, the secret of their survival may be due to their eating *raw* meat, which contains enough vitamin C to prevent scurvy, or nibbling on a piece of liver, which is rich in vitamin A.

It is well known that beriberi was the scourge of some Asian peoples who ate large quantities of highly milled rice, while other groups who ate rice which had been parboiled prior to milling were not as susceptible to this disease. Processed white sugar and white flour are poor sources of minerals and vitamins in comparison with the unrefined products from which they are made.

Even if someone is eating a variety of fruits and vegetables, grains, etc., they may suffer from deficiencies because certain substances in these foods interfere with nutrient utilization. For instance, vegetables of the cabbage family contain goitrogenic substances, so named because of their interference with the utilization of iodine. Phytates can bind to calcium, magnesium, iron and zinc in some whole grains so that their absorption is reduced. Oxalates from rhubarb and spinach can also reduce the absorption of some trace minerals. Vitamins A, C, E and B1 may be destroyed by cooking foods at high or prolonged temperatures in the presence of oxygen, and some minerals and water-soluble vitamins may be lost when they are extracted from foods by the cooking water, which is often discarded.

NUTRITION STARTS IN THE SOIL

Much recent debate has centered on mineral-deficient soils as a cause of human deficiency diseases other than goiter. This condition is more common in areas where the soil and water have abnormally low levels of iodine. Mineral-deficient soils may also be responsible for lower levels of minerals in certain food plants, and in livestock fed these plants.

Controversy arises because some soils naturally contain an abundant supply of most of the elements needed by plants, animals and man, whereas other soils may have an abundant supply of most required elements and yet be deficient in one or more essentials. In the southwestern United States, the soils are deficient in phosphorus; northwestern and Great Lakes areas are deficient in iodine, and southeastern U.S. soils tend to be deficient in cobalt. Differences between plant species in their tendency to accumulate different elements are often important in determining the mineral status of livestock that eat these plants. In some areas of the U.S., forages such as alfalfa and clover contain adequate levels of cobalt for cattle and sheep—which convert the mineral to vitamin B12—but grass species in the same fields or pastures do not contain enough cobalt to meet the requirements of these animals.[1]

At every step in the chain from soils to man, the essential mineral elements interact with other elements, and these interactions may profoundly affect: 1) the availability of essential elements to plants, animals or man; 2) the amount of the essential element required for normal growth or metabolic function. For example, the availability of zinc to animals and humans may be depressed if their diets are high in calcium, and high levels of molybdenum may interfere with copper metabolism. However, much of the American diet is made up of products from farm animals that have been fed mineral supplements to compensate for mineral deficiencies in their feeds and forages. Often, the minerals present in animal feeds are in forms which are more efficiently utilized by man than the mineral compounds present in the plants. Two examples are the iron in hemoglobin and the chromium in the glucose tolerance factor. Strict vegetarians who eat no animal foods are more likely to develop deficiencies from eating nutrient-deficient plants than people who eat liberal amounts of animal foods.[1]

In the *Canadian Medical Association Journal* in 1991, Ranjit Kumar Chandra, M.D., of Memorial University of Newfoundland in St. John's said that, in Canada, 10 to

28 percent of the elderly are at risk for dietary deficiencies of calcium, beta-carotene, vitamin A, vitamin C and vitamin D. A smaller portion are at risk for deficiencies of protein, zinc, vitamin B1, vitamin B6 and chromium. Concerning blood levels, he added, vitamin B6, vitamin C, vitamin D, zinc, iron and protein are the most common deficiencies in the elderly. However, he said, the major nutritional problems in the elderly in Canada appear to be low energy intake and dietary deficiencies of calcium, zinc, iron, vitamin A, vitamin C, vitamin D and excess intake of dietary fat.[2]

In the U.S., some 6.4 million new cases of eye disease occur each year; at least 11 million people have impaired vision that cannot be corrected with glasses, and 800,000 of them are considered legally blind—usually defined as having vision worse than 20/200, reported Robert B. Nussenblatt, M.D., in the 1993 edition of *Medical and Health Annual*. He continued:

> Animal studies have evaluated the protective potential of a large number of nutrients in the development of cataracts. In general, the experimental approach has been to either remove from the diet or give in large doses the nutrient in question. Preliminary research has focused on certain minerals and vitamins that function as antioxidants. Oxidative processes in the lens of the eye are thought to play an important role in the development of cataracts. Activated forms of oxygen, which can be formed as a result of normal metabolism or certain outside stimuli such as ultraviolet light, are believed to be highly damaging to the lens of the eye in particular. A variety of chemical processes that can counteract oxygen's activation and subsequent harmful effect on the lens are present in the eye.[3]

In animal studies naturally occurring antioxidant enzymes such as superoxide dismutase (SOD), catalase and selenium-dependent glutathione peroxidase have all been implicated in such protective mechanisms. Consequently glutathione, vitamin C, vitamin E, carotenoids, selenium, calcium, zinc, riboflavin (B2) and tryptophan (an amino acid) have all been suggested as supplements that may have the potential to enhance the protection from cataracts.[3] (Tryptophan is no longer available as a supplement in the U.S., since the FDA removed it from the marketplace after a batch of improperly made product in Japan caused a number of deaths.)

In the December 11, 1970 issue of *Science*, Helen L. Cannon of the U.S. Geological Survey in Denver, and Howard C. Hopps of the University of Missouri, said that the possibility of casual relationships between environmental factors and the occurrence of many degenerative diseases is slowly being recognized. The geochemistry of rocks, soil, plants and water—should be further studied carefully and the distribution of minor elements should be compared with geographic patterns of animal and human health and disease. We know that calcium, phosphorus, iron, copper and all the other important inorganic nutrients somehow make their way from a never-ending source in the rocks to the soils and waters, and from there into plants, animals and humans. But there are unanswered questions.

- How is this transport accomplished and how easily do the various elements move into and through the food chain?
- What effects do climate and time have on this movement?
- What sort of interactions go on between the various elements as they come into contact with one another to enhance or hinder this process?
- How are these elements utilized by different kinds of organisms, and . . .
- What effects do even small excesses or deficiencies of any one ion have on the health of plants or animals?

In an article by W. G. Hoekstra of the University of Wisconsin published in the September–October 1964 issue of *Federation Proceedings,* Hoekstra reviewed many of the various relationships between phosphorus and calcium, zinc and calcium, zinc and copper, cadmium, iron and molybdenum. He concluded that: "The complexity of the mineral imbalance problem is apparent. It is apparent that our understanding of the mechanisms of mineral imbalances is fragmentary. New interrelationships are constantly being discovered. It is my firm opinion that we are presently recognizing and correcting only a small fraction of the mineral imbalance problems currently plaguing animals and man."[4]

Since many Americans succumb to malnutrition during a hospital stay, and, unfortunately, many of them die because of improper nutrition, I wondered just how nutritious is the hospital fare that many patients get. I found an answer in the May 1970 issue of the *Journal of the American Dietetic Association,* in which Dr. Annette Gormican of the Department of Medicine and Nutritional Sciences at the University of Wisconsin analyzed 128 foods served at a hospital. Especially noted was the content of calcium, phosphorus, potassium, magnesium, sodium, aluminum, barium, iron, strontium, boron, copper, zinc, manganese and chromium.

Dr. Gormican found that there is a wide range of discrepancies in the trace mineral content of common foods, compared to the official nutrition tables. Iron and copper varied widely. In some cases, they were higher than the official levels and in some cases lower. She also found that home-grown tomatoes used in this hospital were lower in calcium, phosphorus, potassium, sodium and iron than the amounts recorded as official by the U.S. Department of Agriculture. A large amount of aluminum was found in a processed cheese, apparently attributed to an emulsifier, sodium aluminum phosphate. When she compared the hospital diets with those studied by other workers in the field, Gormican said, "Much lower values were observed for magnesium, aluminum, barium, iron, boron, copper and manganese.

The levels of phosphorus, potassium, calcium, sodium and zinc were just about the same as those listed in the 'average American diet' by other scientists. In the case of chromium, the level appeared to be a bit higher."[4]

Magnesium deficiency, also called hypomagnesemia, is a condition in which an organism fails to receive an adequate supply of the mineral. Magnesium is essential to enzyme reactions necessary in the metabolism of ingested carbohydrates and sometimes has the ability to replace a portion of body calcium. Almost three-fourths of the mineral found in the body is associated with calcium in the skeleton and tooth dentine formation, with the remainder contained in soft tissues and body fluids. Its specific function is not certain, but studies indicate magnesium probably serves as a catalyst in other physiological activities. Magnesium forms positive ions (charged particles) in solution and is essential to the electrical breakdown of nutrient and other material within the cells; it is also necessary for the stimulation of muscles and nerves.[5]

Magnesium deficiencies are noted in chronic kidney disease and other conditions of acidosis (pathological excess of acid), including diabetic coma. Symptoms of deficiency include weakness, dizziness, distension of the abdomen and convulsive seizures.[5]

Infants fed whole cow's milk have lower intakes of iron, linoleic acid and vitamin E and excessive intakes of sodium, potassium and protein.[6] Infants fed iron-fortified formulas or breast milk for 12 months generally maintain their iron stores. Research has shown that iron status is significantly impaired when whole cow's milk is introduced into the diet of six-month-old infants. But infants fed partially modified milk formulas with supplemental iron in a highly bioavailable form, such as ferrous sulfate, appear to maintain adequate iron status. The American Academy of Pediatrics recommends that infants be fed breast milk for the first six to 12 months of life. The only alternative is iron-fortified infant formula. Solid foods should be added between the ages of four and six months. The consumption of breast milk or iron-fortified formulas, along with appropriate solid foods and juices during the first 12 months of life, can maintain balanced nutrition.[6]

POOR DIET LINKED TO HEART HEALTH

As I reported in *Program Your Heart for Health,* Jacobus Rinse, Ph.D., a Dutch-American consulting chemist, had an attack of angina pectoris in 1951 when he was 51. This prompted Rinse to investigate the causes of atherosclerosis, ostensibly to improve his own health and thus prolong his life. His observations and experiences were recorded in the July 1973 issue of *American Laboratory.* (Rinse died in 1993 at the age of 92 while attempting to rescue a drowning friend.)

After suffering the heart pains and violent attacks, Rinse was told by his physician that he probably had 10 years to live, providing he avoided all types of physical exercise. What had stunned Rinse was that he did not fit the typical heart attack profile. He did not smoke, he was not obese, he was not under tension, he exercised and there was no family history of the disease. It was first thought that he had gotten too much exercise while clearing trees from a plot where he planned to build a house. But this was later discounted. Being a chemist and used to laborious studies and experiments, he began reading articles, books, abstracts, etc., relating to hardening of the arteries. Of special interest was the *Journal of the American Oil Chemists Society,* because it contained a section of abstracts on "Biochemistry and Nutrition." A useful booklet was *The Pulse Rate* by Arthur F. Coca, M.D.[7]

After reviewing his situation objectively, Rinse theorized that there might be a deficiency of some kind in his diet. Since a chemical plant must have primary and secondary materials in order to operate, he reasoned that the human body must also have secondary materials—minerals, trace minerals, vitamins, enzymes, etc.—to produce energy, to digest proteins, fats and carbohydrates. A chemical plant can operate with shortages because of the reserves and substitutes, but even these are likely to play out, say during wartime. Similarly, he said, the body eventually experiences various disturbances if the metabolism is not working properly. Although some of these body necessities are needed in very small amounts—copper, cobalt, manganese, iron, vitamin B6, vitamin B12, he added, because of these shortages, plus reduced food intake as we grow older, it makes sense to add multivitamin tablets and mixtures of minerals.

In the article, Rinse reviewed some of the literature on hardening of the arteries and some of the companion disorders: angina pectoris, heart infarct, cerebral thrombosis (blockage of a blood vessel in or to the brain), intermittent claudication (blockage in a leg), high blood pressure (by blocking a kidney artery), cataract and xanthomatosis (yellow plaques under the skin). In the final stages, he learned, arteriosclerosis occurs with hardening and finally the calcification of the blood vessels. And he described cholesterol, which serves as an intermediate for the biosynthesis of bile acids, hormones and vitamin D.[7]

In 1951, when his condition worsened, Rinse experienced increasing pressure or light pain (angina) in the breast after exercising. The pain subsided as he rested, but the light pressure continued for several days. His physician prescribed an anticoagulant (Dicumarol), a drug that delays the clotting of blood, and nitroglycerin tablets. Nitroglycerin relaxes the blood vessels, increasing the supply of blood and oxygen to the heart while reducing the work load. He resumed work in a few days, but walking up stairs or a hill reminded him that the angina was still present. His pulse rate increased rapidly and did not subside for about an hour.

Theorizing that a food deficiency might be the cause, Rinse began experimenting with enzyme-rich foods such as raw herring, raw eggs, red meat, uncooked vegetables, yogurt, etc. But he could not tell whether or not there was any change in his condition. But, he said, the use of garlic definitely increased the activity limit. Concurrently, he began taking one gram (1,000 mg) of vitamin C daily. Later he added a multivitamin tablet. His breakfast consisted of a cereal with milk and yogurt, along with wheat germ, brewers yeast and brown sugar (one tablespoon of each), which are rich in vitamins and minerals. After conferring with Drs. Evan and Wilfrid Shute at the Shute Clinic in London, Ontario, Rinse began taking 200 IU of vitamin E after each meal.

Rinse followed this regimen, including other nutrient-dense foods, for several years. By avoiding strenuous exercise, he lived a fairly normal life, although there were occasional warnings that he still had angina pectoris. When the pressure in his breast increased, this was a signal to rest. And, of course, the pulse rate was a reliable guide.

In 1957, Rinse experienced rather severe heart pains, which gradually subsided in about an hour. But the angina pains remained, especially if he walked up stairs. He also observed spasms and an increase of 50 strokes in the pulse rate. He considered an allergy as a cause of the angina, but later ruled that out. About this time, he read that lecithin and safflower oil can reduce cholesterol content in the blood, so he added a tablespoon of each to his breakfast ration. Within a few days, the spasms stopped and the high pulse rate diminished. His health continued to improve and, after three months, all symptoms of angina disappeared, even after exercising. Within a year, he could resume heavy outdoor work and running. At the time of the article in *American Laboratory*—16 years after his initial angina—Rinse said that he had not had a recurrence of angina or other diseases.[7]

Elated with his progress, and eager to discuss his findings with friends, Rinse, at the suggestion of Dr. W. L. Ladenius, a Dutch physician, prepared a booklet which might interest those with atherosclerosis. One friend, who had survived a cerebral thrombosis and a heart infarct at the age of 53, decided to take the food supplements recommended by Rinse. Six months later the man was again working full time and had not had a relapse. (An updated version of the original booklet, *The Rinse Formula*, is available from Keats Publishing, Inc., of New Canaan, Connecticut.)

Another friend, a 69-year-old Dutch executive, had a blood clot in one of his legs. He was placed on anticoagulants and his butter and egg consumption was curtailed. Learning about Rinse's success, the man concocted his own product consisting of safflower oil, palm kernel fat and nitrogen as a substitute for butter. It is widely used in Holland.

Rinse's regimen was soon publicized in the United States, and his diet suggestions began to gain popularity. One 72-year-old man, who suffered from a series of heart attacks and angina pectoris, told Rinse that the regimen had cured his problems within three months, enabling him to take long walks for the first time in six years.

Case Histories Show Improvement

Another man, a Dutch mechanical engineer, 48, had such severe angina pectoris that he had to stop working. Prescribed drugs were of little value. He wrote Rinse that, after beginning the Rinse breakfast, he was back at work in two months. He was able to run again and he could work at times in deep-freeze storage rooms without any bad effects.

A 72-year-old Texan, a consulting chemist, read about Rinse's diet suggestions in *Chemical Week*. The man told Rinse that he had suffered several heart attacks, but with the Rinse breakfast and the diet supplements his health improved rapidly. He was able to give up the prescribed medicines and was soon at work again.

A Vermont woman, 70 years of age, had survived blockage in the neck artery and partial paralysis. She began the Rinse regimen and her health improved rapidly. She did not have recurrences, Rinse reported. Clinical tests showed that all cholesterol deposits had disappeared.

A Dutch internist told Rinse that he prescribed the special breakfast to many of his older patients. Many of them soon resumed their activities, even though they had been invalids for a long time. In another letter, the chemist learned that his breakfast and supplements had halted the progression of cataracts in two elderly women. A colleague regulated his wife's blood pressure with "Rinse's Morning Feed," which will be given later. A chemical engineer found that the Rinse recommendations cured his heart condition; 10 years later he was still in good health. The supplements were used by a Chicago man to cure his arthritis; two friends had the same results with their bursitis.[7]

Rinse believed that the most essential ingredients of his breakfast are the lecithin and the polyunsaturated oil, and he suggested for those who cannot take brewer's yeast (health food stores have a debittered supplement), they should increase their B complex supplements. Those not using milk or yogurt can combine the mixture with fruit juice or soup. The polyunsaturated oil can be used on salads or as margarine. He also recommended bone meal because of its rich source of calcium, magnesium, phosphate and other minerals.[7]

Concerning cholesterol, Rinse said that, although the substance can contribute to hardening of the arteries, it has also been demonstrated[8-10] that many people are healthy even though they have a high cholesterol count. Rinse explained that, if your food contains less cholesterol, your liver will produce more, that is, it will make up the difference in the amount of cholesterol needed by your body.

He added that drugs for removing cholesterol can cause serious side effects (cataracts, loss of hair, etc.). But lecithin, when added to the diet, prevents unwanted deposits of cholesterol from forming; any excess of cholesterol in the bloodstream is removed via the intestines, he said.

If the main problem with hardening of the arteries is to keep cholesterol deposits from forming on the arterial walls, Rinse continued, then lecithin should be taken in sufficient amounts. Lecithin is produced commercially from soybean oil; it is also available in nuts, eggs, seeds and soybeans. He said that the majority of fatty acids in human food are saturated, therefore, the lecithin produced in the liver will contain these fatty acids in larger quantities. And, since the molecular weight of lecithin is about double that of cholesterol, one should consume from four to six grams of lecithin and an equal amount of polyunsaturated oil each day. For more advanced cases of hardening of the arteries, Rinse said, this amount of lecithin and oil should be increased.[7]

Referring to an article by Lester Morrison, M.D. (Geriatrics 13:12, 1958), Rinse noted it was Morrison who had suggested the mixture of lecithin and oil. Some of Morrison's patients could not tolerate this amount three times a day, as he had recommended, and so the amounts had to be reduced for those patients. (Morrison discusses lecithin in more detail in his book, Dr. Morrison's Heart-Saver Program, St. Martin's Press, New York, 1982.)

Rinse added that polyunsaturated oil by itself will not dissolve cholesterol. Therefore, lecithin is a necessary ingredient. In Norway, where the people eat a lot of fish, the addition of polyunsaturated oil to the diet did not help prevent hardening of the arteries appreciably. It is the lecithin that they also need, Rinse said. He quoted Van Buchem as saying that, "The advice to recommend the consumption of polyunsaturated oils by the whole population with the exclusion of saturated fats is insufficiently founded."[7]

Van Buchem discussed a study of 48 men, ranging in age from 40 to 60, done at the Gaubius Institute in Leiden, Holland. Half of the men had complications associated with hardening of the arteries and the other half did not. The men who had a lecithin content of 36 percent or higher in their blood fats did not have hardening of the arteries; those with 34 percent or lower did.[7]

Rinse added that polyunsaturated oils are oxidized easily in the oxygen-rich arterial bloodstream. And he noted that vitamin E and lecithin are natural antioxidants. Oils used for paints, for example, must be dried, but those for human consumption should not oxidize or dry to avoid the formation of free radicals, which may cross-link tissues and cause rigidity and loss of flexibility in the muscles and arteries. If cross-linking occurred, he said, it might result in internal bleeding. For that reason, Rinse recommended the addition of vitamin E and vitamin C. C is a water-soluble antioxidant; vitamin E is fat-soluble. Rinse noted that *both* vitamins help to dissolve cholesterol and both may prevent heart disease.

If these vitamins are used with lecithin and polyunsaturated oil, Rinse believed that the amounts needed are smaller than when the two vitamins are taken alone. He recommended 100 to 200 IU/day of vitamin E and 500 to 1,000 mg/day of vitamin C. He noted that sulfur and its derivatives are also antioxidants. Two good food sources of sulfur are garlic and onions. In France, farmers give their horses these two foods to remove hardening of the artery obstructions in their legs. Sulfur, according to the medical literature, is also useful for arthritis.

A number of other vitamins and minerals may prove useful in the treatment of hardening of the arteries. These include vitamin B6, vitamin B3 (nicotinic acid, one form of this vitamin), iron, calcium, magnesium, manganese, cobalt, zinc, chromium, potassium, copper, vanadium, iodine, phosphorus and selenium.

One study compared the soft water of Glasgow, Scotland, with the hard, calcium-containing water of London, England. There were fewer deaths from atherosclerosis in London. And Dr. Henry A. Schroeder reported that chromium is helpful in reducing cholesterol levels.[7]

The clotting of blood can aggravate hardening of the arteries by closing off the arteries. A familiar anticoagulant is cumarol or its derivatives; this same substance is used for poisoned arrows by some South American Indians. Rinse added that such anticoagulants are often necessary for bedridden patients, but that for those who can move about, the use of cumarol or other substances might be dangerous for people with weakened arteries. He suggested a wider use of vitamin E and vitamin K as anticoagulants. As to whether or not hardening of the arteries can be reversed, Rinse reported in *Chemisch Weekblad* and *Chemical Week* in 1961 that it definitely can be. The chances are better, of course, for those with less severe lesions and those who are younger. In such cases, this regimen has dissolved the cholesterol deposits so that blood could flow freely through the arteries. But Rinse has also reported considerable success with those from 65 to 80. These older people should not overdo physical activities, especially if their arteries have lost their flexibility or contain weak spots or calcium deposits, he cautioned.

Rinse is convinced that food deficiencies are the major cause of hardening of the arteries; that tension, smoking, obesity and heredity are only contributory. These deficiencies are brought about, he said, because of:

1. Refining of our foods, which removes many of the needed vitamins and minerals;
2. Decreased amount of food eaten because of age or less physical activity;
3. Faulty digestion, which means that we do not absorb the nutrients from our foods because of a metabolic dysfunction.[7]

Although many of Rinse's case histories are anecdotal, they serve to suggest that the "fickle finger of fate" doesn't give this person angina pectoris, that person cancer, etc. It is obviously something in their diet, lifestyle or heredity that is contributing to the problem, and nutritional intervention can often return those people to good health.

 DR. RINSE'S MORNING FEED

Mix together one tablespoon of soybean lecithin, debittered brewer's yeast and raw wheat germ, and one teaspoon of bone meal. You may prepare a larger amount for later use: four parts of each of the first three ingredients to one part of the bone meal.

Mix in a bowl:
Two tablespoons of the above mixture.
One tablespoon of dark brown sugar (skip this one if you can).
One tablespoon of safflower oil or other linoleate oil, for example, soybean oil.
Add milk to dissolve sugar and yeast.
Add yogurt (preferably home made) to increase consistency.
Add cold cereal for calories as needed or mix with hot cereal such as oatmeal or porridge. Raisins and other fruits may be added if desired.
For severe cases of hardening of the arteries the quantity of lecithin should be doubled.

To this ration add:
500 mg of vitamin C daily.
100 IU of vitamin E daily.
1 multivitamin-mineral tablet daily.

The rest of the diet can include high-protein foods, including eggs, fruits, vegetables, nuts, seeds, dairy products, including butter, etc. High-melting fats such as regular margarine should be avoided. The linoleate-containing margarines at your health food store are acceptable, but butter is preferred because it contains medium-chain triglycerides (MCT fat).

References

1. Ensminger, Audrey H., et al. *Foods and Nutrition Encyclopedia.* Clovis, Calif.: Pegus Press, 1983, pp. 524ff.
2. Chandra, Ranjit Kumur, M.D., et al. "Nutrition of the Elderly," *Canadian Medical Association Journal* 145:1475–1487, 1991.
3. Nussenblatt, Robert B., M.D. "Eye Diseases and Visual Disorders." In *Medical and Health Annual.* Chicago: Encyclopaedia Britannica, Inc., 1993, pp. 292ff.
4. Adams, Ruth, and Murray, Frank. *Minerals: Kill or Cure?* New York: Larchmont Books, 1974, pp. 29ff.
5. *The New Encyclopedia Britannica,* Chicago, 1993, p. 678.
6. "The Use of Whole Cow's Milk in Infancy: Committee on Nutrition," *Pediatrics* 89(6):1105–1107, June 1992.
7. Murray, Frank. *Program Your Heart for Health.* New York: Larchmont Books, 1978, pp. 51ff.
8. Van Buchem, F.S.P., *Nutr. Dieta* 4:122–147 (1962).
9. Van Buchem, F.S.P., *Ned. Tydschr. v. Geneeskunde* 115:1311 (1971).
10. Pries, C. and Van Buchem, *Ned. Tydschr. v. Geneeskunde* 111:1594 (1967).

5

Should You Drink Mineral Water?

WHEN parasite-infected water caused diarrhea, vomiting and a number of deaths in Milwaukee, Wisconsin in 1993, it focused attention on our aging water systems and whether or not our tap water is indeed safe. Even if water supplies meet Environmental Protection Agency standards, there is still a possibility that some municipal water sources may contain abnormal amounts of lead, pesticides, radon, nitrates and other potential carcinogens.

According to Dr. James M. Symons in *Plain Talk About Drinking Water*, small water systems have the most trouble meeting these standards. "In 1990, in the United States, 9.5 percent of the 51,654 smaller water suppliers—serving populations of 3,300 or less—violated standards for germs in their drinking water. Less than one percent of the larger systems had similar violations. Records are not kept on the quality of private wells."[1]

Over the past 20 years, about 7,700 cases of sickness in the U.S. were traced directly to drinking water each year. These illnesses, characterized by vomiting and diarrhea, were most often caused by the improper treatment of the water.[1]

During the outbreak in Milwaukee, an estimated 281,000 people became ill between March 1 and April 10, 1993, Lawrence K. Altman, M.D., reported in the April 20 issue of *The New York Times*. The outbreak, traced to cryptosporidia parasites, was apparently caused by runoff from farms and animal waste. Heavy rains carried the contaminated water into the Milwaukee River, then into Lake Michigan and the water intake sites in the Milwaukee area.[2]

"Further shaking confidence in water supplies in the country was a scathing report issued last week by the General Accounting Office, an investigative agency of Congress," Altman said. "It found that most state inspection programs to insure the safety of public water supplies are a shambles."[2]

The Congressional report stated that "consumers may be getting their drinking water from systems that have not been inspected in 10 years or more or that may have significant undetected deficiencies."

The cryptosporidium parasite was discovered in animals in 1907, but it was not linked to human disease until 1976, Altman continued. Since then it has been blamed for a number of outbreaks traced to public water supplies, and it qualifies as one of the new and emerging microbes that the National Academy of Sciences believes could threaten the nation's health.

CHLORINE IS NOT ENOUGH

"Because cryptosporidia are resistant to chlorination, filtration is the only way to keep drinking water parasite-free," Altman said. "Many waterworks around the country are aging and vulnerable to breakdown, and experts are urging an increase in research to find new ways to identify and remove dangerous microbes from drinking water."

Cryptosporidiosis tends to affect those with an impaired immune system, Altman added. Such an outbreak might be especially harmful to patients with AIDS, cancer and other immunological disorders.[2]

Four major outbreaks of cryptosporidiosis are known to have occurred in the U.S. and three in the United Kingdom, according to Marilynn Marchione in the April 29, 1993 issue of Medical Tribune. The first outbreak was reported in 1984 in a suburb of San Antonio, Texas; the second in 1987 in Carrollton, Georgia; and the third sometime in the 1980s in eastern Pennsylvania.[3]

During the Milwaukee outbreak, residents were urged to boil their water for at least five minutes, and bottled water sales naturally soared. Prior to the outbreak, at least 45 people had reported poor water quality to the treatment plant, Marchione said.[3]

Major ground water contamination has been found in widespread areas of the country, including New Jersey, Long Island and upstate New York, reported Philip Shabecoff in the August 13, 1981 issue of The New York Times. But that is just the tip of the iceberg. The EPA has identified over 30,000 industrial waste dumps, many containing toxic chemicals but having no safeguards to prevent seepage into water supplies.

"The contamination of ground water is an insidious process, with plumes of chemicals slowly thrusting into aquifers and contaminating water well by well," Shabecoff added. "Unlike surface contamination, which is quickly diluted, chemicals in rock-bound ground water tend to remain highly concentrated in the water that flows from the tap. Ground water pollution is also hard to detect and treat."[4]

The EPA identified more than 160 organic compounds, including a number of confirmed or suspected carcinogens, and a variety of other toxic pollutants in city water systems around the country, according to Peter Gwynne in the February 17, 1975 issue of Newsweek. The chemicals come mostly from petrochemical plants, other heavy industries and agricultural run-off, and some experts expect more of these contaminants will be found.[5]

An example of excessive chemical contamination is in Louisiana, which tops all other states in the amount of toxic chemicals discharged into the air, land and water, reported *Friends of the Earth* in 1992. The EPA estimated that 715 million pounds of toxic chemicals were discharged along "Cancer Alley" in 1988.[6]

With this brief overview of the dangers facing us each time we open the water tap in our homes, is it any wonder that more and more Americans are turning to mineral water, sparkling water and other bottled waters? Many other Americans are turning to bottled water to avoid having to drink fluoridated water. (This is addressed in another chapter.)

Mineral water is generally considered to be water that is drawn from an underground spring or other source which contains dissolved solids or trace minerals in the ratio of 500 or more parts per million. Some mineral waters contain 618 ppm. These water sources are generally well protected, so that there is a minimum amount of contamination from outside sources.

LABELS, TERMS CONFUSING

There are about 475 bottled water plants in the U.S., producing more than 600 different brands, according to the International Bottled Water Association in Alexandria, Virginia. Another 75 brands are imported waters, most of which are in the naturally carbonated mineral water category.[7]

"The Food and Drug Administration, which regulates bottled water as a 'food,' has declined to define 'mineral water' or 'natural,' " the Association said. "The U.S. government does not regulate mineral water in the same way it does other bottled waters, however, mineral water must still meet FDA Good Manufacturing Practices, health and safety standards and labeling requirements."[7]

The Association regards mineral water as bottled water that contains not less than 500 ppm of total dissolved solids. For those mineral waters which are bottled and sold as carbonated or sparkling waters, the following information is declared on the label:

1. "Naturally carbonated mineral water" or "naturally sparkling mineral water" means water whose carbon dioxide content is from the same source as the water;
2. "Carbonated natural mineral water" or "sparkling natural mineral water" means water to which has been added carbon dioxide of an origin other than the water table or deposit from which the water comes;

3. "Carbonated drinking water" means water to which has been added carbon dioxide of an origin other than the source water.[7]

William Carl Clifford in the July 1976 issue of *Weight Watchers Magazine* explained:

The traces of minerals in mineral water may be something that either you or your doctor thinks you need. Many mineral waters are low in sodium—several of them specify this on the label. All are free of sugar, and you can drink any quantity of them without harm. Besides enjoying mineral waters at home, travelers frequently order them in hotels and restaurants. This is a more common practice abroad than it is in America, and many foreign restaurants insist that you buy a bottle of water if you don't order wine. You might like to follow the same rule traveling across America, both to avoid the different sets of bacteria in each place, and to give yourself a little harmless luxury, especially if others are drinking alcohol.[8]

Here is the mineral content of a popular brand of bottled water:

TABLE 5.1

MINERAL CONTENT OF BOTTLED WATER

MINERALS	MILLIGRAMS PER LITER
Bicarbonate	97.5
Calcium	27.4
Chloride	6.5
Fluoride	*
Iron	*
Magnesium	6.0
Nitrate	0.6
Potassium	2.0
Sodium**	13.0
Sulfate	36.7
pH	7.9
Alkalinity	0.0
Hardness	89.2
Total dissolved solids/liter	165.0

* Below detectable limits.
** Sodium free. The FDA classifies sodium free as less than 20.5 mg/liter.

Another reason for drinking bottled water is to avoid the potential risks of consuming too much chlorine, which is used in *all* water supplies to kill bacteria.

"When added to drinking water, chlorine interacts with trace chemicals in the water to form cancer-causing byproducts," according to Daniel Wartenberg, Ph.D., and Caron Chess in the 1994 edition of *Medical and Health Annual.* "Previous studies comparing the cancer rates of populations with and without chlorination have had equivocal results."[9]

They added that, on the basis of a statistical appraisal, they found significantly increased risks of rectal and bladder cancer in people who drank chlorinated water.[9]

"It is possible to overdose on chlorine and fluoride from drinking tap water, especially if you are a heavy drinker of coffee and tea, or if you use other fluoridated products like toothpaste and mouthwash," reported James Braly, M.D., in *Dr. Braly's Food Allergy and Nutrition Revolution.* "Excessive chlorine elevates serum cholesterol and has been reported to damage the walls of arteries. Excess fluoride can discolor one's teeth and cause brittle bones."[10]

In the July 11, 1992 issue of *Science News,* K. A. Fackelmann discussed a statistical analysis of 22 studies by Robert D. Morris of the Medical College of Wisconsin in Milwaukee. His extensive research found that those who drink chlorinated water run a 21 percent greater risk of bladder cancer and a 35 percent greater risk of rectal cancer than those who drink little or no chlorinated water.[11]

Franz H. Rampen, et al., reported in the May 1992 issue of *Epidemiology* that the worldwide pollution of rivers and oceans and the chlorination of swimming pool water may be contributing to increases in melanoma, a deadly skin cancer, and that more studies are needed.[12]

In *The Federal Veterinarian,* August 1992, researchers said that standard chlorinated water can destroy polyunsaturated fatty acids, which might alter DNA.[13]

Chlorine also destroys vitamin E and many of the intestinal flora that are necessary for digesting food, according to *Foods and Nutrition Encyclopedia.*[14]

Roughly 200 million U.S. residents drink water disinfected with chlorine, said J. Raloff in the June 3, 1989 issue of *Science News.* Decades of research have demonstrated chlorination's benefits in limiting outbreaks of typhoid fever and other acute diseases from microbial contaminants, Raloff added, but four groups of federal researchers report that these benefits may come at the expense of a small added risk of chronic disease—mostly heart disease or cancer.[15]

For those who can afford bottled water, it would seem to be a wise investment in good health.

REFERENCES

1. Symons, Dr. James M. *Plain Talk About Drinking Water*. Denver, Colorado: American Water Works Association, 1992, pp. 5ff.
2. Altman, Lawrence K., M.D. "Outbreak of Disease in Milwaukee Undercuts Confidence in Water," *The New York Times*, April 20, 1993, p. C3.
3. Marchione, Marilynn. "Milwaukee Outbreak Linked to Parasite-Infected Water Source," *Medical Tribune*, April 29, 1993.
4. Shabecoff, Philip. "Toxic Chemicals Loom as Big Threat to the Nation's Supply of Safe Water," *The New York Times*, August 13, 1981, p. B6.
5. Gwynne, Peter. "How Pure Is Your Water?" *Newsweek*, February 17, 1975, pp. 89–90.
6. "Come Along on a Cancer Alley Tour," *Friends of the Earth*, October 1992, pp. 8ff.
7. "20 Questions About the Bottled Water Industry," International Bottled Water Association, Alexandria, Virginia, 1989.
8. Clifford, William Carl. "Turn Off the Tap and Turn On to Mineral Water," *Weight Watchers Magazine*, July 1976, pp. 16ff.
9. Wartenberg, Daniel, Ph.D., and Chess, Caron. "Environmental Health." In *Medical and Health Annual*. Chicago: Encyclopaedia Britannica, Inc., 1994, pp. 287ff.
10. Braly, James, M.D., and Torbet, Laura. *Dr. Braly's Food Allergy and Nutrition Revolution*. New Canaan, Conn.: Keats Publishing, Inc., 1992, p. 244.
11. Fackelmann, K. A. "Hints of a Chlorine-Cancer Connection," *Science News* 142:23, July 11, 1992.
12. Rampen, Franz H., et al. "Is Water Pollution the Cause of Cutaneous Melanoma?" *Epidemiology* 3(3):263–265, May 1992.
13. "Radical Concerns Over Drinking Water," *The Federal Veterinarian*, August 1992, p. 4.
14. Ensminger, Audrey H., et al. *Foods and Nutrition Encyclopedia*. Clovis, Calif.: Pegus Press, 1983, p. 406.
15. Raloff, J. "Chlorination: Residues Cloud Water Safety," *Science News* 135:342, June 3, 1989.

6

The Chelation Therapy Controversy

ALTHOUGH the medical establishment generally frowns on chelation therapy, this procedure is being used by a number of holistic physicians to treat a wide variety of conditions:

- Heart and artery problems
- To enhance memory
- To prevent cholesterol deposits in the liver
- To dissolve kidney stones
- To minimize the effects of intermittent claudication (a cramping exercise-induced pain caused by an inadequate supply of blood to muscles).
- Chelation therapy is also used to purge the body of toxic metals such as lead and mercury.
- To decrease macular degeneration

. . . And many other health complaints.

WHAT IS CHELATION THERAPY?

As explained by Morton Walker, D.P.M. in his book, *The Chelation Answer,* chelation therapy consists of injections of a synthetic amino acid, such as ethylenediamine tetra-acetic acid (EDTA), which is introduced into the body through an intravenous infusion. This protein-like material ties up or "chelates" various minerals that are in the bloodstream. Since calcium is one of the most prevalent minerals in the bloodstream, a chelating agent has a profound effect on calcium metabolism and the availability of the mineral, since it locks onto the ionic calcium and removes it from the body, mainly via urine.[1]

Medical science recognizes that a major component of circulatory impairment is spasm or constriction of the arteries. Although the origin of the arterial spasm is not known, blood vessel specialists believe that the major problem involves some disturbance of calcium metabolism in the cardiovascular system. Sidney Alexander, M.D., Chief of Cardiology at the Lahey Clinic and Professor of Medicine at the Harvard Medical School, said that medicine's recognition of calcium's role in blocking arterial blood flow is bringing about "a pharmacological revolution" in cardiovascular treatment. Walker theorizes that chelation (pronounced key-lay-shun) therapy may soon begin to be recognized as the leader in that revolution. In fact, EDTA chelation therapy is the first of an entirely new class of medicines known as calcium channel blockers. Walker explained:

> This new understanding about the underlying involvement of excess accumulation of heart and blood vessel calcium has been tied to the aging process. It is known that if a person could avoid an excessive calcification of the cells in the arteries, he or she would avoid loss of arterial elasticity. The blood would circulate more effectively, bringing nutrition to all the body cells and taking away their waste products. Research evidence from both living animals and human cadavers indicates that EDTA chelation therapy partially eliminates or reverses the formation of atherosclerotic plaque. While the reversal of plaque formation in human arteries has not been proven to the satisfaction of everyone in medicine, much documentation exists confirming that intravenous EDTA infusion does increase the circulation in most people having this chelation treatment.[1]

Tests reveal that infusions of EDTA help to pull calcium from atherosclerotic plaque and other areas of the body where it is abnormally deposited, such as in tendons, joints and ligaments. Fortunately, this procedure does not appear to significantly remove the mineral from bones and teeth.[1]

"Chelation therapy has worked extremely well for more than 300,000 victims of hardening of the arteries," Walker said. "A patient's blood pressure usually becomes normal, hands and feet grow warm with improved blood flow, kidney problems are averted and the chances of stroke or heart attack are greatly reduced. Remarkable circulatory improvement takes place through all the blood vessels. Yet, for many reasons—mostly political—chelation therapy is seldom recommended by an orthodox physician as the treatment of choice for a person's impaired cardiovascular system. As it stands now, someone who is suffering from hardening of the arteries generally receives grossly incomplete information about his exact circulatory condition and all of the different therapies available."[1]

USES OF CHELATION THERAPY

William J. Mauer, D.O. of Zion, Illinois is a Diplomate in Chelation Therapy of the American Academy of Medical Preventics. He believes that EDTA chelation therapy is useful because it:

- Eliminates heavy metal toxicity.
- Makes arterial walls more flexible.
- Manages excess quantities of fat in the blood.
- Prevents osteoarthritis.
- Causes rheumatoid arthritis symptoms to disappear.
- Has an anti-aging effect.
- Smooths skin wrinkles.
- Offers psychological relief.
- Assures the presence of adequate zinc in the blood.
- Lowers insulin requirements for diabetics.
- Dissolves large and small thrombi.[1]

In *Minerals: Kill or Cure?*, Ruth Adams and I reported the EDTA forms compounds that are very stable, thus holding on to the metal until it can be dispatched out of the body. EDTA can be used against cadmium, chromium, cobalt, copper, lead, manganese, nickel, radium, selenium, tungsten, uranium, vanadium and zinc. Another chelating agent, dimercaprol, is used by physicians to detoxify people who have accumulated too much antimony, arsenic, bismuth, gold, lead, mercury, nickel and tungsten in their bodies. Dimercaprol and EDTA are used to chelate lead. For those who accumulate too much iron, the drug deferoxamine is used. An overdose of thallium, which is used in rat, ant and roach poisons, can be removed from the body with dithiocarb or dithizon.

A disease called polycythemia involves the making of too many red blood cells in the body. Too much cobalt can cause this disorder in rats, mice, guinea pigs, dogs, ducks, chickens and human beings. A number of years ago a number of heavy beer drinkers suffered severe heart damage because the beer was contaminated with cobalt. EDTA was given to them to remove the metal from their bodies.[2]

Chelating agents are also used to make essential minerals more available to plants, animals and human beings. EDTA is used to make iron in soil more available to plants, for example. The chelates of iron can be put in the soil or sprayed on the plants. Chelated minerals can also be used in animal feed to increase the animals' absorption of iron, copper, zinc, etc. Casein (a protein in milk) and liver extract contain chelates which improve the absorption and utilization of zinc. And chelated minerals are available in health food stores to help in the absorption of the supplements.[2]

"Because a few of the chelated minerals are made in such a way as to provide a dramatic increase in mineral absorption, many people have expressed concern about getting an overdose," reported H. Dewayne Ashmead, Ph.D., in *Conversations on Chelation and Mineral Nutrition*. "While some forms of chelated minerals do increase the chances of mineral toxicity, a lot depends on how naturally the chelate is processed. In other words, how closely does the manufacturing of the chelate conform to the way the body would build that same chelate under ideal conditions? The question of toxicity revolves around the idea that ingestion of certain chemicals that are used in the growing or processing of foods is harmful to the body because of the abnormal reactions which these chemicals may cause."[3]

The same problem is associated with nonchelated minerals, Ashmead added. Magnesium sulfate, an inorganic form of the mineral, produces diarrhea. Iron sulfate can cause gastric upset (diarrhea or constipation) and should not be taken with vitamin E, since it has a destructive effect on the vitamin. These toxic reactions, he continued, do not occur if these same minerals which cause constipation, diarrhea, gastric upset, etc., are *ionized*, that is, removed from their carriers such as carbonate, sulfate and gluconate, and properly chelated with amino acids from hydrolyzed protein.[3]

Writing in the *Journal of the National Medical Association* in 1990, Efrain Olszewer, M.D. said that chelation therapy is safe and that it has been utilized by over 500,000 patients without a reported incidence of renal failure or death since 1960. He said that the reported kidney side effects occurred prior to 1960, before the advent of routine biochemical screening and also in patients receiving more than three grams of EDTA per infusion and/or those who had lead poisoning, which can form lead complexes in the kidney. When intracellular calcium is chelated by EDTA, there is an increase in vascular diameter and blood flow, decreased vascular tone and contractility and a decrease in peripheral resistance by removing intracellular calcium from ischemic tissue.[4] Olszewer's research team, from Tulane University School of Medicine in New Orleans, made their observations after doing a double-blind study with 10 male patients with Type II (LaFontaine) peripheral vascular disease. Although 20 intravenous infusions (EDTA, magnesium, B-complex vitamins and vitamin C) or a placebo were planned, clinical and laboratory tests showed a dramatic improvement in the treatment group after 10 infusions and the code was broken. There was no change in the placebo group.[4]

W. Blumer, M.D., a Swiss physician, has used a calcium-EDTA chelation injection for 30 years to treat patients with lead intoxication, especially those who live near roadways or who are exposed to lead at work, such as garage employees or chauffeurs. He also uses oral doses of vitamin C, which enhances the effect of EDTA, and vitamin B1 (thiamine), which is important for the penetration of EDTA into the central nervous system. Blumer reported that two-thirds of the patients treated with this therapy are completely cured of their psychological symptoms and that 20 percent are clearly improved. For those whose symptoms resurface in several months or years, the same therapy is prescribed and positive results are reported.[5]

Dementia Reversed

In March, 1985, Abram Hoffer, M.D., Ph.D., writing in *Orthomolecular Medicine for Physicians,* told how he had interviewed an elderly man one month after he had received his last of 20 chelation treatments. He had had Alzheimer's disease, and, according to his wife, he had deteriorated to such a degree he could no longer speak intelligently; he was disoriented and could not be left alone in a city for even a few seconds, as he wandered away and became lost.[6]

"After 10 treatments," Hoffer said, "he was no longer disoriented in space. About this time he seemed to awaken from a sleep. I asked him what was his memory of the condition he had been in. He replied he could not remember what it was like, but he recalled that sometime during the last 10 treatments he had awakened. When I saw him he spoke well, tended to be garrulous, but showed no evidence of any Alzheimer's speech disorder. Here is an objective measure of the value of chelation. I was very impressed. I hope any critic will not immediately demand a double-blind controlled experiment until he is prepared to direct me to the literature that shows the spontaneous recovery rate is more than 0 percent. One recovery in a disease where there have been none before is surely very significant. What we must know is what proportion of Alzheimer's sufferers will respond; is this related to metal intoxication, and, if it is, which element is most significant?"[6]

A number of reports have shown that many American children, especially those in the inner cities, are suffering from lead poisoning, which hinders their growth. Lead seems to inhibit thyroid stimulating hormone, which helps to regulate growth. However, a study reported in *Science News* in 1992 found that the children given chelation therapy experienced a rapid growth spurt. In one child, bone growth rate almost tripled.[7]

W. Blumer, M.D., the Swiss physician previously mentioned, reported in *Environmental International* in 1990 that 231 people living near a road had a higher incidence of cancer than those living in a traffic-free section of the same town. Fifty-nine of those living near the road were treated with EDTA to eliminate lead and only one of them died of cancer. Thirty of those who were not given chelation therapy died. He and his colleagues believe that lead in automobile gasoline, combined with other carcinogens in automotive exhaust, increases the incidence of cancer. Other carcinogens along the roadway included nitrosamines, epoxides, tetraethyl-lead and asbestos.[8]

"Chelation therapy is another alternative to surgery for treatment of atherosclerosis," reported Jonathan V. Wright, M.D., in *Dr. Wright's Guide to Healing with Nutrition*. "Starting as simply a series of intravenous infusions of EDTA, chelation therapy has grown to include attention to diet and vitamins and minerals as well. Although ignored and put down by established medical organizations, physicians who practice chelation therapy have helped many individuals with atherosclerosis and serious symptoms regain their health without surgery. Many practitioners of chelation therapy are members of the American Academy of Medical Preventics, whose headquarters is in Beverly Hills, California. It's been my observation that a disproportionately large number of individuals with hardening of the arteries at a relatively young age have problems with nutrient malabsorption."[9]

For those with heart and artery complications, memory lapses and other complications listed at the beginning of this chapter, chelation therapy may be beneficial. Even with the 20 to 30 treatments that are usually recommended, chelation therapy costs only a fraction of what a heart bypass or other surgery would cost.

REFERENCES

1. Walker, Morton, D.P.M. *The Chelation Answer*. New York: M. Evans and Co., Inc., 1982, pp. 10ff.
2. Adams, Ruth, and Murray, Frank. *Minerals: Kill or Cure?* New York: Larchmont Books, 1974, pp. 271–273.
3. Ashmead, H. Dewayne, Ph.D. *Conversations on Chelation and Mineral Nutrition*. New Canaan, Conn.: Keats Publishing, Inc., 1989, p. 32.
4. Olszewer, Efrain, M.D., et al. "A Pilot Double-Blind Study of Sodium-Magnesium

EDTA in Peripheral Vascular Disease," *Journal of the National Medical Association* 82(3):173–177, 1990.

5. Blumer, W., M.D. "Treatment of Subjective Central Nervous Symptoms with Intravenous CaNA$_2$-EDTA Injections," *Proceedings, Trace Elements in Man and Animals/Chelation of Trace Elements.* Chapter 24 (Tema7) 24(1): 24, 1991.

6. Hoffer, Abram, M.D., Ph.D. *Orthomolecular Medicine for Physicians.* New Canaan, Conn.: Keats Publishing, Inc., 1989, p. 154.

7. "Why Lead May Leave Kids Short," *Science News,* August 29, 1992, p. 14.

8. Blumer, W., and Reich, T. H. "Leaded Gasoline—A Cause of Cancer," *Environmental International* 3:465–471, 1990.

9. Wright, Jonathan V., M.D. *Dr. Wright's Guide to Healing with Nutrition.* New Canaan, Conn.: Keats Publishing, Inc., 1990, pp. 244–245.

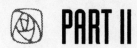

PART II

Minerals You Cannot Live Without

7

Some Drugs Can Destroy Minerals

JUST as some minerals have a love-hate relationship (such as copper and zinc) an equally ominous situation arises when certain drugs interact with minerals. This can result in a potentially violent interaction, somewhat akin to two angry bull elephants during the rut. This is especially critical for many senior citizens, who often take a handful of drugs every day without knowing how each drug will affect the other. It is common knowledge that when two drugs combine, say in the gut, they create a third potentially dangerous substance. When you consider the many possible interactions between all the drugs a person is taking, this can lead to a life-threatening situation. Even such a seemingly benign substance as aspirin kills several hundred Americans annually; tranquilizers have been documented as responsible for the deaths of several thousand people in the U.S. each year.[1]

C. P. Chien, et al. reported back in 1978 that 83 percent of all individuals over 60 years old take two or more drugs. Of the total medications used by this population, 40 percent are over-the-counter (OTC) drugs. In another study, P. Guttman said that 61 percent of the elderly take OTC drugs, 31.7 percent take analgesics and 7.1 percent take laxatives. And analgesics and laxatives, along with antacids, are the major classes of OTC drugs that can cause nutritional deficiencies. The significance of these nutrient losses depends upon the overall nutritional status of the patient. OTC drug-induced nutrient losses can cause serious disorders in the elderly individual who is marginally nourished or suffering from subclinical malnutrition, Guttman added. The nutritional effects of these OTC preparations can impact minerals and other nutrients. As an example, aspi-

51

rin can cause iron deficiency and folic acid depletion; acetaminophen can result in sodium depletion; laxative use and abuse can cause a potassium deficiency; antacid use and abuse is related to aluminum toxicity, folic acid malabsorption, magnesium overload, milk-alkali syndrome, phosphate depletion and sodium overload.[2]

All drugs must be detoxified or undergo biotransformation in order to be excreted, according to Robert H. Garrison, Jr., M.A., R.Ph., and Elizabeth Somer, M.A., R.D. in *The Nutrition Desk Reference*. The biochemical reactions involved are mainly enzymatic and require certain vitamins and minerals as co-factors. Those who are at risk for vitamin and mineral adequacy, especially the elderly on poly drug therapy, may have an impaired ability to metabolize certain drugs. Most drugs are metabolized in two phases. First, if they are not water-soluble, they are converted into water-soluble products to enable transport and excretion. They must then be conjugated to facilitate removal from the body. Vitamin C, calcium, copper, glycine, iron, magnesium, nicotinic acid (B3), pantothenic acid, protein, riboflavin (B2) and iron play key roles in the first step of drug detoxification or biotransformation. If any of these nutrients are deficient, incomplete drug metabolism is possible, which leads to prolonged drug action or side effects from incomplete drug metabolites.[2]

In the second step of drug biotransformation, the authors explained, vitamin B12, nicotinic acid, folic acid, lipoic acid and pantothenic acid, along with carbohydrates, fats and amino acids play a key role. Researchers are still studying the effects of large doses of single nutrients on drug metabolism:

> Many drugs, especially the cardiovascular drugs, can cause mineral deficiencies. Because of the delicate interrelationships among minerals, drug-induced mineral depletion may cause greater imbalances than the drug-induced vitamin deficiencies. It is not uncommon for patients, especially the elderly, to be taking several drugs at the same time that can cause serious mineral imbalances. Hypokalemia with potassium depletion is a well-recognized side effect of diuretics (water pills). The thiazides, furosemide and ethacrynic acid can all cause potassium depletion. Other drugs that may cause hypokalemia and/or potassium depletion include levodopa, amphotericin B, phenolphthalein, senna, bisacodyl, corticosteroids, gentamicin and salicylates at excessive dosages.[2]

Diuretics can also cause serious magnesium imbalances. Most practitioners and pharmacists are aware of diuretic-induced potassium deficiencies and frequently prescribe potassium supplements. Since diuretic-induced magnesium deficiencies are less well known, this consequence of diuretic therapy may be more serious.

Thiazide diuretics are a major class of drugs that can induce a magnesium deficiency. This popular drug, which is used to treat high blood pressure, may increase the risk for cardiac disorders by inducing a magnesium deficiency.

Mildred Seelig, M.D. said that Americans are at risk for magnesium *adequacy*, not necessarily because of inadequate intake, but because of excessive phosphate, fat, sugar and alcohol consumption. Therefore, drugs such as the thiazide diuretics increase the risk of magnesium deficiency. Magnesium supplementation in patients taking thiazide can play a significant role in decreasing some of the untoward effects of these popular diuretics. Other medications that can induce a magnesium deficiency, Somer and Garrison noted, include furosemide, ethacrynic acid, gentamicin, cisplatin, neomycin and colchicine.[2] Magnesium supplements should be prescribed with these drugs.

The other mineral most frequently involved in drug-nutrient interactions is calcium. This, of course, can impact on osteomalacia or osteoporosis by inducing calcium imbalances through mechanisms other than malabsorption. Some of the drugs that affect calcium malabsorption include: Prednisone and other glucosteroids, for allergic and collagen disease; diphosphonates for Paget's disease; glutethimide, a sedative; and these anticonvulsants—phenobarbital, diphenylhydantoin and primidone.[2]

With all of the potential interactions between minerals and drugs, as well as other nutrients, it is easy to see why physicians are often at a loss as to why a patient died. The death certificate may indicate that the patient succumbed to a heart attack or other common ailment, when in fact they may have died from malnutrition or other unsuspected complications.

REFERENCES

1. Hughes, Richard, and Brewin, Robert. *The Tranquilizing of America*. New York: Harcourt Brace Jovanovich, 1979, pp. 8ff.
2. Garrison, Robert H., Jr., M.A., R.Ph., and Somer, Elizabeth, M.A., R.D. *The Nutrition Desk Reference*. New Canaan, Conn.: Keats Publishing, Inc., 1990, pp. 279ff.

8

Why You Must Have Calcium

COMPRISING from 1.5 to 2 percent of an adult's body weight, calcium is essential for the clotting of blood, the action of certain enzymes, as well as the control of the passage of fluids through the cell walls. The right proportion of calcium in the blood is responsible for the alternate contraction and relaxation of the heart muscle. And calcium, in a complex combination with phosphorus, another mineral, gives rigidity and hardness to bones and teeth. A person who weighs 154 pounds would have 2.3 to 3.1 pounds of calcium and 1.2 to 1.7 pounds of phosphorus in his body. Since the two minerals are so closely related, it is important that our diet not contain an overabundance of one mineral and a short supply of the other one, according to *Food, the Yearbook of Agriculture, 1959.*[1]

A hormone secreted by the parathyroid glands (which are embedded in the thyroid gland) plays an important part in the body's use of calcium and an indirect part in the use of phosphorus. The parathyroid hormone keeps the amount of calcium in the blood at a normal level of about 10 milligrams per 100 milliliters of blood serum, which is the watery part of the blood that separates from a clot. Any significant deviation is dangerous to health, since the hormone can shift calcium and phosphorus from the bone into the blood. If the blood levels are too high, it can increase the excretion of these minerals by the kidneys. If anything reduces the secretion of the parathyroid hormone, the calcium in the blood drops quickly, the phosphorus rises, and severe muscular twitching results.

Between 10 and 50 percent of the calcium that we take in is not absorbed but is excreted in the feces. The calcium that is absorbed makes its way in the blood to areas where it is needed, especially bones. Any calcium that is unused is then excreted by the kidneys into the urine. Obviously, healthy kidneys are necessary for the metabolism of calcium and other minerals. Vitamin D is also essential for the proper absorption of calcium from the gastrointestinal tract.

Another disturbance in calcium metabolism is the milk-alkali syndrome. If there is excess calcium in the blood, calcium is deposited in the soft tissues, and the kidneys may not function properly. Vomiting, gastrointestinal bleeding and high blood pressure may also be present. This disturbance occurs chiefly in people with ulcers who for many years have used an almost exclusively milk diet with large amounts of antacids to neutralize the excess acid of the gastric juice. Recovery generally depends on changing the diet under medical supervision to rid the body of the excess calcium. No cases have been reported on a diet of milk without the antacids.

Ninety-nine percent of the calcium of the body is present in the bones and teeth, where calcium salts—chiefly calcium phosphate—held in a cellular matrix provide the rigid framework of the body, according to *Foods and Nutrition Encyclopedia*. It has been estimated that in an adult male about 700 milligrams of calcium enter and leave the bones each day. Although teeth are somewhat similar to bone in chemical composition, tooth enamel is much harder and is lower in water content—only about 5 percent. Unlike that of bone, calcium in teeth cannot be replaced and therefore teeth cannot repair themselves.[2]

Calcium salts are more soluble in an acid solution. Therefore, calcium absorption occurs mainly in the upper part (duodenal area) of the small intestine, where the food contents are still somewhat acidic after being digested in the stomach. An increase in the passage of food through the gastrointestinal tract also decreases the percentage of absorption.[3]

NEEDS CHANGE

Calcium absorption is dependent on the calcium needs of the body, the type of food and the amount of calcium ingested. Growing children and pregnant and breast-feeding women utilize calcium most efficiently, roughly 40 percent. The body's need is greatest and the absorption of calcium is relatively more efficient following long periods of low calcium intake and body depletion and during healing of bone fractures.

In addition to the amount of calcium in the diet, a number of factors influence the absorption of the mineral. These include:

1. An adequate supply of vitamin D, either from the diet or exposure to ultraviolet radiation from the sun. The vitamin (or its metabolite, 25-hydroxycholecalciferol), increases calcium absorption by inducing synthesis

of a calcium-binding protein that helps transport the mineral through the intestinal walls.

2. The amount of protein in the diet increases the rate of calcium absorption from the small intestine. This is probably because amino acids or links of protein, such as lysine and arginine, which are liberated in the course of protein digestion, form soluble calcium salts which are more easily absorbed. Of course, increased absorption may be offset by the increased urinary loss of the mineral with high-protein diets.

3. Lactose, the sugar in milk, increases the rate of calcium absorption from the small intestine. Since milk is the only source of lactose, the improved absorption of the mineral is dependent on the availability of intestinal lactase, the enzyme that hydrolyzes lactose.

4. Absorption of calcium is enhanced by an acid medium (a lower pH), since it keeps the mineral in solution. And, as previously mentioned, most of the absorption takes place in the duodenum, the first section of the small intestine, which is located between the stomach and the jejunum.

At the same time, a variety of dietary factors can interfere with calcium absorption.

1. An insufficient supply of vitamin D decreases the amount of the calcium-binding protein. In northern climates or smoggy cities, where UV radiation is limited or blocked, the dietary source of vitamin D becomes very important.

2. An excess intake of calcium or phosphorus inhibits the absorption of both minerals and the increased excretion of the lesser mineral. That is why the calcium to phosphorus ratio is so important. This ratio in typical American diets has been variously reported to be 1:1.5 to 1:1.6. The most desirable ratio is thought to be 1.5:1 for infants; decreasing to 1:1 at one year of age; and remaining at 1:1 for the rest of life.

3. Phytic acid, which is found in the outer hulls or bran of many grains, forms an insoluble salt with calcium (calcium phytate) thus preventing the absorption of the mineral. This is thought not to be a major problem unless a person's diet is composed mostly of whole-grain cereals and/or the amount of calcium in the diet is low. Phytin can be separated by the enzyme phytase, which is found in several grains. The presence of this enzyme may explain why the mineral is more available in leavened than unleavened breads.

4. Oxalic acid, which is found in spinach, beet tops, swiss chard, cocoa, rhubarb and other foods, can prevent the absorption of calcium because of the formation of calcium oxalate, which is a relatively insoluble compound.

5. The fiber in plants with small amounts of phytate bind with calcium in proportion to its uronic acid content. Uronic acids can be digested by bacteria in the colon, which may explain why calcium absorption is increased slowly after a change from a low-fiber to a high-fiber diet.

6. Excessive fat in the diet, especially saturated fat, decreases calcium absorption, since the fats interact with calcium to form insoluble soaps, a process called saponification. These insoluble soaps are excreted in the feces, taking with them some calcium and possibly fat-soluble vitamin D. This is why patients with chronic intestinal complaints, such as celiac sprue and celiac disease, are known to have steatorrhea (increased fat in the feces) and may develop osteomalacia later on. Osteomalacia is characterized by a softening of the bone due to a deficiency in calcium and vitamin D.

7. Since calcium is insoluble in an alkaline medium, it is poorly utilized under these conditions.

8. People who are under extreme stress or who do not exercise sufficiently often have negative calcium balances, even though the diet may contain a great deal of the mineral. Aging is also thought to inhibit the rate of calcium absorption.

"Prolonged bed rest during convalescence from illness makes bones weaken, and after a few weeks of being propped up, idle, a bone in the leg loses a substantial proportion of its bone/calcium content," according to *ABC's of the Human Body*. "The same sort of thing happened early in the space program; prolonged missions in the weightlessness of outer space kept the astronauts immobile. The lack of exercise contributed to the bone loss. Now, astronauts follow an exercise regimen while orbiting the Earth and their bones fare much better. Certainly, there is plenty of evidence that exercise causes bones to grow sturdier and increases their capacity to store minerals and manufacture blood cells."[4]

As you grow older, your body's supplies of calcium begin to dwindle, and, if the calcium level in your blood should fall below its normal range, the body begins to draw on the supply in your bones. This is especially critical for older people, who tend to be careless about their diets and they often neglect eating enough calcium-rich foods. In addition, older people tend to exercise less, and they are apt to spend more time indoors. This prevents them from absorbing enough vitamin D from the sun. After menopause, women tend to lose the protective effect of the hormone estrogen, which often results in a rapid loss of bone calcium. This paves the way for osteoporosis and a spate of broken bones.

"Bones are among the most perfect creations of nature," reported *ABC's of the Human Body*. "Each one can withstand four times the weight resisted by a comparable amount of reinforced concrete and about the same weight resisted by aluminum or light steel. The key to the bones' extraordinary strength-lightness ratio is the way atoms of calcium and phosphorus are densely packed together inside the bone in regular, crystalline patterns. Diamonds, which are the hardest of all natural substances, owe their great density to similar crystalline structures."[4]

STRONG, BUT VULNERABLE

As perfect as they are, a bone's crystalline patterns are somewhat flawed, in that they often develop tiny fissures or cracks somewhat akin to the crystalline dislocations that cause "fatigued" metal to collapse. If these cracks are not contained, by healing, they can widen and seriously weaken the bone. A sharp blow to a bone can cause somewhat the same effect as a whack to a diamond, which can crack along its lines of cleavage.

"Another hazard is the fact that under certain circumstances, radioactive substances, such as radium, can accumulate in bone," the publication added. "Once radium is present, even tiny amounts of it become 'the enemy within,' destroying the surrounding marrow and bone tissue with 'tracer bullet' radiation. This occasionally causes fatal tumors. So, ironically, your body's enormously strong inner scaffolding, the skeleton, can become one of its most vulnerable points."

Although the bony framework of the body weighs only about 20 pounds, the bones do much more than allow you to stand and walk. For example, they protect your internal organs: the skull safeguards the brain, while the rib cage shields the heart and lungs. The marrow inside some of the bones produces red blood cells that carry oxygen and nutrients throughout the body, while the marrow in other bones makes millions of white cells that destroy harmful bacteria. In addition, bones have the ability to repair themselves after an injury without leaving a scar.

In understanding the internal scaffolding of the body, we find that the skull, spine and rib cage account for 80 of the body's 206 bones, thus forming the "axial" skeleton. The others are known as the "appendicular" skeleton and include the shoulder, arms, hands, hips, legs and feet. The skull contains 28 bones, with eight of them fused to cover the brain. At the bottom of the skull is a hole that surrounds the top of the spinal cord. The shoulder group includes the shovel-shaped scapula (from the Greek meaning "dig"), and the key-shaped clavicle, which translates from Latin as "little keys." The 24 ribs are anchored to the spine to protect the heart and lungs. Also included are the thick breastbone. The lower half of the skeleton begins with the pelvis and ends with the 26 bones in the ankles and feet.[5]

REFERENCES

1. *Food, the Yearbook of Agriculture*. Washington, D.C.: U.S. Government Printing Office, 1959. (Out of print.)
2. Ensminger, Audrey H., et al. *Foods and Nutrition Encyclopedia*. Clovis, Calif.: Pegus Press, 1983, p. 291.
3. Ibid, p. 292.
4. Guinness, Alma E., editor. *ABC's of the Human Body*. Pleasantville, N.Y.: The Reader's Digest Association, Inc., 1987, p. 182.
5. Ibid, pp. 106–161.

9

Which Foods Contain Calcium?

ALTHOUGH 99 percent of the calcium in the body is used to build strong bones and teeth, the mineral is also essential for the clotting of blood; muscle contraction and relaxation (including the heart); nerve transmission; the secretion of hormones; cell-wall permeability; and for enzyme activation. Therefore, calcium is one of our most important minerals and studies suggest that many of us are not ingesting the daily Recommended Dietary Allowance.

When you ask nonlacto-ovo vegetarians where they are getting their calcium, they invariably say that it comes from spinach. But, according to *Composition of Foods*, Agriculture Handbook No. 8, a serving of spinach (100 grams) contains only 93 mg of calcium.[1] That means that if you are relying on spinach as your source of calcium, you would have to ingest almost nine servings of spinach daily to meet the RDA. Plus, because of the oxalic acid in spinach, very little of the calcium is actually being absorbed.[1]

LIMITATIONS OF VEGETABLES

"Women cannot get sufficient calcium from spinach," Robert P. Heaney, M.D., John A. Creighton University Professor, Creighton University, Omaha, Nebraska, told me. "For reasons not entirely understood, but partly explained by the oxalic acid content of spinach, the calcium of spinach is not available to the body. That has been thoroughly tested and is now a solidly established fact. However, the calcium from other vegetable sources is available. We have tested intrinsically labeled kale, which can serve as a surrogate for all of the *Brassica sp.* vegetables (which includes turnip, mustard and collard greens, among others). It is, however, unlikely that people will eat enough greens in contemporary society to get their full calcium requirement. If a person were doing heavy farm labor, and greens were a major component of the diet, then things would be different. But that is not the way things are today."[2]

Other poor sources of calcium, because of their oxalic acid content, are beet tops, rhubarb, swiss chard and cocoa. The oxalic acid converts the calcium into calcium oxalate, a relatively insoluble compound, and removes it from the body without it being absorbed.[3]

In a study reported in the *American Journal of Clinical Nutrition,* Heaney and colleagues Connie M. Weaver, Ph.D., of Purdue University, and Robert R. Recker, M.D., of Creighton University, tested the absorbability of calcium from spinach and milk in 13 healthy adults in a randomized crossover study. The absorption of calcium from milk was higher in every case, with the mean absorption from milk averaging 27.6 percent and 5.1 percent from spinach. Because of the variability of mechanisms used to measure the results, it is possible that the calcium absorption from spinach may be even lower, they added.

"Despite the conflicting data from many calcium-balance studies in humans extending back over 60 years, it would seem that the observations reported (in our study) conclusively establish that the calcium in spinach has very limited bioavailability."

They added that spinach contains appreciable quantities of magnesium, which would be expected to compete with calcium for complexing with the oxalate. Magnesium oxalate is about two orders of magnitude more soluble than calcium oxalate, so the spinach magnesium would not be expected to bind very much oxalate. Nevertheless, they continued, it is difficult to say exactly what might happen under the extremely complex conditions that exist in the intestinal contents and they could, therefore, not exclude some small contribution from this source.[4]

In another study, involving 11 healthy women ranging in age from 20 to 45, Heaney and Weaver reported in the *American Journal of Clinical Nutrition* in 1990 that calcium is absorbed slightly better in kale than in milk. However, they added, "The somewhat higher absorbability found for kale relative to milk is probably of little practical nutritional importance."

The researchers said that many dark-green leafy vegetables are known to have relatively high calcium nutrient densities and, spinach excepted, have been presumed to be good sources of calcium. Animal studies have generally supported this assumption as have a few balance studies in humans. But balance studies in humans are prey to large errors, and hence the question of absorbability of calcium from these sources has remained open, they said. Their study is thought to be the first that describes in humans the absorbability of calcium from kale by use of modern isotope methods and an intrinsically labeled food source.

"We selected kale specifically because it was a low-oxalate vegetable that nevertheless contains some of the pectins and other plant fibers that might be typical of other greens," the researchers said. "For example, the total fiber content of kale (2.6 g per 100 g) is similar to that of spinach (2.3 g per 100 g). Kale also has approximately the same uronic acid content as spinach."[5]

Kale seemed a suitable choice because it is one of the varieties of *Brassica oleracea,* several of the members of which are known to be rich in calcium and are commonly recommended to the general public as good calcium sources (e.g., broccoli). Further, they said, turnip, collard and mustard, the greens of which are also rich in calcium, are also members of this same Brassica genus. Hence kale seemed a good surrogate for a large class of low-oxalate, high-calcium vegetable greens.[5]

In yet another study, published in *Calcified Tissue International,* Heaney, Recker and Weaver reported that, in studying four food calcium sources, kale was slightly better than 2-percent milk and bone meal, with spinach a distant fourth. And bone meal was substantially better absorbed than hydroxyapatite, a synthetic chemical that resembles the mineral salt of bones and teeth.[6]

An article in *Osteo Forum* in 1989 said that, in addition to effective calcium intake to maintain bone health, other factors are also involved, such as absorption efficiency, the level of obligatory losses, mechanical loading (exercise) and normal gonadal hormone levels. Other factors which are also of critical importance to all women, since they impact on bone mass, include smoking, alcohol abuse, corticosteroid therapy and prolonged use of aluminum-containing antacids.

"While some people can conserve calcium efficiently and maintain balance on relatively low intakes, many cannot," Heaney said. "For a population, the best strategy seems to be to assure rather higher intakes than had previously been thought sufficient. Several converging threads of evidence suggest that intakes in the range of 1,000 to 1,500 mg/day—and possibly even higher—may be optimal."

Over 10 years ago Matkovic et al., in a cross-sectional study, reported a 60 to 75 percent reduction in hip fracture in Yugoslav women who had calcium intakes in the range of 1,000 to 1,100 mg/day, compared with women who had intakes about half that level. Later, Holbrook et al., in the United States, reported a 60 percent reduction in hip fractures in individuals with habitual calcium intakes above 765 mg/day when compared with those who got under 470 mg/day.[7]

"Many longitudinal studies have shown either slowing or cessation of bone loss when persons on previously average-to-low intakes are raised to 1,500 to 2,500 mg/day of calcium," Heaney continued. "For example, two recently completed randomized trials lasting from two to four years, demonstrated complete cessation of bone loss in osteoporotic women on intakes at or above 1,500 mg/day. These studies complement many other reports that have also shown a substantial effect of high calcium intakes on the rate of bone loss in normal postmenopausal women."[7]

SUPPLEMENTS ARE ESSENTIAL

If you are still not convinced that daily calcium intake from foods and/or supplements, is not a deterrent to bone problems, consider the study by M. Andon, et al., of the University of California at San Diego, and reported in the *American Journal of Clinical Nutrition* in 1991. The study, involving postmenopausal women between the ages of 57 and 72, tabulated the calcium intake, which averaged 606 mg/day of calcium; the intakes ranged from 304 to 906 mg/day. Those who got less than the average calcium intake exhibited significantly reduced bone mineral density when compared to women whose daily intake of the mineral was above the average.[8]

In fact, it is never too late to increase calcium intake to strengthen mineral-deficient bones, according to M. Thomas, et al., of the University of Texas Medical Branch at Galveston, in *Bone Mineral* in 1991.[9]

As we know, dairy products are rich sources of calcium. Depending on the type of yogurt, you can obtain between 274 to 452 mg of calcium from one cup of yogurt.[10] See Table 8.1 for foods rich in calcium.

"While drinking plenty of skim milk would seem to be an obvious solution (for getting more calcium in your diet), many people don't like its taste or can't digest the lactose most dairy products contain," reported the March 12, 1988 issue of *Science News*. "Many who could eat cheese are reluctant to make [this] their primary calcium source because of the calories, cholesterol and fat it contains. But two alternatives that might warrant consideration include tofu and lime-treated corn tortillas, according to new animal research at the University of Illinois in Urbana-Champaign."

Researchers Angela Poneros-Schneier and John Erdman say that tortillas' main calcium source is the lime, an alkaline compound added to soften the corn as it is boiled. Not only is the tortilla's calcium "highly bioavailable"—almost equivalent to that in milk—but the lime treatment enhances protein quality. The Illinois team measured the leg bones of rats after they had been eating tortillas for 27 days and found that they can provide up to almost 300 mg/day of calcium per 100 g (3.5 ounces).[11]

TABLE 9.1

FOODS RICH IN CALCIUM

A serving of any of the following foods provides at least 10 percent of the U.S. Recommended Daily Allowance of calcium for adult men and women. (The USRDA is 1,000 milligrams.)

FOOD	SERVING SIZE	MILLIGRAMS OF CALCIUM
Plain, low-fat yogurt	8 ounces	415
Canned sardines, with bones	3 ounces	371
Part skim-milk ricotta cheese	½ cup	334
Skim milk	1 cup	302–316
Two-percent low-fat milk	1 cup	297–313
Swiss cheese	1 ounce	272
Soft-service ice cream	1 cup	236
Nonfat dry milk	¼ cup	209
Cheddar, Muenster, or part skim-milk mozzarella cheese	1 ounce	203–207
Fried oysters, dipped in egg, milk, bread crumbs	4 oysters	196
Slivered almonds	½ cup	179
Cooked, chopped collards	½ cup	178
Pasteurized process American cheese	1 ounce	174
Canned salmon, with bones	3 ounces	167
Feta cheese	1 ounce	140
Cooked broccoli	¾ cup	132
Tofu	1 piece (2½×2¾×1 inch)	108

From *FDA Consumer,* October 1986, p. 36. Taken from The U.S. Department of Agriculture's "Nutritive Value of Foods," Home and Garden Bulletin No. 72.

More unexpected was a finding that the calcium in the soybean-based tofu they studied was 12.6 percent more bioavailable than that in nonfat milk, *Science News* continued. It had generally been assumed, said the researchers, whose study was initially published in the January/February 1988 issue of the *Journal of Food Science*, that milk products provide a more bioavailable source of calcium than do plant products.

However, the Illinois scientists pointed out that the type of calcium used is important. For example, tofu, in which calcium sulfate is used to coagulate soybean "milk" during processing, provides about 128 mg of calcium per 100 g. Tofu made with magnesium chloride instead of calcium sulfate offers only about one-tenth as much of the mineral.[11]

REFERENCES

1. *Composition of Foods,* Agriculture Handbook No. 8. Washington, D.C.: U.S. Government Printing Office, 1975, p. 59.
2. Heaney, Robert P., M.D. Personal letter, June 21, 1990.
3. Ensminger, Audrey H., et al. *Foods and Nutrition Encyclopedia.* Clovis, Calif.: Pegus Press, 1983, p. 293.
4. Heaney, Robert P., M.D., et al. "Calcium Absorbability from Spinach," *American Journal of Clinical Nutrition* 47:707–709, 1988.
5. Heaney, Robert P., and Weaver, Connie M. "Calcium Absorption from Kale," *American Journal of Clinical Nutrition* 51:656–657, 1990.
6. Heaney, Robert P., et al. "Absorbability of Calcium Sources: The Limited Role of Solubility," *Calcified Tissue International* 46:300–304, 1990.
7. Heaney, Robert P., M.D. "Calcium Intake and Bone Health," *Osteo Forum,* Excerpta Medica, Amsterdam 2(3):1, 1989.
8. Andon, M., et al. "Spinal Bone Density and Calcium Intake in Healthy Postmenopausal Women," *American Journal of Clinical Nutrition* 54:927–929, 1991.
9. Thomas, M., et al. "Calcium Metabolism and Bone Mineralization in Female Rats Fed Diets Marginally Sufficient in Calcium: Effects of Increased Dietary Calcium Intake," *Bone Mineral* 12:1–14, 1991.
10. Kleiner, Susan M., Ph.D., R.D., L.D. "Yogurt: A Culture in Itself." In *Medical and Health Annual.* Chicago: Encyclopaedia Brittanica, Inc., 1994, p. 463.
11. "Need Calcium? Try Tofu and Tortillas," *Science News* 133:174, March 12, 1988.

10

Calcium May Reduce the Risk of Getting Colon Cancer

STATISTICALLY, 80 percent of cancers are caused by environmental agents; the remaining 20 percent are genetically transmitted. Cancer of the colon and rectum is the third leading incidence of cancer in males, accounting for 77,000 cases annually. Prostate and lung lead the incidences of cancer among males. For females, colon and rectum cancer ranks second only to breast cancer, resulting in 75,000 cases each year, according to Mukti H. Sarma, Ph.D., in the 1994 issue of *Medical and Health Annual*.[1]

The genetic defects resulting in cancer can be detected in the DNA obtained from blood samples, Sarma reported. In inherited colorectal cancer, for example, some patients are prone to develop polyps that are benign (harmless) at the beginning but can develop into malignant tumors in the course of time. These are called familial adenomatus polyposis. Bert Vogelstein and Kenneth Kinzier of Johns Hopkins University School of Medicine in Baltimore, Yusuke Nakamura of the Tokyo Cancer Institute, and Ray White of the University of Utah in Salt Lake City have identified the gene responsible for this type of colorectal cancer, Sarma said. The gene is located in a discrete portion of chromosome 5, which is mutated in patients who are found to have inherited the disease.

"In May 1993," Sarma continued, "an international team of scientists headed by Vogelstein in the United States and Albert de la Chapelle at the University of Helsinki in Finland, provided evidence of the presence of a gene located on chromosome 2 that could carry the inherited susceptibility to a much more common form of colon cancer in which there is no development of polyps. These patients have what is known as hereditary nonpolyposis colorectal cancer and are also prone to develop other malignancies such as cancer of the ovary, uterine lining and kidney."

66

Although colorectal cancer is very common, its cause has been difficult to detect. Now the chromosome 2 satellite DNA can be used as a marker and a blood test developed to identify high-risk individuals. Once this person has been identified as a carrier, preventive measures can be recommended, and the patient can be closely monitored for the first sign of malignancy.[1]

BENEFICIAL BEYOND BONES

Increasing dietary calcium may help to prevent colon cancer, even in patients with a familial history of the disease, according to Michael Herring in the January 29, 1986 issue of *Medical Tribune*. The study, headed by Martin Lipkin, M.D., and Harold Newmark of Memorial Sloan-Kettering Cancer Center in New York City, found that high calcium intake is accompanied by decreased cell proliferation in colonic epithelial cells.

Herring also reported that the study found that "supplemental dietary calcium had the effect of restoring the crypt epithelium to a more normal, quiescent equilibrium in proliferation" in all subjects. Lipkin said "this is the first demonstration in humans of an induced reversal of an abnormal proliferative state of the lining of the colon known to be associated with an increased incidence of colon cancer." The finding, originally reported in the *New England Journal of Medicine* (313:22, 1985), parallels results gleaned from animal studies and also dovetails with epidemiologic evidence that added calcium reduces the risk of colon cancer.

With the use of rectal biopsies, the researchers examined the frequency and distribution of proliferating colonic epithelial cells in 10 asymptomatic subjects, whose families had an increased incidence of colon cancer. Before calcium supplementation, the proliferative profile of the epithelium resembled that of patients who had actually had colon cancer. Two to three months after calcium supplementation (Western-style diets with 1.25 g of calcium carbonate, which is about one and one-half times the RDA) the researchers observed a decrease of more than 40 percent in the proportion of epithelial cells.

"Before calcium," Herring added, "the study group's colonic epithelium resembled that of 12 patients in whom familial colon cancer had been resected. After calcium, the profile was much closer to that of 29 controls who were Seventh-Day Adventist vegetarians, a group known to be at comparatively lower risk for the disease."

As to how calcium is beneficial in preventing colorectal cancer, Lipkin was quoted as saying that it apparently acts as a "biological response modifier" on the colonic cells. Without calcium, he added, colonic cells in general may tend to have an expanded proliferation rate. This can be due to the irritating effects of bile acids and fatty acids in the colon. But the addition of the mineral tends to quiet proliferation by binding these acids in the colon, thus inhibiting their irritating effect on epithelial cells, which may multiply in an attempt to protect themselves.[2]

J. Silberner stated in the December 7, 1985 issue of *Science News* that the calcium and colon cancer connection has long been suspected. Colorectal cancer incidence is higher than normal among people who drink soft water, which is low in calcium. And people eating diets high in calcium and vitamin D have a lower-than-normal incidence of the cancer.[3]

Calcium above the RDA—for example, 1,500 to 2,000 mg—may be necessary to protect the colon against cancer-producing chemicals, according to the September 1990 issue of *U.S. Pharmacist*. Animal studies at the Memorial Sloan-Kettering Cancer Center show that by reducing dietary calcium intake, we speed up the rate at which cells in the lining of the colon proliferate and are replaced. When this is permitted to continue the animals develop polyps, which eventually results in cancers of the colon.

The researchers, who discussed their study in more detail in *Medical World News* (31(4):22, 1990), explained that animals exhibiting excessive colon cell turnover in response to calcium deprivation quickly return to normal when adequate calcium is restored to the diet.

"In humans," *U.S. Pharmacist* added, "a similar effect on colon cell turnover was recently demonstrated in the M. D. Anderson Cancer Hospital at the University of Texas in Houston. Thus, while it has not been proved beyond doubt that supplemental calcium will help to prevent human colon cancer, the evidence to date points in that direction. Furthermore, since a high fluid intake seems to have somewhat the same beneficial effect, one might consider taking calcium and fluid at the same time by drinking more milk (skimmed or low-fat) and calcium-enriched orange juice."[4]

Researchers at Motala Hospital and the University Hospital in Linkoping, Sweden, reported in *Cancer* in 1992, that patients with colorectal cancer are more apt to consume diets low in calcium, fiber, vitamin B2 (riboflavin) and phosphorus than those who do not have the disease. The researchers came to their conclusions after tabulating results from a study of 41 patients with colorectal cancer and the same number of matched controls. Dietary intakes were studied for the previous 15 years. The researchers added that total fiber and cereal intake were inversely related to rectal cancer risk, while cancer risk went up as alcohol intake increased.[5]

A research team at the University of Kentucky at Lexington reported in *FASEB*

Journal in 1991 that tumor incidence was 50 percent lower in a group of laboratory rats getting the highest amounts of calcium and vitamin D, compared to the other groups in the study. The study lasted for 32 weeks, during which time the incidence of colon tumors was analyzed. Serum levels of calcium and vitamin D were checked throughout the study.[6]

Supplementation with 1,250 mg/day of calcium for two or three months in those who are at high risk for colon cancer showed a reduction of thymidine-labeling index from 16 to 10 percent following supplementation, according to Bernard Levin, M.D., in *Cancer* in 1992. In another study, 30 first-degree relatives of eight patients with colonic cancer and eight patients with colon polyps were treated with 1,250 mg of calcium carbonate. Colonic proliferation was reduced by 30 percent during the calcium treatment and rebounded during the placebo treatment, stated Levin, who is professor of medicine, gastrointestinal oncology and digestive diseases, at the M. D. Anderson Cancer Center of the University of Texas.[7]

In a study reported in *Lancet* in 1985, which involved 1,954 men, those with the lowest combined index of calcium and vitamin D were two and one-half times as likely to develop colorectal cancer as the male volunteers who had the highest index. That was even after age, alcohol consumption, smoking, body mass index and fat intake were evaluated.[8]

The suggestion that calcium might help deter colon cancer got a boost when researchers noticed that the disease seemed to strike more frequently in latitudes far from the equator—places with less sunshine, according to *The Complete Book of Vitamins and Minerals for Health.* The hypothesis was that since sunlight helps the body make vitamin D, and vitamin D enables the body to absorb calcium, it was this nutritional pair that reduced colon cancer.[9]

On top of this, scientists reported that in Scandinavia colon cancer occurs least where consumption of milk is greatest. And a 19-year-study in Chicago revealed that men with the lowest intake of vitamin D and calcium had about three times the risk of colorectal cancer as those who had the highest intake.[9]

REFERENCES

1. Sarma, Mukti H., Ph.D. "Cancer." In *Medical and Health Annual.* Chicago: Encyclopaedia Britannica, Inc., 1994, pp. 253ff.
2. Herring, Michael. "Calcium Supplements May Prove Hedge Against Colon Cancer," *Medical Tribune,* January 29, 1986, p. 6.

3. Silberner, J. "Colorectal Cancer: Calcium a Key?" *Science News* 128:362, December 7, 1985.
4. "Calcium and Cancer of the Colon," *U.S. Pharmacist,* September 1990, p. 102.
5. Arbman, G., et al. "Cereal Fiber, Calcium, and Colorectal Cancer," *Cancer* 69:2042–2048, 1992.
6. Beaty, M., et al. "The Effect of Dietary Calcium and Vitamin D on Colon Carcinogenesis Induced by 1.2-Dimethylhydrazine," *FASEB Journal* 5:926A, 1991.
7. Levin, Bernard, M.D. "Nutrition and Colorectal Cancer," *Cancer* 70(6):1723–1726, Suppl., September 15, 1992.
8. Garland, C., et al. "Dietary Vitamin D and Calcium and Risk of Colorectal Cancer: A 19-Year Prospective Study in Men," *Lancet* 1:307–309, 1985.
9. Editors of *Prevention* Magazine. *The Complete Book of Vitamins and Minerals for Health.* Emmaus, Pa.: Rodale Press, 1988, p. 298.

11

Calcium Versus High Blood Pressure

AN estimated 60 million Americans—almost one in three—suffer from hypertension or high blood pressure. This condition is often called "the silent killer" because there are few clues as to what causes it. Among black Americans, 28.2 percent are thought to have hypertension, compared with about 16 percent for whites. In any event, the economic burden on the nation from this condition is tagged at about $10.7 billion annually.

WHAT IS HIGH BLOOD PRESSURE?

High blood pressure or hypertension develops when the force of blood against the walls of the arteries that carry blood throughout the body is greater than it should be. This continuous strain on the cardiovascular system, over time, can cause a number of serious and life-threatening illnesses, such as heart attacks, strokes, kidney failure and damage to the blood vessels that nourish the retinas of the eyes.

There are two types of high blood pressure, essential hypertension and secondary hypertension. In essential hypertension, there is no apparent reason for elevated blood pressure. In secondary hypertension, the cause has been identified by a physician. These causes include kidney disease, hormonal disorders such as Cushing's disease, aldosteronism (an overproduction of the hormone aldosterone), the use of oral contraceptives or pregnancy.[1]

According to *The American Medical Association Family Medical Guide*:

A tendency toward essential hypertension seems to run in families. In other words, blood pressure appears to be influenced by heredity as well as by life-

71

style. It also seems likely that people who are overweight when they are young are more apt to have high blood pressure in middle age than their lean contemporaries, and that there is a link between high blood pressure and high salt intake. In most cases of hypertension, the blood pressure rises steadily over a number of years unless it is treated. Occasionally, however, an exceedingly high blood pressure develops very quickly. This dangerous condition, which can be either essential or secondary, is known as malignant hypertension. It is most often found among smokers.[1]

Blood pressure varies from person to person and even in different parts of your body. As an example, it is higher in your legs than in your arms. For the sake of convenience, however, it is usually measured in one of the large arteries of one or both arms.

There are two types of pressure, systolic and diastolic. Systolic pressure, taken from the Greek word *systole,* meaning contraction, is the peak pressure when your heart contracts to pump blood. This is the first number on your blood pressure reading chart. Diastolic pressure, the second number, is the pressure when your heart is resting between beats. It is named after the Greek word *diastellin,* meaning "to expand."

Blood pressure is measured with the familiar sphygmomanometer, in which a cuff is applied to your arm and tightened. It is hooked up to a column of mercury and a gauge. The physician uses a stethoscope to listen for the various sounds made as blood moves through the arteries. If the physician says your blood pressure reading is 120/80, it is expressed in terms of millimeters of mercury, that is, 120 mm Hg/80 mm Hg. (Hg is the chemical symbol for mercury.)

As explained in *The Physicians' Manual for Patients:*

Everyone's blood pressure varies during the course of a day. As would be expected, it is usually lower when resting or engaged in quiet activities, and it may spurt up during a sudden burst of activity, such as running to catch a bus or exercising. Age also affects blood pressure; it is generally lower in children and gradually rises as we grow older. Although there is some disagreement over how high is too high, the average normal blood pressure for healthy children is about 90/60, while the normal adult average ranges from 100/85 to 135/90. A diastolic pressure over 85 in an otherwise healthy adult is regarded as suspiciously high, and a reading of 140/100 usually would be diagnosed as hypertension and should be treated. Many experts feel that any diastolic pressure that is consistently over 95 should be treated.[2]

Although physicians use a variety of drugs to treat hypertension—diuretics, vasodilators, beta-blockers, adrenergic inhibitors, angiotensin-converting enzyme or ACE inhibitors, etc.—our purpose here is to focus mainly on the role of calcium in lowering blood pressure.

Speaking at a meeting of the American College of Cardiology in Dallas in 1984, Lawrence M. Resnick, M.D., assistant professor of medicine at the Cornell University Medical College in New York, said that diastolic blood pressure dropped significantly in 16 of 26 patients with mild essential hypertension treated only with dietary calcium supplements for six months. According to the May 14, 1984 issue of *Medical World News* that reported on the study, the mean blood pressure for the group dropped from an initial 161/94 mm Hg to 154/89 mm Hg after six months, or a mean diastolic pressure drop of 5 mm Hg. But among the 16 responders, diastolic pressure went down 10 mm Hg or more. The decline was greatest in patients with low initial serum ionized calcium levels and, for the most part, with low-renin hypertension.[3] Renin is an enzyme formed in the kidneys and not the same as rennin, the enzyme that curdles milk. Some researchers have suggested that high amounts of renin (pronounced REE-nin) may be more indicative of a heart attack than the usual so-called risk factors. In fact, studies have shown that at least half the heart attacks occur in individuals with normal cholesterol and blood pressure levels, who don't smoke or have diabetes.

Patients were excluded from the Cornell trial if they had a history of kidney stones or basal hypercalciuria (excreting large amounts of calcium in the urine). This left 26 people who were treated with two grams (2,000 mg) of calcium carbonate given daily in four divided doses. They did not reduce their salt intake or otherwise modify their diet during the six-month study. The average age of the volunteers was 56.

"The Cornell results appear more striking than those obtained by an Oregon Health Sciences University team, which were reported to the western section of the American Federation for Clinical Research earlier this year," *Medical World News* added. "In a double-blind, randomized, crossover study of 30 controls and 28 patients with mild to moderate hypertension treated with 1,000 mg of calcium daily for eight weeks, hypertension chief David A. McCarron and his team detected a significant systolic pressure drop in 46 percent of the patient group."

McCarron told the magazine that Cornell's apparently better response rate may be attributable to the larger dose of calcium and longer duration of therapy. He added that blood pressures among his patients were still dropping at the end of the eight-week trial, and subsequent analysis of a larger group completing the trial gave a response rate closer to the New York results. He added that the New Yorkers had more responders probably because their population was skewed toward low-renin hypertensives and blood renin activity reflects serum ionized calcium levels.[3]

The precise mechanism by which calcium can lower blood pressure in responders isn't clear, but the Cornell team believes calcium acts as a calcium blocker by competing with the hormone 1,25-dihydroxyvitamin D. Resnick added that, "We've found that 1,25-dihydroxyvitamin D administration will undo calcium effects on blood pressure, so we think that calcium is suppressing the hormone."[3]

A research team at Purdue University and the Indiana University School of Medicine, headed by Roseann M. Lyle, Ph.D., found that 1,500 mg/day of calcium for 12 weeks lowered blood pressure in a group of white and black men. This study was reported in the April 3, 1987 issue of the *Journal of the American Medical Association*. The volunteers, ranging in age from 19 to 52, who did not have especially high blood pressure, were assigned to one of the racial groups or to a placebo group. The researchers said:

> This study demonstrates that a calcium supplement of 1,500 mg/day produced a modest but significant decrease in blood pressure in both white and black normotensive men, compared with a placebo. The experimental protocol and statistical design minimized the possibility that the response observed was due to observer bias or sampling error. The calcium carbonate supplement was well tolerated, and no participants were withdrawn from the calcium therapy because of any adverse signs, symptoms or electrolyte abnormalities. Although there is no clear explanation of the mechanisms involved with the decrease in blood pressure demonstrated by this study, it adds to evidence from previous investigations in support of the blood pressure-lowering effect of supplemental calcium. There were no differences in the blood pressure response to calcium supplementation between the white and black men, but further research is warranted to investigate the relationship of calcium intake to blood pressure in the high-risk black population group.[4]

CERTAIN RACES FACE HIGHER RISKS

At a conference held at Emory University and the Morehouse School of Medicine in Atlanta in 1987, researchers found that calcium supplements can reverse the effects of salt on hypertensive African-Americans, reported *The New York Times,* March 6, 1987.[5]

Neil Shulman, M.D., an associate professor at Emory and coordinator of the conference, said that black Americans have abnormally high blood pressure twice as often and seven times more severely than white Americans. Hypertension kills an estimated 60,000 black Americans each year.

In the calcium study, conducted by Michael B. Zemel, M.D., and James Sowers, M.D., of Wayne State University in Detroit, black adult volunteers were given salt with varying amounts of calcium during a two-week period. Some of the people had high blood pressure and some did not.

"When a high level of salt and a low level of calcium were given, the blood pressure rose for all the people tested," the *Times* reported. "But when a higher level of calcium was added to a high-salt diet, the blood pressure was lowered among those who suffered from hypertension. The increase of calcium with a high-salt diet resulted in a slightly higher level of blood pressure among people who did not have the disease, although that increase was not so high as the one recorded on a high-salt, low-calcium diet."

Zemel told the conference that, in most cases, they had succeeded in reducing blood pressure, often down to the normal range, with only 1,000 mg/day of calcium.[5]

In another presentation at the conference, Gerald S. Berenson, M.D., of the Louisiana State University Medical Center, said that there are certain warning signs of high blood pressure, especially among black children, that can be detected earlier than previously thought. His study, lasting 15 years, involved 8,000 black and white children in Bogalusa, Louisiana.

Berenson and his colleagues found that black children, in addition to having hypertension, tend to have less body fat and slower heart rates than white children. They also have higher insulin levels, lower renin and dopamine beta-hydroxylase levels and lower excretion of urinary potassium than their white counterparts. The lower sugar level, impeded electrolyte production and potassium excretion contribute to high blood pressure, he said.

"Once we can identify these factors, along with high blood pressure levels and family history—even if the child is not yet displaying clinical symptoms—we'll be able to better control or even prevent the onset of hypertensive disease," Berenson added.[5]

Researchers at Boston University School of Medicine selected boys and girls, ages three to six, from the Framingham Children's Study, and recorded their food habits for one year. Up to five blood pressure readings were taken at the beginning of the second year of the study. Systolic blood pressures averaged 95.9 mm Hg with the range being from 73 to 129 mm Hg. Diastolic pressures averaged 54.6 mm Hg, with the range being from 37 to 78 mm Hg. The research team said that dietary calcium is inversely correlated with blood pressure in children as it is in adults. As an example, for every 2.5 mmol of dietary calcium there was a 2.27 mm Hg reduction in systolic blood pressure. However, in this study, there was no association between calcium intake and diastolic pressure, reported the *Journal of the American Medical Association.*[6]

At a meeting of the American Heart Association in New Orleans in 1992, James H. Dwyer, Ph.D., of the University of Southern California School of Medicine at Los Angeles, said that people under the age of 40, who are moderate drinkers and who are not overweight, may be able to significantly reduce their risk of developing high blood pressure by eating more calcium-rich foods, according to the December 10, 1992 issue of *Medical Tribune.* While studying the diets of over 6,600 men and women, the researchers noted that the risk of developing hypertension was lowered by an average of 12 percent for each 1,000 mg of calcium consumed per day. But for those who are under 40, who are not overweight and who do not drink alcohol daily, they can lower their risk of developing high blood pressure by 40 percent for each 1,000 mg/day of calcium they ingest.[7]

In a 20-week study at Auburn University in Alabama, researchers studied the blood pressure of 30 pregnant women with normal blood pressure and 20 hypertensive pregnant women, ranging in age from 18 to 28, reported the *American Journal of Clinical Nutrition* in 1992. The women were given either 1,000 mg/day of calcium or a placebo. The researchers found that the added calcium reduced diastolic blood pressure and serum ionic calcium levels in the women who had high blood pressure, but there was no change in the pregnant women with normal blood pressure readings.[8]

In *Nutrition Reports International* in 1987, Marvin L. Bierenbaum, M.D., of the Kenneth L. Jordan Research Group, Montclair, New Jersey, and his colleagues reviewed the relevant literature concerning whether or not milk can lower blood pressure and cholesterol and triglyceride levels. Work in their laboratory in 1965 first demonstrated that increased calcium ingestion for three weeks caused a decrease in serum lipids in humans. This research was reported in the *British Medical Journal* by H. Yacowitz, et. al in 1965.[9]

Subsequent long-term studies by Bierenbaum and co-workers (reported in *Lipids* in 1972) showed that after one year supplemental calcium had a beneficial effect on both high cholesterol and high triglyceride levels in patients with abnormal blood lipids. Bierenbaum said:

As to the mechanism involved, work in our laboratory has added much clarification. In an early rat study, it appeared that lowering the blood cholesterol level by increasing dietary calcium was mediated by increased excretion of sequestered bile acids. A longer term study confirmed these findings and revealed no associated side effects. One further beneficial effect of supplemental calcium was an increased fecal excretion of some potentially deleterious trace metals, i.e., cobalt and cadmium. Supplementing the diet with vitamin D increased absorption of calcium without significantly decreasing its fat-lowering effects, raising the possibility of simultaneously treating both calcium deficiency and hyperlipidemia with a single agent.

In their study of milk, the New Jersey team used 200 healthy volunteers, both male and female, who worked at the New Jersey Bell Telephone Company in Newark. Their aim was to determine what affect skim milk and 2 percent fat milk, both fortified with milk solids to bring the calcium content to 1,400 mg per quart, might have on blood pressure. The volunteers began by drinking one quart of the fortified milk, in four separate feedings per day, for three months. They were then switched over to the fortified two-percent fat milk, also for three months. The volunteers ranged in age from 21 to 65.

After analyzing the data, the researchers found that systolic blood pressure in the volunteers went from about 126 to about 119 mm Hg at six months; diastolic readings decreased from about 82 to 76 mm Hg. It was noted that a greater decrease occurred in subjects with blood pressures over 140/90. Cholesterol levels dropped from about 209 to 204. There was no appreciable change in blood sugar, triglycerides, high-density lipoprotein cholesterol (the good kind), or potassium levels.

"The finding of one clearly and one marginally beneficial effect following increased calcium intake with a milk-solid fortified milk supplement is very encouraging," Bierenbaum and colleagues said. An additional epidemiological study by M. R. Garcia-Palmieri, et al. in *Hypertension* in 1984 (6(3):322–328), revealed that a two-fold incidence increase in high blood pressure could be found in subgroups who drank no milk as compared to those who consumed one quart of milk a day, confirming the inverse association between calcium intake and hypertension.[9]

In *The Calcium Connection*, Cedric Garland, M.D., and Frank Garland, M.D., reported that several studies have shown that those who take 1,200 mg/day of calcium have lower blood pressure and fewer health problems than people who consume smaller amounts. They added that adults getting 500 mg/day or less of calcium had twice the risk of high blood pressure as those consuming 1,500 mg or more daily. The Garlands reported:

The connection between calcium and blood pressure was backed by a Rancho Bernardo, California study, a 15-year-study of adult residents of a suburban community near San Diego, initiated by Elizabeth Barrett-Connor and her colleagues at the University of California at San Diego. It showed that men who drank three or more glasses of milk a day had average blood pressures of 134/78, while those who consumed two glasses or less per day had average pressures of 137/81. This is a difference of three points in the systolic and diastolic blood pressure. A clinical trial of blood pressure medication by the Medical Research Council in Britain reported in the *British Medical Journal* in 1985 that a 10-point drop in blood pressure cut the risk of stroke virtually in half.[10]

Vitamin D, which aids in the body's ability to absorb and use calcium, may play a role in regulating blood pressure, the authors continued. They quoted a study by MaryFran Sowers and colleagues at the University of Iowa in 1985, who found that women under 35 who took in 400 IU/day of vitamin D had systolic blood pressure six points lower than those who took in smaller amounts—an average of 111/69 compared to 117/69. Sowers attributed one point of the blood pressure drop to intake of calcium and the rest to vitamin D.[10]

Several mechanisms for lowering blood pressure with the aid of calcium have been proposed, according to John A. McDougall, M.D., in *McDougall's Medicine: A Challenging Second Opinion*. More calcium taken into the body through the diet causes the kidneys to excrete more sodium, the primary ingredient in table salt that raises blood pressure. And, he added, calcium will also dilate the blood vessels and lower the resistance in the peripheral blood system, thus lowering blood pressure.[11]

In a study at Wayne State University in Michigan, six noninsulin-dependent diabetics with high blood pressure were taken off of their hypertension medication and supplemented with 600 mg/day of calcium for three months, reported *Hypertension* in 1988. The researchers reported that forearm blood flow increased, left ventricular mass was reduced and blood pressure decreased following the calcium therapy.[12]

Researchers at the Netherlands Institute of Dairy Research reported in the *International Journal of Medicine* that the calcium and potassium in milk can lower blood pressure. In the study, 60 females with normal blood pressure drank either regular milk (1,180 mg calcium, 1,650 mg potassium and 110 mg magnesium) or mineral-poor milk (95 mg calcium, 580 mg potassium and 10 mg magnesium) while eating a low-calcium diet. The volunteers drinking the normal milk had the greatest reduction in systolic pressure—minus 4.1 percent versus 1.3 percent.[13]

In a study by Jiang He, et al., in the March 1991 issue of *Hypertension*, the researchers evaluated the ingestion of calcium, potassium, sodium and magnesium and their relation to blood pressure in four different groups of men in China and controls in other areas of the nation. Their research confirmed other studies which show that a diet low in sodium and high in potassium, calcium and magnesium prevents the development of high blood pressure.[14]

REFERENCES

1. Kunz, Jeffrey R. M., M.D., editor-in-chief. *The American Medical Association Family Medical Guide.* New York: Random House, 1982, pp. 382–383.
2. Subak-Sharpe, Genell J., editor. *The Physicians' Manual for Patients.* New York: New York Times Books, 1984, pp. 33–34.
3. "Study Builds Support for Calcium as Therapy for Some Hypertensives," *Medical World News,* May 14, 1984, pp. 18–20.
4. Lyle, Roseann, M., Ph.D., et al. "Blood Pressure and Metabolic Effects of Calcium Supplementation in Normotensive White and Black Men," *Journal of the American Medical Association* 257(13):1772–1776, April 3, 1987.
5. "Conference Assesses the Role of Calcium in Blood Pressure," *The New York Times,* March 6, 1987, p. A29.
6. Gillmann, M., et al. "Inverse Association of Dietary Calcium with Systolic Blood Pressure in Young Children," *Journal of the American Medical Association* 267:2340–2343, 1992.
7. "Calcium Averts Hypertension," *Medical Tribune,* December 10, 1992, p. 5.
8. Knight, K., et al. "Calcium Supplementation on Normotensive and Hypertensive Pregnant Women," *American Journal of Clinical Nutrition* 55:891–895, 1992.
9. Bierenbaum, Marvin L., M.D., et al. "The Effect of Dietary Calcium Supplementation on Blood Pressure and Serum Lipid Levels: Preliminary Report," *Nutrition Reports International* 36:1147–1157, 1987.
10. Garland, Cedric, M.D., and Garland, Frank, M.D. *The Calcium Connection.* New York: G. P. Putnam's Sons, 1988, pp. 52ff.
11. McDougall, John A., M.D. *McDougall's Medicine: A Challenging Second Opinion.* Piscataway, N.J.: New Century Publishers, Inc., 1985, p. 189.
12. Zemel, M., et al. "Dietary Calcium Supplementation Increases Forearm Blood Flow and Reduces Left Ventricular Mass in Hypertensive Non-Insulin Dependent Diabetics," *Hypertension* 12:344, 1988.
13. Van Beresteijn, E., et al. "Milk: Does It Affect Blood Pressure? A Controlled Intervention Study," *Journal of International Medicine* 228:477–482, 1990.
14. He, Jiang, et al. "Relationship of Electrolytes to Blood Pressure in Men: The Xi Peoples Study," *Hypertension* 17(3):378–385, March 1991.

12

Children Must Have Plenty of Calcium

Aт a meeting of the American Society for Bone and Mineral Research in Anaheim, California in 1986, Charles Chestnut III, M.D., professor of medicine and radiology at the University School of Medicine in Seattle, spoke about children's calcium requirements. He said that since so many youngsters are not building maximum bone mass today, that tomorrow's problem with osteoporosis will be even greater than "the epidemic" being witnessed today. He added that perhaps we have been targeting the wrong age group—notably older women—for developing osteoporosis. As reported in the September 24, 1986 issue of *Medical Tribune*, Chestnut said studies show that from age 11, American women consistently fail to consume enough calcium—even at current recommended levels, which many researchers consider to be too low.

Chestnut's study involved 31 healthy Caucasian females, all 14 years of age. Eighteen of the volunteers were enrolled in two weeks of calcium balance studies at calcium intakes ranging from 270 to 1,637 mg/day. Calcium balance was positive at a calcium intake of 575 mg/day or greater, and there was a significant linear correlation between calcium intake and calcium retention, with the largest calcium retention recorded at an intake level of 1,506 mg/day. The girls in the treatment group averaged around 1,000 mg/day of calcium, which, of course, is below the Recommended Dietary Allowance of 1,200 mg/day. Since the volunteers were from a fairly affluent group, they were likely to consume more calcium than the general population. However, almost one-fourth of the girls consumed only between 300 and 400 mg/day of calcium, Chestnut said.

"Our preliminary data support the hypothesis that the teen years could be a critical period for peak bone mass formation due to the ability of young skeletons to store extra amounts of calcium," Chestnut added. "We really do feel that we're dealing with a calcium-deficient female population in this country. Not only are they calcium-deficient, they often substitute carbonated soft drinks for milk and the higher phosphorus content of these drinks further impedes calcium absorption in the body."[1]

In 1988, a seminar, part of a "National Conference on Women's Health Series," was sponsored by the Food and Drug Administration in Bethesda, Maryland. Chestnut and Robert P. Heaney, M.D., the John A. Creighton University Professor at Creighton University in Omaha, Nebraska, spoke about an "osteoporosis epidemic" on the horizon.[2]

EPIDEMIC OF BRITTLE BONES?

Heaney suggested that there is a "ticking time bomb" in the form of a 21st-century osteoporosis epidemic that will manifest when the baby-boomer and younger generations reach old age. He added that already-poor calcium-intake levels, especially among young women, are apparently declining further as diets become overloaded with soft drinks and processed food instead of dairy products and vegetables.[2]

By increasing daily calcium intake from 80 percent of the recommended daily allowance to 110 percent with calcium supplements, there was a significant increase in total body and spinal bone density in adolescent girls, reported Tom Lloyd, Ph.D., and colleagues in the August 18, 1993 issue of the *Journal of the American Medical Association*.[3]

Lloyd and his colleagues at the M. S. Hershey Medical Center in Hershey, Pennsylvania, said that the increase of 24 g of bone gain per year among the calcium-supplemented group translates into an additional 1.3 percent skeletal mass per year during adolescent growth, which may provide protection against future osteoporotic fracture.

The 18-month randomized, double-blind, placebo-controlled study involved 94 girls with a mean age of almost 12 years. In the test group, the girls were supplemented with 500 mg/day of calcium citrate melate, while the controls received identical placebo or "nothing" pills.

"The increase in the age-adjusted incidence of osteoporosis in Western countries has led to an examination of how bone growth and maintenance are affected by diet, exercise and modern lifestyle factors," the research team said. "General consensus is that peak bone mass of premenopausal women is a major determinant of osteoporosis later in life. Cross-sectional studies of bone density in children and young adults have documented that rapid increases occur during puberty in both sexes, and that peak bone density in the spine and hip of females is achieved near the age of 20 years."

During the study, the average calcium intake from dietary sources in both the test and placebo groups was about 960 mg/day or 80 percent of the Recommended Dietary Allowance. This is somewhat greater than the national survey data that show mean calcium intakes for 12- to 14-year-old girls to be about 850 mg/day or 71 percent of the RDA. The researchers added that the additional calcium received by the supplemented group brought their average total daily intake to 115 percent of the current RDA, which is 1,200 mg/day. They said that it is unclear whether greater gains in bone density could have been achieved with greater calcium intake, and they were not sure whether gains in bone density will persist in the absence of a continued greater intake of the mineral.

They added that other researchers have pointed out that calcium balance, and presumably skeletal calcium retention, increase during adolescence with intakes of up to about 1,500 mg/day of calcium. This suggests that intakes somewhat greater than the RDA will result in increased peak bone density and mass. And, they continued, calcium supplementation for a group of 12-year-old girls resulted in significant gains in total body and spinal bone density. The increase may ensure optimal development of peak bone mass, which could lower the risk of osteoporotic fractures later in life.[3]

In a study by Matti J. Valimaki, et al. at Helsinki University Central Hospital in Finland, and reported in the July 23, 1994 issue of the *British Medical Journal,* it was found that both genetic and environmental factors determine peak bone mass. For example, bone mineral density at the femoral neck was 7.6 percent to 10.5 percent higher in those with the most regular exercise, compared to those with the least exercise. In men, regular smoking reduced femoral neck bone mineral density by 9.7 percent, compared to nonsmokers. For women, consumption of 800 to 1,200 mg/day of calcium increased bone mineral density at the femoral neck by 4.7 percent, compared to those who consumed less.[4]

"Osteoporosis has many causes, but insufficient calcium intake is certainly one of them," said Robert P. Heaney, M.D., of Creighton University, speaking at a seminar, "Building Strong Bodies for Life," held February 9, 1994 in New York City. The seminar was sponsored by the Continental Baking Company in St. Louis, to introduce their calcium-enriched bread.[5]

Heaney added that calcium intakes in the United States have been going down during the last 20 years, rather than up, and that this is certain to make the osteoporosis problem worse. He added that "We need to do something to turn that around, and we need to do it now." While Caucasian teenage boys generally get sufficient amounts of calcium, African-American teenage males fall considerably short of the 1,200 mg/day, he continued.[5]

"While African-Americans can adapt better to deficient calcium diets than can whites, African-Americans pay an unacceptably high price in terms of high blood pressure, which is a major health problem for them generally. Low calcium diets make that worse," he said.[5]

Another speaker, Connie M. Weaver, Ph.D., professor and department head, Department of Foods and Nutrition, Purdue University, Lafayette, Indiana, said that, "Osteoporosis is not just a women's disease. Approximately 20 percent of individuals suffering from the affliction are men. However," she added, "new research shows that calcium intakes higher than the current RDA—five servings of calcium-rich foods rather than four—increase bone mass of adolescents. Every five percent increase in bone mass maintained through adulthood translates into a 40-percent reduction in risk of bone fractures."[5]

MOST AMERICANS LACKING IN CALCIUM

Writing in *Nutrition Notes,* a publication of the American Institute for Cancer Research, Washington, D. C., for November 29, 1993, Karen Collins, M.S., R.D., said that surveys find that many people get less calcium than they really need or realize they're getting. Without dairy products, she continued, an average diet provides only 300 mg of calcium per day; high-calcium vegetables such as broccoli can't really compensate. Since each cup of milk provides about 300 mg of calcium, adults need almost two cups of milk daily, while adolescents need three cups, with the RDA total met through other dietary sources of calcium.[6]

In the Total Diet Study, headed by Jean Pennington, Ph.D., of the Food and Drug Administration in Washington, D. C., dietary intakes of calcium, sodium, potassium, phosphorus, magnesium, iron, zinc, selenium, iodine, copper and manganese were tabulated in eight age- and sex-matched groups from 1982 to 1989. The daily intakes were compared to the RDAs to see how those groups were doing nutritionally.

Some of the results showed that Americans are consuming too much sodium (salt) and too little copper. Teenage girls are deficient in calcium, magnesium, iron and manganese. And adult women are getting insufficient amounts of calcium, magnesium, iron and zinc. Pennington also found that infants' diets were low in calcium and zinc, while teenage boys and men consumed inadequate amounts of magnesium. She also reported that the minerals typically low in female diets are those most closely associated with anemia and osteoporosis. As for males, low amounts of magnesium put them at risk for developing high blood pressure and heart attacks.[7]

At the University of Utah School of Medicine in Salt Lake City, Gary M. Chan, M.D., evaluated bone mineral status of children ages two to 16 and correlated this with their calcium intake. Calcium intake was adequate for most of the children 11 and younger, but below the RDA in most older children. Evaluating 164 healthy children using photon absorptiometry showed that 70 percent of the children younger than 11 consumed the RDA for calcium (800 mg/day), but only 37 percent of the children older than 11 were getting the recommended 1,200 mg/day.[8]

Writing in the *Canadian Journal of Public Health* in 1991, Robert G. McCulloch, Ph.D., and colleagues at the University of Regina, in Regina, Saskatchewan, Canada, said that if maximizing peak bone density in early childhood is a goal to prevent osteoporosis, then efforts should be made to prevent smoking, especially heavy smoking in young women. They noted that smoking prevention and cessation efforts should be directed at younger women, who are developing this habit at increasing rates.[9]

Using a study by Gary Chan, M.D., of the University of Utah, as background, researchers at the Department of Public Health in Palma de Mallorca, Spain, and the National Institute of Health in Mallorca, reported that bone fractures in children are related more to the calcium content of the diet than to childhood accidents. They reached their conclusion after studying 1,308 children, ranging in age from 11 to 14, who lived in three Spanish towns—Andraitx, Palma and Felanitx. The calcium content of public water supplies played a role in the extent of fractures, reported the *American Journal of Diseases in Children* in 1992.[10]

BONE FORMATION PEAKS EARLY

Studies with girls age 5 through 16 show that most bone-forming activity occurs in the years just before and just after the start of puberty, according to Steven A. Abrams, M.D., of the Children's Nutrition Research Center, Agricultural Research Service, USDA in Houston. He added that the first signs of puberty in U.S. girls usually begin between the ages of eight and 11, with the average around 10. Menstruation follows two to three years later, with age 12.5 being average, he said.[11]

"The current recommendations for increasing calcium intake to 1,200 mg/day in 11- to 24-year-olds may need to be adjusted to start and end at an earlier age," said Abrams, who was speaking at the annual meeting of the Federation of American Societies for Experimental Biology in Washington, D. C., on April 27, 1994.

Abrams' studies show a rapid drop in bone-forming activity within two years after menstruation begins. By age 15, there was very little bone being formed, since the girls excreted nearly as much calcium as they absorbed. He added that there's no reason to think you can't start to emphasize calcium intake around age 5. The primary prevention of osteoporosis begins before puberty, he said.[11]

REFERENCES

1. McGuire, Rick. "Are Calcium-Deficient Teeners Setting Up An Osteoporosis Epidemic?" *Medical Tribune,* September 24, 1986, p. 6
2. Haglund, Keith. "Osteoporosis Epidemic Seen Ahead," *Medical Tribune,* February 25, 1988, p. 9.
3. Lloyd, Tom, Ph.D., et al. "Calcium Supplementation and Bone Mineral Density in Adolescent Girls," *Journal of the American Medical Association* 270(7):841–844, August 18, 1993.
4. Valimaki, Matti J., et al. "Exercise, Smoking and Calcium Intake During Adolescence and Early Adulthood as Determinants of Peak Bone Mass," *British Journal of Medicine* 309:230–235, July 23, 1994.
5. Wolford, Lisa. "Building Strong Bodies for Life." Seminar held by Continental Baking Co., February 9, 1994, in New York City.
6. Collins, Karen, M.S., R.D. "Teen Diets May Lack Vital Calcium," *Nutrition Notes,* November 29, 1993.
7. Pennington, Jean, Ph.D., et al. "Total Diet Study Nutritional Elements, 1982–1989," *Journal of the American Dietetic Association* 91:179–183, 1991.
8. Chan, Gary M., M.D. "Dietary Calcium Affects Bone Mineral Status in Children, Adolescents," *Journal of Musculoskeletal Medicine,* February 1992, pp. 58, 59.
9. McCulloch, Robert G., Ph.D., et al. "The Effect of Cigarette Smoking on Trabecular Bone Density in Premenopausal Women," *Canadian Journal of Public Health* 82:434–435, November/December 1991.
10. Verd, S., et al. "Dietary Calcium and Bone Health," *American Journal of Diseases in Children* 146:660–661, 1992.
11. McBride, Judy. "Extra Calcium Before Age 10 May Help Stem Osteoporosis After 50," USDA Agricultural Research Service, April 28, 1994.

13

Calcium Helps to Prevent Osteoporosis

"SHE fell and broke her hip" is a typical comment after an older woman has had such an accident. What usually happens is that the pelvic bone or femur, the long bone of the leg, weakened by osteoporosis, breaks due to the stress of walking or moving around and then the woman falls. Signs of osteoporosis are the familiar dowager's hump and a bent-over posture, in which the body steals calcium from bones because of a calcium-poor diet. Although there are no other major signs of osteoporosis as the disease progresses, an early clue is the loss of teeth in middle-age. Deterioration of the jaw bone, which results in loosened teeth, is a warning sign that osteoporosis is in its early stages.

We often think of bones as solid, inanimate objects, but, for growth and maintenance, living bone tissue undergoes continuous remodeling throughout a person's life. One group of cells breaks down the bone tissue and another group builds it back up. A process known as mineralization gradually puts calcium and phosphorus into a framework made by the bone-forming cells. Thus, the body's total bone mass continues increasing until the skeleton reaches maturity as a person reaches his or her mid-30s. Unfortunately, after about age 30 or a little beyond, more bone tissue from the spine is lost than is gained. And, at about age 40, bone loss begins to exceed bone gain in other areas of the skeleton.[1]

Some decrease in bone density—osteopenia—is thought to be normal with aging and inevitable for everyone. But it's abnormal and not necessarily inevitable for so much bone tissue to be lost that fractures occur, as is evident in the type of osteopenia called osteoporosis or brittle bone disease.

"Men and black women are at less risk than Caucasian women of developing osteoporosis," Dixie Farley said in *FDA Consumer*. "One reason may be that they generally have more bone mass at maturity. Men have about 30 percent more bone mass than women; blacks about 10 percent more than whites. People with greater bone mass presumably must lose more bone than people with smaller bone mass before the fractures of osteoporosis occur."

In the initial phase of bone loss, most women lose slightly less than one percent of bone mass a year. Following menopause, they lose one to two percent a year. Spinal bone loss is said to be even greater during the first few years. when women reach their 70s, their bone loss diminishes at the same rate as males, which is about 0.5 percent a year.

Decreased estrogen, the female sex hormone, has been strongly associated with postmenopausal bone loss. For some women, bone loss may increase so significantly that the fractures of osteoporosis occur. The first bones to become dangerously porous are the weight-bearing lower vertebrae. Their obvious weakened condition makes them highly vulnerable to crushing. Coughing, bending or other moderate movement—such as turning in bed—may be all that's required for a fracture. As the vertebrae collapse and wedge together, they cause the rib cage to tilt forward toward the hipbones, forcing the stomach to protrude and the upper spine to curve outward in the familiar dowager's hump.

There are basically two types of bone tissue: the inner bone of spongy, honeycomb-like tissue called *trabecular* bone; and the outer, compact *cortical* bone tissue. Roughly 80 percent of the body's total bone is the cortical type, but the vertebrae are mostly trabecular, with only a thin cortical-bone wall. Trabecular bone begins diminishing 10 years before cortical bone.

"In osteoporosis," Farley said, "the earliest fractures are usually in the vertebrae. Fractures are also common in the armbones at the wrist and the thighbones at the hip. In terms of health threat as well as dollars, fractures are the most costly."[1]

THE RAMIFICATION OF HIP FRACTURES

At an international conference, "Research Advances in Osteoporosis," held in February 1990 in Washington, D.C., participants learned that osteoporosis affects an estimated 24 million Americans. The most life-threatening type of osteoporosis-related fractures are hip fractures, which cause approximately 50,000 deaths annually. Hip fractures are responsible for the majority of osteoporosis-related deaths because they increase vulnerability to illnesses such as pneumonia and sometimes result in fatal complications. For example, if a blood clot dislodges from the site of the fracture and is carried throughout the body, the risk of stroke or heart attack increases dramatically.

Those attending the conference, sponsored by the National Osteoporosis Foundation (NOF), the American Society for Bone and Mineral Research and the National Institutes of Health, also learned that hip fractures account for about 25 percent of fractures or about 300,000 each year. Approximately one-quarter of those who break a hip after age 55 do not heal well enough to be able to walk without help, and 12 to 20 percent are in long-term institutions one year after the injury.

The burden of osteoporosis, in addition to its associated pain and suffering, often involves long-term physical, psychological and financial complications. Following a fracture, the patients' immobility or inactivity can increase the rate of bone loss and contribute to other health conditions. The cost of long-term care and related expenses can be financially crippling, and resultant lifestyle changes can have serious psychological consequences. The annual cost of treating osteoporosis is about $10 billion annually. Treatment of hip fractures accounts for about $7 billion each year.

The frequent fractures, pain and limitation of activity related to osteoporosis often cause patients to feel depressed, hopeless and not in control, the conference attendees were told. Patients may perceive the disorder as a threat, loss or challenge, and they often react by denying or avoiding the problem. This can lead to additional harm, especially if the patient does not take necessary precautions or comply with a prescribed exercise regimen.

The financial costs of osteoporosis are enormous and growing, making it a leading public health problem. The average annual cost for hip fracture patients needing hospitalization and institutionalization is about $26,000, not including physicians' fees. Because of the growing elderly population in the United States, annual costs related to osteoporosis are expected to increase from the current $10 billion to $30 billion within the next 30 years.[2]

Risk Factors

Although the precise cause of osteoporosis is not yet fully understood, there are a number of risk factors that have been clearly defined. These include:

1. Age. There is a twofold increase in risk for each 10-year increase in age beyond 65.
2. Female gender.
3. Caucasian or Asian race. Physicians are still not sure why white women over 60 years of age have twice the risk of fractures as African-American women.
4. Thin or slender build.

5. Family history of osteoporosis.
6. Early menopause (before 45), either natural or artificial, as a result of removal of ovaries or abnormal menstrual cycle due to excessive exercise or anorexia.

   For women, the rate of bone loss is dramatically increased by the loss of estrogen production associated with menopause. Although menopause usually occurs at about age 50, it can occur in women as early as their 30s and as late as their 60s. After menopause, the ovaries no longer produce sufficient amounts of estrogen. This hormone is thought to slow down bone loss and improve the absorption of dietary calcium in the intestine. An estimated 50 percent of bone loss in women occurs during the first seven years after menopause.
7. A calcium-deficient diet.
8. Lack of exercise. Of special importance is weight-bearing exercise which makes the muscle work against gravity, such as weight training, low-impact aerobics and tennis.
9. Cigarette smoking and excessive alcohol consumption seem to interfere with calcium absorption. These habits may also impact on vitamin D absorption, as well as on various minerals needed for strong bones.
10. Medications. These include the corticosteroids, which can lead to the loss of bone tissue.[2]

"Each year, osteoporosis causes about 1.3 million fractures and leads to more than 50,000 deaths," said William A. Peck, M.D., vice chancellor for medical affairs and dean of the Washington University School of Medicine, St. Louis, Missouri, co-chairman of the Washington conference and president of the NOF. "We expect to come out of this conference with clear direction for use of newer therapies, guidelines for the use of existing therapies and precise objectives for continued research to help overcome the disorder."

Peck said that newer therapies being evaluated include nasal calcitonin and diphosphonates, both of which may provide significant options for treating osteoporosis. Several studies have shown that nasal calcitonin slows the rate of bone loss, with only minimal side effects, including nausea. Calcitonin is a naturally occurring hormone secreted by the thyroid gland which inhibits bone resorption. Salmon-calcitonin, which is a synthetic formulation, is being used to slow the bone resorption rate in patients with osteoporosis. Diphosphonates, now being investigated in a multicenter trial, may inhibit bone removal and permit bone formation, with gastrointestinal side effects occasionally seen. Diphosphonate is a chemical compound said to bind to bone tissue and impede resorption by inhibiting the formation and activity of osteoclasts, the bone-resorbing cells.

Also on the conference agenda was a discussion of the National Osteoporosis Foundation's Scientific Advisory Board Task Force regarding the use of bone mass measurement. This is a noninvasive diagnostic technique which provides unprecedented accuracy in the early detection of osteoporosis and can be used to determine fracture risk.

"Bone mass measurement devices are currently available but are underutilized because they are not covered by Medicare," said C. Conrad Johnston, Jr., M.D., professor of medicine, Indiana University School of Medicine, Indianapolis, who co-chaired the NOF Task Force. "In the near future, we hope to see adequate reimbursement for these valuable diagnostic tools, since they can help reduce the devastating physical and emotional effects, as well as the costs, associated with osteoporosis."

"There are effective therapies available today to prevent or treat osteoporosis, such as improved calcium intake in young and old adults, estrogen replacement therapy in postmenopausal women and calcitonin for women more than 15 years postmenopausal," Peck concluded. "However, with 24 million Americans affected by osteoporosis, it's clear that these therapies are being underutilized. Improved understanding of prevention, treatment and diagnosis in osteoporosis will help millions of patients and—as is our goal—decrease the impact of the disorder for future patients and their families. This conference will help the medical community focus its continuing research efforts and give direction for improved osteoporosis management into the next century."[3]

A study of 283 elderly patients with hip fractures in a Dayton, Ohio hospital indicated that 14.8 percent of them died within a year, reported Rita Lazarony in the February 18, 1987 issue of *Medical Tribune*. The expected mortality rate for a normal population of a similar age is around 9 percent, added Drs. Stephen B. Sexson and James T. Lehner of the Miami Valley Hospital in Dayton.

The Ohio researchers presented their findings at the annual meeting of the American Academy of Orthopaedic Surgeons in San Francisco, and confirmed a risk equation reported by other professionals. Their data included the type of fracture, age of the patient, sex, general medical condition and the ability to walk after the fracture.

Age was significantly and directly related to mortality, especially for the patients who were 80 and older, Sexson explained. As an example, the expected mortality for those between 60 and 69 is two percent. But in the Ohio study, the mortality rate for that age group was 8.6 percent. For those between 70 and 79, the expected annual death rate is five percent, but in the Ohio study it was 13.9 percent. For patients between 80 and 89, the expected death rate is 11 percent annually, but in the Ohio study of those over 80, mortality was 20.7 percent.

Those who are more ambulatory at discharge tend to have a higher survival rate, Sexson said. For example, the one-year survival rate for persons using a walker was 93.3 percent (180 of 193 patients); the survival rate for those using a wheelchair was 73.4 percent (52 out of 70 patients); and the survival rate for persons who were bedridden when they were discharged was 31.3 percent (five out of 16).

Those in reasonably good health at the time of the fracture were more likely to survive for a longer time, Sexson continued. The higher survival rate generally corresponded to a smaller number of perioperative medical conditions, such as cardiovascular, pulmonary, metabolic, musculoskeletal, gastrointestinal and genitourinary ailments, anemia, cancer or cerebral dysfunction. Those who had no medical problems had 100 percent one-year survival; those who had three preexisting medical conditions had a 73.5 percent survival time.

Sexson went on to say that the number of hours that elapsed from the time of the fracture to the time of corrective surgery had a bearing on the patients' survival rate. The one-year survival rate is somewhat higher if surgery is performed within 24 hours (91 percent) than if it is delayed until after 24 hours (83 percent), he said. But again the survival time is dependent on the number of preexisting medical conditions. For those who had only one or two medical conditions, the survival rate was 97 percent. If the patient had three or more medical problems, the survival time was reduced to 67 percent. Based on their study, Sexson and Lehner recommend that healthy patients should undergo surgery within 24 hours of admission, while less healthy people can be stabilized medically before their operation without adding increased risk.[4]

A study of human bones unearthed after two centuries in a London church crypt suggest a possible clue as to why so many elderly women today suffer hip fractures associated with osteoporosis, according to an article in the March 16, 1993 issue of The New York Times.

"Previous studies have shown that osteoporotic hip fractures are much more common today than would be expected, even with increased life expectancy," the Times reported. "In Britain, the incidence of hip fractures in women and men has doubled in the last 30 years. Fractures have increased in the United States and Canada as well. One possible explanation is that modern women's bones are weaker than those of their ancestors."[5]

During the restoration of Christ Church Spitalfields in the East End of London, scientists from the Wynn Institute for Metabolic Research, Britain's Natural History Museum and University College in London, examined the thigh bones of

87 women buried in the crypt from 1729 to 1852. After comparing their findings with bone-density measurements of 294 present-day women, the scientists, whose original study appeared in *Lancet,* found that the older bones were stronger than contemporary ones.

Although the scientists obviously could not compare dead bones with living ones, since muscle tissue and fat play an active part, they did look at the bone density of postmenopausal women—those 45 and older—compared with pre-menopausal women in both groups. They reported that the rate of bone loss was significantly greater in postmenopausal women today than in women of the same age group who lived 200 years ago. They added that even young women now show some bone loss when contrasted with their older counterparts.

"We don't know why this is," said Belinda Lees, a scientist who specializes in metabolic bone disease at the Wynn Institute in London. "But one factor may be the lower degree of physical activity in present-day women."

EXERCISE IS A FACTOR

The researchers said that church records and diaries document that many of the women in the Spitalfields sample worked 14 hours a day as silk weavers and walked a great deal. By contrast, the women in the present-day sample lead more sedentary lives.

"Studies have shown that weight-bearing exercise not only builds bone, but also increases muscle mass, which can protect against fractures by absorbing the shock of a fall," the *Times* said.

Added Jonathan Reeve, M.D., head of bone disease research for the Medical Research Council in London, previous studies have shown the strongest support that physical activity protects against osteoporosis-related fractures. But, he said, bone is just one of the important things that determines how strong bones are. The internal architecture is important as well, and bones need to be connected properly. Like scaffolding, a few missing pieces will dramatically weaken the structure, he added.[5]

Although calcium plays an important role in building strong, healthy bone, osteo-porosis is not simply a calcium-deficiency disease. Instead, it is a complex disorder involving the process by which healthy bone is constantly broken down and rebuilt. This process, known as bone remodeling, is carried out by bone cells called *osteo-clasts* (which resorb or break down bone) and *osteoblasts* (which are responsible for bone building and deposition), according to research presented at a meeting of the American Academy of Family Physicians in New Orleans in 1988.[6]

Basic research over the past 20 years has shown that groups of osteoclasts and osteoblasts form "packets" called basic multicellular units (BMUs), within which resorption and formation activity is joined and controlled by chemical signals. Some of the chemicals in the body involved in this process include cacitriol (a form of vitamin D), calcitonin (a hormone secreted by the thyroid gland), parathyroid hormone (PTH), prostaglandins and bone growth factors (proteins).[6]

TYPES OF OSTEOPOROSIS

Within BMUs, the remodeling cycle starts with resorption of bone by osteoclasts, which creates pit-like depressions. When the osteoclasts have done their job, the osteoblasts begin to lay down new bone tissue in these pits. At any given time, some BMUs are in the resorption phase, some are involved in formation, while others are temporarily inactive. This complete cycle takes about three months. Osteoporosis develops when resorption exceeds formation, resulting in a loss of bone mass and density. As to how this happens, researchers are still in the dark.

Primary osteoporosis has been classified into two types. Type I, postmenopausal osteoporosis, occurs usually in 25 percent of women between the ages of 50 and 75 who have gone through menopause. It may also occur in younger women who, for a variety of reasons, have had their ovaries surgically removed. The development of this type of osteoporosis is related to the loss of estrogen that was produced by the ovaries. It is not yet known whether the accelerated bone loss associated with menopause is directly due to the fall in estrogen levels or whether more complex biochemical mechanisms are at work. Type II primary osteoporosis occurs as a result of bone loss due to the natural aging process in both men and women over the age of 70.

Secondary osteoporosis may result from treatment with steroid drugs (cortisone, prednisone, etc.) or heparin, an anticoagulant. It may also occur as a result of other disorders, such as multiple myeloma (a malignant tumor of the bone marrow), kidney disease, leukemia, hyperthyroidism (excessive activity of the thyroid gland) and impairment of calcium absorption in the gastrointestinal tract.

Osteoporosis prevention should begin early in life. Children, especially girls, should begin to build as much bone mass as possible by engaging in regular weight-bearing exercise (running, walking, aerobics, etc.) and by eating foods that contain sufficient amounts of calcium and vitamin D.[6]

The American Academy of Family Physicians' daily calcium recommendations for those in the United States, Canada and Europe is shown in Table 13.1.

However, there is much debate about the proper amount of calcium that is needed to replace losses in women at risk. Current recommendations are 1,500 mg/day of calcium for these women. This should be obtained through calcium-rich foods and calcium supplements.[6]

TABLE 13.1

DAILY RECOMMENDED CALCIUM INTAKE

	UNITED STATES mg/day	CANADA mg/day	EUROPE mg/day
Adolescents	1,200	700 to 1,000	600 to 1,000
Non-osteopenic women	800	700	500 to 800
Postmenopausal women	1,500	800	500 to 800

Although researchers are still debating whether or not calcium and vitamin D supplements can deter bone loss in postmenopausal women, the two nutrients did just that, according to Ian R. Reid, M.D., and colleagues in the February 18, 1993 issue of The New England Journal of Medicine. The research team, from the University of Auckland in New Zealand, found that calcium supplementation significantly slowed axial (vertebral) and appendicular (arms and legs) bone loss in normal postmenopausal women.[7]

In the study, the researchers studied 122 women with no appreciable health problems for three years after they had reached menopause and who were getting at least 750 mg/day of calcium. For the following two years, the women were randomly assigned to a test group given either 1,000 mg/day of calcium or a placebo.[7]

Every six months, the research team, using dual-energy X-ray absorptiometry, analyzed the bone mineral density of the whole body, lumbar spine and femur. Blood and urine metabolism and excretion of the mineral were measured after three, 12 and 24 months. The women in the test group were given 1,000 mg/day of calcium as an effervescent tablet containing 5.24 grams of calcium lactate-gluconate and 0.8 gram of calcium carbonate, which was dissolved in water. The placebo group took effervescent tablets containing sugar.

At the conclusion of the study, the researchers determined that, in the calcium group, the loss of total body bone mineral density was reduced by 43 percent when compared with the placebo group. In addition, the rate of loss of bone mineral density was reduced by 35 percent in the legs in the calcium group. Calcium was of significant benefit in the lumbar spine and in the Ward's triangle (neck of the femur), since the rate of loss was reduced by 67 percent.

The New Zealand researchers concluded: "The results of this study are generally consistent with previously published results. We confirmed that appendicular bone loss slows with calcium supplementation."[7]

In an editorial accompanying the study, Robert P. Heaney, M.D., of Creighton University in Omaha, Nebraska, said that, "although we do not know everything there is to know about calcium intake and age-related bone loss, or the mechanisms by which vitamin D impacts on calcium absorption, we do know enough to act now."[8]

He noted that the growing body of controlled trials, all showing a benefit of calcium, vitamin D, or both, lends persuasive evidence that some portion of age-related bone loss in elderly women in Europe and North America is due to insufficient intake of calcium and vitamin D, and that some portion of osteoporotic fractures could be prevented by ensuring higher intakes of both nutrients. European studies suggest that it is never too late to start treatment and that reductions in fractures can occur in as little as 18 months.[8]

"Even a 20-percent reduction in the rate of hip fractures would mean 40,000 to 50,000 fewer hip fractures each year in the United States, for an average annual savings of $1.5 to $2 billion," Heaney said. "It, therefore, seems prudent to increase the intake of calcium and vitamin D in most postmenopausal women—calcium to at least 1,000 mg/day and preferably to 1,500 mg/day, and vitamin D to 400 to 800 IU/day—without waiting for more information."[8]

In a European study recorded in the December 3, 1992 issue of *The New England Journal of Medicine,* Marie C. Chapuy, Ph.D., and colleagues in Lyon, France, studied 3,270 women ranging in age from 69 to 106. In the treatment group, the women were given 1,200 mg/day of calcium and 800 IU/day of vitamin D. For those who completed the 18-month study, the number of hip fractures was reduced by 43 percent, and the number of nonvertebral fractures was 32-percent lower when compared to the placebo group.[9]

In an earlier issue of the same medical journal, Bess Dawson-Hughes, M.D., and colleagues studied bone loss in 361 postmenopausal women, ages 40 to 70. They were consuming less than the Recommended Dietary Allowance for calcium.[10]

In the treatment group, the women were given an extra 500 mg/day of calcium combined with citric and malic acids (CCM), two natural fruit acids, the same amount of calcium carbonate or a placebo.

"The positive effects of CCM were obtained without the use of estrogen and are the first to show that a form of calcium can prevent bone loss at the hip and spine," Dawson-Hughes said.

A Japanese study, reported in the *International Journal of Vitamin and Nutrition Research* in 1991, found that a high salt intake resulted in a loss of calcium in both men and women. Thus, said the researchers at the National Institute of Health and Nutrition in Tokyo, high-sodium diets may increase the risk factor for bone loss.[11]

The importance of calcium, copper, zinc and manganese in the prevention and/or treatment of osteoporosis was detailed by P. Saltman in the *Journal of the American College of Nutrition* in 1992. During the two-year, double-blind, placebo-controlled trial, over 200 postmenopausal women received either: 1) A placebo; 2) 1,000 mg/day of calcium in a supplement plus placebo; 3) A placebo plus 15 mg/day of zinc, 2.5 mg/day of copper and 5 mg/day of manganese; or 4) 1,000 mg/day of calcium plus the three trace minerals. The research team at the University of California at San Diego reported that bone loss was significantly greater in the placebo group than in the calcium plus placebo and in the calcium plus mineral groups. There was no significant bone loss in the calcium plus placebo group, while there was a strong suggestion of increased bone mineral density in the calcium citrate-malate plus trace mineral group.[12]

Bone loss can apparently be reversed with a mineral-rich supplement known as microcrystalline hydroxyapatite concentrate (MCHC), According to O. Epstein in the *American Journal of Clinical Nutrition* in 1982. MCHC is an extract of whole, raw, young animal bone that contains calcium, phosphorus, magnesium fluoride, zinc, copper, manganese, organic constituents such as protein and other nutrients. It is reportedly absorbed well and has been shown to arrest trabecular bone loss.[13]

At a meeting of the American Academy of Orthopedic Surgeons in San Francisco in 1993, speakers promoted the increased consumption of calcium and vitamin D, along with exercise, especially weight-bearing exercises such as walking, jogging and biking.[14]

"Older individuals who exercise regularly have one-half the fracture risk of those who do not exercise," said William Robb III, clinical assistant professor at Northwestern University in Chicago. "In addition to slowing bone loss at all ages, exercise likely increases balance skills and better maintains protective reflexes."[14]

He added that, "Older individuals taking medications that alter balance or alertness should be assessed to minimize dosages or modify medication usage. Of particular concern are the long-acting sedatives, such as benzodiazepines, which significantly increase fracture risk—shorter-acting medications can effectively reduce fracture risk."[14] (Benzodiazepines, which are prescribed for anxiety, include such products as Valium, Librium, Xanax, Tranxene, Serax, Ativan, Centrax, etc.)[15]

In a three-day diet survey of 108 premenopausal female recreational runners and 34 female controls, Tom Lloyd, Ph.D., and colleagues at The Milton S. Hershey Medical Center in Pennsylvania, reported that 80 percent of the runners did not meet the RDA for calcium, iron and zinc.[16]

An increase in dietary calcium protects middle-age and older men and women from hip fractures, according to researchers at the University of California at San Diego. The association between calcium and fracture rate remained after the data were adjusted for cigarette smoking, alcohol intake, exercise and obesity.[17]

"Low-trauma fractures in the elderly, as is true for all fractures, are the result of force and fragility; the more fragile the bone, the less force will be required to produce a fracture," reported Robert P. Heaney, M.D., in the May/June 1990 issue of the *Journal of the American Medical Association.* "But fracture-producing force itself is usually a result of some fall or other injury, or the application of bad body mechanics."[18]

He added that the force a bone actually experiences is influenced, as well, by such factors as soft tissue mass, which absorbs energy in falls and hence lessens the force directly applied to bone. This last point helps to explain why overweight women have only about one-third the expected risk of developing osteoporotic fractures. Skeletal fragility, he added, is a multifactorial affair, with some of the contributing causes probably extending back to childhood.[18]

"Only two to six percent of falls in the elderly result in fracture, but the risk of fracturing as a result of a fall is greater with a fragile skeleton than with a strong one," Heaney continued. "Hence causes of falls, such as environmental hazards, poor vision, postural instability, central nervous system dysfunction, syncopal [fainting] attacks, as well as various medications that may lead to such problems, must all be considered as part of a comprehensive fracture context. Some investigators consider these factors to be more important than low bone mass for some fractures, such as the hip."

Delicate Balance

The relationship between intake, excretory loss and retention of calcium is complicated, Heaney admitted, since both absorption and excretion are related to intake, to some extent in a nonlinear manner. In other words, as calcium intake goes up, both urinary and fecal losses go down, while absorption fraction falls. Since some of the absorbed calcium will be excreted in the urine, the relation of intake to retention is even less efficient. Studies by Heaney and his colleagues and others show that roughly 10 percent of an intake increment is absorbed and

6 percent excreted in the urine, while only about 4 percent will be retained (exclusive of dermal losses). He added that dermal losses of calcium, such as through sweating, amount to at least 15 to 25 mg/day under sedentary conditions and even more when people exercise. Combined with other secretory losses (hair, nails, etc.), these combined losses may total up to 60 mg/day. At the prevailing adult levels of absorption efficiency, Heaney said, this level of nonexcretory loss, all by itself, demands as much as 420 to 550 mg/day of intake.

Heaney added that from birth to age 10 to 12, bone loss increases from an average of 25 grams to about 390 to 450 grams. Since the increase is about linear, daily retention must average about 100 mg of calcium. Isotope-based studies have shown that the absorption efficiency for children averages between 35 and 45 percent. Using a conservative estimate for aggregate excretory and dermal losses of between 100 and 150 mg/day of calcium, it would seem that an intake of between 550 and 650 mg/day of calcium should meet the needs of bone growth during childhood. And, while allowing for interindividual variation, he said, this leads to an estimated Recommended Dietary Allowance value close to the present U.S. figure—800 mg/day for children up to age 12—which would seem to be adequate.

To absorb enough calcium both to mineralize the growing skeleton of adolescents, and to offset known excretory losses, requires, at prevailing absorption efficiencies, a mean intake close to 1,200 mg/day of calcium throughout adolescence. But this is the value for the present RDA, and, allowing for population variance, the adolescent RDA should be higher still, perhaps 1,400 to 1,500 mg/day. This conclusion is supported by the balance studies of Matkovic, et al., in which increasing dietary calcium from 250 to 1,600 mg/day in adolescent females produces a nonsignificant increase in urine calcium. This finding strongly suggests that, even at an intake of 1,600 mg/day, the capacity of the growing skeleton to utilize dietary calcium has not been saturated. Since the average daily retention rate during adolescence is at least twice that during childhood, it makes good sense to suggest that the adolescent RDA also should be at least twice the childhood level.[18]

Absorption efficiency in young adults has been extensively studied and is known to average about 32 percent, Heaney added. If obligatory losses average around 200 mg/day, and using a conservative estimate for skeletal retention of 20 mg/day, a mean intake of 900 to 1,000 mg/day for this age group should suffice, he said. But, making allowance for population variation in absorption and excretion, the RDA should probably be 1,200 mg/day through age 30.

"In the absence of pregnancy and lactation, a woman's requirement from age

30 to menopause is probably the lowest since childhood," Heaney said. "Absorption averages 30 to 35 percent and extraintestinal excretory losses—150 to 200 mg/day—values that translate to a mean requirement of 600 to 700 mg/day. Nordin's balance data point to an only slightly lower figure of 500 to 600 mg/day. Hence the two estimates are essentially congruent. Both lead to a calculated RDA for this age of 800 to 1,000 mg/day of calcium."[18]

"Obtaining 1,000 to 1,400 mg/day of calcium from dietary sources becomes difficult unless a large percentage of calorie requirements are consumed as dairy products," said Lindsay H. Allen, Ph.D., R.D., of the University of Connecticut in Storrs, in the July/August 1986 issue of *Clinical Nutrition*. She added that women in the United States consume on average 530 to 570 mg/day of calcium after the age of 35. Therefore, she said, many older adults should consider the use of calcium supplements.[19] Allen continued:

There has been insufficient systematic evaluation of the relative absorbability of calcium from the available commercial supplements. The usual recommendation is to choose those with the highest percentage of calcium to minimize the size and/or number of doses that must be consumed. Side effects are uncommon, but large amounts of calcium carbonate may cause constipation, and calcium gluconate occasionally causes diarrhea. Since calcium carbonate is cheap and contains the highest percentage of calcium, this is often the supplement of choice. Some antacids, and oyster shell, are basically calcium carbonate. Unfortunately, there is increasing evidence that this form of calcium might not be as well absorbed as others. In particular, this salt is not well absorbed by persons with poor gastric acid production, and some degree of achlorhydria (absence of hydrochloric acid in the gut) is not uncommon in elderly persons. Such persons can absorb calcium citrate well and some of the calcium from calcium carbonate if it is consumed with meals, when gastric acid production is stimulated.[19]

The American diet of processed foods, carbonated soft drinks, caffeine and high protein, sugar and salt consumption can promote osteoporosis, according to John R. Lee, M.D., a practitioner in Sebastapol, California, in *Alternative Medicine: The Definitive Guide*. The processed foods lead directly to calcium loss because these foods are nutrient deficient. This, he said, stimulates the need for protein, which, when eaten in very large amounts, can cause the body to lose calcium.[20]

"This relationship between protein intake and calcium loss has been known to researchers since 1920," Lee continued, "but protein continues to be considered synonymous with being well-fed. But the body cannot store protein, and the excess is metabolized and excreted in urine. Excess protein creates an excess of the waste products that result from the breakdown of protein, including ammonia and acids. Ammonia prevents calcium from being reabsorbed by the kidneys. The acids, which need to be buffered by calcium, also deplete bones of this mineral. Vegetarians seem to have a definite advantage in calcium balance. In one study involving 1,600 women, lacto-ovo vegetarians (vegetarians who eat milk and eggs) had only 18-percent bone loss, as compared to omnivores (people who eat all types of food), who had lost 35 percent."

A high-salt diet depletes the body of calcium. For example, women eating 3,900 mg/day of sodium excreted 30 percent more calcium than those eating 1,600 mg/day. And he said, sugar has been linked to a loss of calcium and a high-sugar diet can cause metabolic problems that can contribute to mineral imbalances.

In addition, soft drinks and caffeine are detrimental to bones. Large amounts of soft drinks, high in phosphorus, can lead to high levels of phosphorus in the blood. And, since the body must maintain the calcium-phosphorus ratio in almost equal amounts, high phosphorus causes calcium to be drawn from the bones to meet the demand. Caffeine is known to cause calcium excretion in the urine as well as in the gastrointestinal tract. Those who drink more than three cups of coffee a day increase their risk of osteoporosis by 82 percent, Lee said.

Alan R. Gaby, M.D., a Baltimore physician, said that calcium may be receiving more attention than it deserves concerning osteoporosis. By that he meant that many other nutrients may be equally critical to the prevention of the soft-bone disease. "Vitamin K, silicon, boron, folic acid (the B vitamin), magnesium and manganese all play a role in bone building and need to be consumed through diet or supplements," Gaby said.[20]

As we have seen, the balance of calcium and phosphorus is critical in preventing osteoporosis. Although this ratio is debated by nutritionists, it is believed the optimal ratio between the minerals should be calcium: phosphorus 1:1. From all the indications, the typical American diet yields 1:2 to 1:4. Ratios more than 1:2 enhance bone resorption, regardless of how much calcium the individual is ingesting, according to H. H. Draper, et al. in Federal Proceedings in 1981.[21]

In a National Institutes of Health Concensus Conference, reported in the Journal of the American Medical Association in 1984, the authors concluded that an increase in calcium intake to 1,000 to 1,500 mg/day, well before menopause, will reduce the incidence of osteoporosis in postmenopausal women. And, they added, increased calcium consumption may well prevent age-related bone loss in men as well.[22]

WHO IS AT RISK?

Writing in *Natural Prescriptions*, Robert M. Giller, M.D., reiterates the types of women who are more susceptible to osteoporosis, namely: Asian women, blond and redheaded women of Northern European ancestry; postmenopausal women; underweight women; women with small bone structure; heavy alcohol users; heavy caffeine users; smokers; women on a high-protein diet; women with a family history of osteoporosis; women who have experienced menopause before age 40; women who are diabetic; women with thyroid disease; women with asthma or other lung diseases; women who take glucocorticoids, such as cortisone and prednisone prescribed for rheumatoid arthritis.

"If you fit several of these descriptions, you should be all the more vigilant about taking steps to prevent osteoporosis," Giller said. "The key to avoiding it is prevention—every woman should monitor her calcium intake throughout her life. Beginning in her teens, she should consume at least 1,200 mg of calcium daily. When she reaches menopause—or if she's nursing—she should increase her intake to 1,500 mg. The reason calcium intake is affected by menopause is that the process of depositing calcium in the bone is very much dependent on the female hormone estrogen, which is diminished after menopause."

Giller added that one reason osteoporosis has become such a problem today is that the major source of calcium, dairy products, are also high in calories and saturated fat. Therefore, many people, especially women, are avoiding these foods for the sake of weight control and cholesterol.[23]

"When the diet is deficient in calcium," Giller explained, "the body 'steals' the essential mineral from the bones for other metabolic processes, making them brittle and thin. When a woman is consuming under 500 mg of calcium a day—half of what her body needs—which describes one quarter of American women, she simply doesn't have enough of the mineral present in her body to carry on normal functions. Every day, her bones are losing a degree of strength and resiliency."

He also pointed out that magnesium, which is involved in calcium metabolism, also plays a critical role in helping to avoid osteoporosis. One study, he said, demonstrated this by supplementing postmenopausal women with half the recommended amount of calcium and twice the recommended amount of magnesium. These women gained bone density at a rate of 16 times greater than women who had nutritional counseling with no added supplements. And, he added, deficiencies of vitamin D can promote bone loss.[23] (The RDA for magnesium for women 15 to 18 is 300 mg/day; for those 19 and over, it's 280 mg/day; for pregnant women, 320 mg/day; for lactating women breast-feeding one to six months, 355 mg/day; those breast-feeding six months or longer, 340 mg/day.)

A PRESCRIPTION FOR PREVENTION

To prevent osteoporosis, Giller makes these recommendations to his patients:

1. Increase foods containing calcium, such as nonfat or low-fat dairy products. Dry, powdered milk can be added to some recipes.
2. Limit protein intake to six ounces daily; use the salt shaker sparingly at table and in cooking.
3. Eliminate caffeine, sugar and alcohol from your diet, stop smoking.
4. Adopt a regular exercise program.
5. In addition to your usual supplement program, make these additions: 1,200 mg of calcium citrate at bedtime; 400 mg/day of magnesium; 2 mg/day of boron. This mineral seems to reduce the loss of calcium from the body. Take a multiple vitamin supplement that provides 400 IU of vitamin D.[23]

Baby Comes First

Although most mothers should breast-feed their infants, there is some concern as to whether or not breast-feeding reduces the mother's supply of calcium. After all, the infant has first choice in taking nutrients from the mother. For example, in one study, women who breast-feed three or more children for 10 months or longer per child had reduced trabecular wrist-bone density and increased their susceptibility to osteoporotic fractures.[24]

Using single-photon densitometry, nutritionists Gordon W. Wardlaw and Anne M. Pike found that ultradistal bone mass was about 18 percent below normal in 11 mothers who had nursed for an average of 10.7 months per child, compared with readings within 2 percent of normal in 10 mothers who had breast-fed three or four children for an average of 2.8 months per child. Volunteers in the study were 21 healthy women between the ages of 30 and 35, who were free of factors influencing bone density, such as the use of alcohol or cigarettes, excessive physical activity, premature menopause, obesity or estrogen supplementation.

"The current findings indicate that even when women consume more than 90 percent of the recommended daily allowance for calcium, long-term lactation can deplete ultradistal bone mass in the forearm," stated *Medical World News*. "Moreover, the researchers note that it is 'unclear if these losses can be reduced by increasing the RDA for calcium,' as some of the women in the long-term group had calcium intakes considerably above the RDA but didn't have a concomitant reduction in bone loss."[24]

Women who nurse their infants for six months or more lose a significant amount of the mineral calcium from their bones, according to the June 26, 1993 issue of *Science News*. Epidemiologist MaryFran R. Sowers and colleagues at the University of Michigan in Ann Arbor said that, although most women make up for that loss after they stop breast-feeding, there is still the possibility that such bone loss may put some new mothers in jeopardy of potentially crippling fractures later in life.[25]

The researchers, whose study was originally reported in the June 23/30, 1993 issue of the *Journal of the American Medical Association*, recruited 98 healthy women during the last months of their pregnancy. Bone density was measured two weeks after delivery and again at various points after the birth of their baby. The researchers found that women who had nursed their babies for six months or longer showed an average loss of bone density of 5.1 percent from the lower spine and a loss of 4.8 percent from the top of the leg bone. There was no loss for the women who bottle-fed their infants or who breastfed for less than a month.

"The average U.S. woman nurses her baby for just three months and thus is unlikely to lose significant amounts of bone," *Science News* added. "Yet Sowers worries that teenage mothers and women who are malnourished may lose a critical mass of bone during lactation. This might put them at risk of developing osteoporosis after menopause."[25]

Stephen P. Heyse of the National Institute of Arthritis and Musculoskeletal and Skin Diseases in Bethesda, Maryland, said, "This isn't to say that women shouldn't breast-feed. Young women should make sure they get enough calcium to build strong bones before they get pregnant."

Abnormally high levels of glucocorticoids interfere with bone and calcium metabolism in a number of ways, according to David W. Dempster, Ph.D., director of the Regional Bone Center, Helen Hayes Hospital, West Haverstraw, New York, and associate professor of clinical pathology at Columbia University in New York City. These drugs decrease the amount of calcium absorbed from food and increase loss of calcium in the urine. This results in an overproduction of another hormone, parathyroid hormone, which attempts to restore the blood calcium levels by removing calcium from bone, he reported in *The Osteoporosis Report*.[26]

In addition, he said, glucocorticoids also exert direct effects on the cells responsible for bone maintenance, stimulating the cells that destroy bone (osteoclasts) and inhibiting those that form new bone (osteoblasts). And the production of estrogen in women and testosterone in men is reduced by glucocorticoids, which may also contribute to bone loss.

Dempster explained that glucocorticoids are hormones produced by the adrenal glands, located above the kidneys. In healthy people, these hormones play an active role in the regulation of blood sugar levels, retention of salt and water, as well as in metabolism and growth. They also have inhibitory effects on the body's immune system and are instrumental in suppressing allergic reactions. When glucocorticoids are produced in abnormal amounts, they can result in Cushing's syndrome or Cushing's disease, which was first described by Dr. Harvey Cushing in 1932. This disorder results in a number of symptoms, such as obesity, muscle wasting and thinning of the skin. One of the most serious complications of Cushing's syndrome, however, is accelerated bone loss which can produce osteoporosis and fractures.

"Cushing's syndrome is so rare that initially glucocorticoid-induced osteoporosis did not represent a clinical problem of public health significance," Dempster continued. "But this changed in the late 1940s when synthetic glucocorticoids were introduced as potent anti-inflammatory and immuno-suppressive medications. These drugs, often simply referred to as steroids (not to be confused with anabolic steroids which some athletes use to build muscle) are still widely used today for the treatment of a number of disorders, such as rheumatoid arthritis, asthma, or psoriasis. While glucocorticoids are very effective in the management of these diseases and greatly improve the patient's quality of life, the potentially serious side effect of osteoporosis might cause considerable pain and disability, and must be carefully monitored."

Glucocorticoids, which are administered in a number of ways, inhibit skeletal growth and development in children and can result in rapid and severe bone loss in adults. The synthetic hormones are administered as tablets or injections into the joints (for arthritis); by inhaler (for asthma); as creams (for skin diseases); or intravenous injection (for multiple sclerosis or after organ transplantation). Although all of these forms can lead to osteoporosis, oral administration and intravenous injection are likely to cause the most damage. The adverse effects of steroids on the skeleton are cumulative, so that even intermittent use of these drugs can cause osteoporosis, Dempster said.

> If you are currently taking steroid medications or are about to start a course of treatment which is likely to last more than a few weeks, the first priority is to talk to your physician about the treatment plan and the risk of osteoporosis. The best way to assess your risk is to have your bone mass measured. The rate and degree of bone loss is proportional to the dose and duration of steroid treatment. Therefore, it is crucial that your physician prescribe the minimum dose required to control your symptoms and that the steroids be discontinued as soon as possible. If steroid use cannot be discontinued, it may be possible to switch from an orally administered drug to a less damaging topical route of administration, such as an inhaler.[26]

Since glucocorticoids impair the body's ability to absorb and retain calcium, Dempster urges those using these drugs to ensure an adequate supply of calcium, either through dietary sources such as dairy products, or by a calcium supplement.

Dietary intake of calcium can be easily estimated and should be supplemented to achieve a level of 1,000 mg/day or 1,500 mg/day in the case of postmenopausal women who are not taking hormone replacement therapy. Postmenopausal women who are on hormone replacement therapy should have 1,000 mg/day of calcium. When you increase your calcium intake, you should have the calcium level in your urine measured because some people have very high concentrations of calcium in the urine when taking steroids. This could lead to the development of kidney stones. In addition to calcium, you should also make sure that your vitamin D intake is sufficient. This is particularly important in people who are housebound and get little exposure to sunlight. These individuals should take a daily supplement of vitamin D, containing at least 400 IU, but not more than 800 IU.[26]

AVOID HOUSEHOLD INJURIES

Although brittle bones are obviously the cause of many falls, the elimination of hazards in the home can be a great deterrent for keeping people out of the hospital. In addition to the diet and lifestyle changes discussed in this chapter, the American Academy of Orthopaedic Surgeons, 6300 North River Rd., Rosemont, Illinois 60018, offers these tips for making the home safe in a booklet, *Live It Safe!* Since many falls and injuries occur in the home, the Academy offers these safety tips:[27]

Stairways
- Provide enough light to see clearly each step and the top and bottom landings.
- Repair loose stairway rugs or boards immediately.
- Do not leave objects on the stairs.
- Do not use patterned or dark carpeting on stairs.
- Install full-length handrails on both sides of the stairway.

Bathrooms
- Place a slip-resistant rug next to the bathtub for safe exit and entry.
- Place nonskid textured adhesive strips on the bathtub and shower floor.
- Install grab bars on the walls around the bathtub.

Bedrooms
- Keep the floor clear of clutter.
- Place a lamp and flashlight near your bed.
- Install a night-light along the route between the bedroom and the bathroom.

Living Areas
- Arrange furniture to provide a clear pathway between rooms.
- Remove low-rise tables, magazine racks, footrests and plants from pathways.

- Keep electrical and telephone cords out of pathways.
- Secure loose area rugs and runners with double-faced tape, tacks or slip-resistant backing.
- Do not stand on unsteady stools, chairs, ladders, etc.

Kitchen
- Clean up spills, dropped food, etc., from floors immediately.
- Use nonskid floor wax.
- Use step stools with an attached handrail.

On June 6–8, 1994, the National Institute on Arthritis and Musculoskeletal and Skin Diseases, as well as other Institutes of the National Institutes of Health (NIH), convened an expert panel to make recommendations concerning how much calcium Americans should be getting to avoid osteoporosis. The findings were reported in the Fall 1994 issue of *Osteoporosis Report,* a quarterly publication of the National Osteoporosis Foundation in Washington, D.C. The panel was chaired by John Bilezikian, M.D., of the Columbia University College of Physicians and Surgeons in New York City, and included 14 nationally known scientists, nutritionists and physicians.[28]

During the two days of deliberations, the panel concluded that millions of Americans are not getting enough calcium in their diets to build strong bones and reduce the risk of osteoporosis. The experts also called for a unified public health strategy to ensure optimal calcium intakes in the population. This prompted the National Osteoporosis Foundation to concur with the conclusions of the panel and to urge federal health officials to increase the current RDAs for calcium, based on the panel's recommendations.

"Over the past 10 years, the public has been exposed to conflicting and confusing information regarding the amount of calcium needed to build and maintain healthy bones," stated Sandra C. Raymond, the Foundation's executive director. "One of the problems has been the failure of the RDAs to keep pace with new scientific information. If we are to adhere to the consensus panel's recommendations for a unified public health strategy to optimize bone health, federal officials must now act to incorporate this panel's findings into the RDAs."

The panel's recommendations are similar to recommendations made by NIH and the Foundation as early as 1987, which suggested 1,000 mg/day of calcium for adult men and women and 1,500 mg/day for postmenopausal women not on estrogen therapy.

"The higher recommendations for children and for adults aged 65 and older reflect new data on optimal calcium intakes in these age groups," said C. Conrad Johnston, Jr., M.D., the Foundation's vice president. "Current research suggests that a greater amount of bone mass accumulates in children and young adults who have a higher calcium intake. The long-term benefit of this higher calcium intake may be a higher peak bone mass, resulting in fewer fractures later in life."

The Foundation's newsletter added that population surveys indicate that girls and young women tend to have a calcium intake of 800 mg/day, well below the recommended 1,200 to 1,500 mg/day. Higher calcium intakes in older adults, especially when coupled with an increased intake of vitamin D, can slow bone loss and prevent fractures.

"The consensus panel felt that age-related losses necessitate a higher calcium intake in women and men ages 65 and over, including older women on estrogen therapy," the newsletter said. "Presently, calcium intakes less than 600 mg/day are common in older adults. In addition, intestinal calcium absorption in the elderly is often impaired and vitamin D levels can be low, contributing to bone loss. The consensus panel suggested vitamin D intakes of 600 to 800 IU/day."[28]

REFERENCES

1. Farley, Dixie. "The Buildup and Breakdown of Bone Tissue," *FDA Consumer,* October 1986, p. 34.
2. Seggev, Michael. "International Osteoporosis Experts Convene in the United States." Recap of the "Research Advances in Osteoporosis" conference, Washington, D.C., February 26, 1990.
3. Ibid.
4. Lazarony, Rita. "Hip Fractures Hasten Death of Frail and Less Mobile," *Medical Tribune,* February 18, 1987, p. 29.
5. "Women's Bones Appear to Have Become Weaker," *The New York Times,* March 16, 1993, p. C4.
6. Torres, Ovidio. "Advances in Postmenopausal Osteoporosis." Seminar conducted by the American Academy of Family Physicians, New Orleans, October 3, 1988.
7. Reid, Ian R., M.D., et al. "Effect of Calcium Supplementation on Bone Loss in Postmenopausal Women," *The New England Journal of Medicine* 328(7):460–464, February 18, 1993.
8. Heaney, Robert P., M.D. "Thinking Straight About Calcium." Ibid, pp. 503–504.
9. Chapuy, Marie C., Ph.D., et al. "Vitamin D3 and Calcium to Prevent Hip Fractures in Elderly Women," *The New England Journal of Medicine* 327(23):1637–1642, December 3, 1992.

10. Dawson-Hughes, Bess, M.D., et al. "A Controlled Trial of the Effect of Calcium Supplementation on Bone Density in Postmenopausal Women," *The New England Journal of Medicine* 323:878–883, September 27, 1990.

11. Itoh, R., et al. "The Interrelation of Urinary Calcium and Sodium Intake in Healthy, Elderly Japanese," *International Journal of Vitamin and Nutrition Research* 61:159–165, 1991.

12. Saltman, P. "The Role of Minerals and Osteoporosis," *Journal of the American College of Nutrition* 11(5):599/Abstract 7, October 1992.

13. Epstein, O. "Vitamin D, Hydroxyapatite and Calcium Gluconate in Treatment of Cortical Bone Thinning in Postmenopausal Women with Primary Biliary Cirrhosis," *American Journal of Clinical Nutrition* 36:426–430, 1992.

14. Phillips, Pat. "As Population Ages, Orthopedists Gird for Increasing Number of Hip Fractures," *Medical Tribune,* March 11, 1993, p. 16.

15. Edelson, Edward. *The ABCs of Prescription Drugs.* Garden City, N.Y.: Doubleday and Co., Inc., 1987, pp. 40–41.

16. Lloyd, Tom, Ph.D., et al. "Nutritional Characteristics of Recreational Women Runners," *Nutrition Research* 12:359–366, 1992.

17. Hollbrook, T., et al. "Dietary Calcium and Risk of Hip Fracture: A Fourteen-Year Prospective Population Study," *Lancet* 2:1046–1049, 1988.

18. Heaney, Robert P., M.D. "Calcium Intake and Bone Health Throughout Life," *Journal of the American Medical Women's Association* 45(3):80–86, May/June 1990.

19. Allen, Lindsay H., Ph.D., R.D. "Calcium and Age-Related Bone Loss," *Clinical Nutrition* 5(4):147–152, July/August 1986.

20. Goldberg, Burton/The Burton Goldberg Group. *Alternative Medicine: The Definitive Guide.* Puyallup, Wash.: Future Medicine Publishing, Inc., 1993, pp. 773ff.

21. Draper, H. H., et al. "Calcium, Phosphorus and Osteoporosis," *Federal Proceedings* 40(9):2434–2438, 1981.

22. "NIH Consensus Conference: Osteoporosis," *Journal of the American Medical Association* 252(6):799–802, 1984.

23. Giller, Robert M., M.D., and Matthews, Kathy. *Natural Prescriptions.* New York: Carol Southern Books, 1994, pp. 264ff.

24. "Osteoporosis Risk in Lengthy Breast-Feeding?" *Medical World News,* December 22, 1986, p. 37.

25. Fackelmann, K. A. "Prolonged Nursing and the Risk of Bone Loss," *Science News,* June 26, 1993, p. 407.

26. Dempster, David W., Ph.D. "Gluocorticoid-Induced Osteoporosis," *The Osteoporosis Report* 8(2):2, 10, Summer 1992, National Osteoporosis Foundation, Washington, D.C.

27. "Live It Safe!" American Academy of Orthopaedic Surgeons, Rosemont, Ill., 1992.

28. "Expert Panel Recommends Higher Calcium Intake," *Osteoporosis Report* 10(3):1, 10, Fall 1994.

14

Calcium and Vitamin D: The Dynamic Duo

VITAMIN D deficiency among the elderly, especially those who live in northern climates, may be a major unrecognized public health problem, according to Judy McBride in the October 1986 *USDA News*, a publication of the U.S. Department of Agriculture in Beltsville, Maryland.

Studies by Michael F. Holick, M.D., an endocrinologist with the Human Nutrition Research Center on Aging at USDA/Tufts University in Boston, Massachusetts, bear this out.

"The elderly are not getting enough of the vitamin from their diets—especially milk—or from brief exposures to the summer sun," Holick said. "To avoid risk of skin cancer, sun exposure should be brief."

THE SUNSHINE VITAMIN

Vitamin D helps the body absorb calcium from the intestinal tract and maintains blood levels essential for proper mineralization of the bone. A deficiency in the two nutrients in adults leads to softening of the bone (*osteomalacia*), compounding the problem of bone loss or osteoporosis in the elderly. And a vitamin D deficiency in those with osteoporosis may significantly increase the risk of bone fractures.

In a study of 142 patients entering Boston's Massachusetts General Hospital with fractured hips, Holick noted that 30 to 40 percent of the patients had little or none of the circulating form of vitamin D in their blood. Other studies, both in the United States and Great Britain, indicate a similar 30 to 40 percent of men and women with hip fractures are deficient in the vitamin, he said.

109

"The major cause of age-related vitamin D deficiency is a decrease in milk consumption," Holick continued. "Relatively few other foods contain vitamin D. Unfortunately, a substantial number of elderly develop an intolerance to milk, and others believe that milk is only for children. Four 8-ounce glasses of milk a day provides 400 IU of vitamin D. Depending on the fat content, 32 ounces of milk supplies about 1,200 milligrams of calcium."

For those who can't tolerate milk, a vitamin D supplement should be taken and/or they should spend more time in the summer sun, Holick advised. But, as people age, the ability of the sun to stimulate and manufacture vitamin D on the skin progressively decreases. In northern latitudes, vitamin D synthesis stops completely in the winter.

In order to get the benefits of summer sunlight and minimize its detrimental effects, Holick suggests that light-skinned elderly people restrict exposure to five to 10 minutes around mid-day in June, when the sun's rays are most direct. When the angle of the sun is lower, exposure can be longer. However, dark-skinned people require five to 10 times longer in the sun, depending on the amount of pigmentation. In one laboratory test, for example, it took a dose of radiation that would produce a severe sunburn in Caucasians to increase vitamin D levels in black skin. And he pointed out that sunblocks do exactly that. The products with a high protection index completely prevent the skin from producing the vitamin.[1]

Another researcher at USDA/Tufts, Elizabeth A. Krall, Ph.D., said that the Recommended Dietary Allowance for vitamin D may be too low to protect older women from losing bone calcium during the winter months, according to the January 30, 1990 issue of *Scientific Research News*. In a study involving 333 women past menopause, Krall found that those who consumed at least 10 percent more vitamin D than the RDA did not have the seasonal see-saw of hormones that regulate blood calcium levels. The RDA is 200 IU/day after age 21; it was lowered from 400 IU/day in previous editions of the *Recommended Dietary Allowances*.[2]

Krall added that an inadequate intake of vitamin D during the sun-starved days of winter, when the skin produces little or no vitamin D, can mean less calcium for the bones. As vitamin D levels dip, another hormone rises to help maintain a constant blood calcium level, probably by borrowing calcium from the bones, she said.

A more pressing issue is that many women don't even come close to getting the RDA for vitamin D. Vitamin intakes in their study ranged from zero to nearly 1,700 IU. But the average intake was only 112 IU or slightly more than half of the RDA.

"Vitamin D inadequacy may be more widespread in the healthy population than recognized," Krall said. "The signs of inadequacy are not well defined. For instance, in normal, healthy people, blood levels of the major circulating form of vitamin D vary six- to seven-fold because of the wide range of dietary intakes and seasonal fluctuations. This form of vitamin D is the precursor to its active, or hormone, form."

Although the RDA has a built-in safety margin to cover most Americans, it is based primarily on studies of younger people. The women in the USDA/Tufts study averaged 58 years old. They were generally healthy and had no problems that might reduce vitamin and mineral absorption. Still, it appears that they need at least 220 IU/day. However, those with absorption difficulties or kidney disease or older people, who have less capacity to absorb and manufacture vitamin D, would need to have even higher levels.

Other studies have confirmed that the women's vitamin D levels peaked during late summer and early fall and hit their lowest levels in late winter and early spring, after the summer reserve has been depleted. At the same time, blood levels of parathyroid hormone, the hormone thought to raise blood calcium by pulling it from the bones, were at their highest. As for food sources of vitamin D, fatty fish, such as herring, salmon and sardines, are the richest sources.[2]

Insiders at Risk

Writing in the *Journal of the American Geriatrics Society* in 1991, F. Michael Gloth, III, M.D., of the Johns Hopkins University School of Medicine and The Francis Scott Key Medical Center in Baltimore, and colleagues from other facilities, said that at the present time there is no specific recommendation for people over 65 years of age. In a normal population, with adequate exposure to sunlight, the current dietary recommendations for adults, in general, may be sufficient for the elderly as well. But, they added, this is not true for that population of elderly who are confined indoors and do not benefit from the sun's ultraviolet radiation.

"The results of [our] study would support the notion that the current RDA is too low for many of those older individuals who get no direct sunlight exposure," the researchers said. "Currently, studies are underway to evaluate how much over 400 IU/day of vitamin D is advisable for those frail elderly who do not get vitamin D from the sun."[3]

Researchers at the University of Tennessee and Baptist Memorial Hospital in Memphis reported that vitamin D, calcium and calcitonin (a hormone) reduced the effects of osteoporotic fractures and may be helpful in treating postmenopausal women with osteoporosis, according to *Clinical Research* in 1988. Thirteen Caucasian women with osteoporosis were involved in the study. Each was given 1,000 mg/day of calcium; 50,000 IU of vitamin D three times weekly; plus the hormone.

The research team, headed by G. Palmieri, et al., stated that trabecular bone volume (the honeycomb-like inner structure of bones) increased 43 percent during the two to six years that the patients were studied. They noted that the large amounts of vitamin D, moderate dosage of calcium and the hormone brought clinical improvement, increased bone volume and a reduction in the expected frequency of bone fractures.[4]

Vitamin D status is most commonly assessed by measuring serum concentrations of 25-hydroxyvitamin D, the major circulating metabolite of vitamin D in the blood. The *American Journal of Clinical Nutrition* reported in 1990 that:

"Many studies have shown that these concentrations decrease with age, because both exogenous and endogenous means of supply tend to be reduced. The absorption of vitamin D from the gut is not impaired by aging, but dietary intake is often reduced. The lowest serum concentrations of the vitamin D metabolite have been found in institutionalized elderly people in countries that do not routinely fortify foods with vitamin D. In the United States the major dietary source of the vitamin is milk that is fortified with either ergocalciferol or cholecaliciferol—the use of the term vitamin D represents either or both forms. Natural sources are fatty fish, fish liver oil and, to a lesser extent, eggs."[5]

When exposure to sunlight is reduced, as in the case of the nursing home population, an additional form of the vitamin, from foods or supplements, may be advisable. In their study, at least 30 percent of the unsupplemented volunteers had low-normal values of the vitamin D metabolite circulating in their blood in September and February.

"The basic diet did not provide the RDA of vitamin D for many of the elderly subjects," researchers noted, "primarily because of their lack of milk intake. A daily vitamin supplement containing 400 IU of vitamin D proved to be sufficient to maintain normal serum (vitamin D metabolite) concentrations throughout the entire year. Seasonal changes in sunlight exposure provided a small fluctuation superimposed on the adequate baseline amount provided by supplementation."[5]

An article in the *Israeli Journal of Medical Science* in 1981 reported that 15 out of 82 elderly people were deficient in vitamin D and the 28 others had borderline levels. Since many of the elderly were farm workers and thus spent a great deal of time in the sun, the study suggests that these seniors had an impairment in vitamin D metabolism, rather than having an inadequate source of the vitamin.[6]

In another study, involving 109 randomly selected elderly women, ranging in age from 65 to 74, each volunteer received either 15,000 IU of vitamin D2 (calciferol) weekly or a placebo. After two years on this therapy, vitamin D therapy significantly reduced the rate of cortical bone loss as revealed by hand radiographs, reported the *American Journal of Clinical Nutrition* in 1985.[7]

PREVENT BONE LOSS EARLY ON

"Bone loss is a slow process occurring over many years, and any protective effect of vitamin D might be concealed if therapy were started too late," reported the April 22, 1987 issue of *Medical Tribune*. "Until these points have been clarified and, in particular, the issue of whether vitamin D supplementation reduces hip fracture incidence has been resolved, the case for routine supplementation in all elderly people remains unproven. Nevertheless, the increased frequency of vitamin D deficiency among certain groups, together with the ease and safety with which normal vitamin D status can be restored, strongly favor supplementation for high-risk patients."[8]

Researchers have confirmed that vitamin D increases calcium absorption from the small intestine, and that a deficiency in the vitamin results in abnormal calcium losses in the feces. A sufficient amount of vitamin D in the diet enhances the absorption of phosphorus through the intestinal wall, independent of calcium absorption, as well as the absorption of phosphates from the small tubes leading from the kidneys. If there is a vitamin D deficiency, urinary excretion of phosphate increases and blood levels go down. The maintenance of a satisfactory phosphate level, as well as the balance between calcium and phosphorus in the blood, is imperative to the process of bone calcification and to the prevention of tetany, which is the abnormal contraction of muscles.

The growth and proper mineralization of the bones and teeth require vitamin D. Lack of the vitamin or lack of exposure to sunlight of children results in weak bones and overgrowth of the softer tissue (cartilage) at the ends of the bones. This can result in enlarged joints, bowed legs, knock knees, beaded ribs and skull deformities. A vitamin D deficiency in adults can cause osteomalacia, the soft-bone disorder, in which there are changes in the shafts of bones as the bones become soft. The vitamin is also necessary in preventing congenital malformations of the newborn and injury to the skeleton of the mother. A vitamin D deficiency will also affect the enamel and dentin of the teeth, since they are both composed mostly of calcium and phosphorus.[9]

Phosphates, which are salts of phosphoric acid, are common ingredients in our food supply. Phosphoric acid is used as a flavoring in soft drinks, bakery products, some cheese products, jellies, candy, frozen dairy products, etc. As explained elsewhere in this book, many people—especially teenagers—are consuming too many phosphate-rich foods. This can send the calcium-phosphorus ratio out of kilter and can lead to osteoporosis later in life.

REFERENCES

1. McBride, Judy. "The Sunshine Vitamin Isn't Just Kid Stuff," *USDA News*, October 1986.
2. McBride, Judy. "Older Women May Need More Vitamin D Than Recommended," *Scientific Research News*, U. S. Department of Agriculture, January 30, 1990.
3. Gloth, F. Michael, III, M.D., et al. "Is the Recommended Daily Allowance for Vitamin D Too Low for the Homebound Elderly?" *Journal of the American Geriatrics Society* 39:137–141, 1991.
4. Palmieri, G., et al. "Effect of Calcitonin and Vitamin D in Osteoporosis," *Clinical Research* 36:A884, 1988.
5. Webb, Ann R., et al. "An Evaluation of the Relative Contributions of Exposure to Sunlight and of the Diet to the Circulating Concentrations of 25-Hydroxyvitamin D in an Elderly Nursing Home Population in Boston," *American Journal of Clinical Nutrition* 51:1075–1081, 1990.
6. Weisman, Y., et al. "Inadequate Status and Impaired Metabolism of Vitamin D in the Elderly," *Israeli Journal of Medical Science* 17(1):19–21, 1981.
7. Nordin, N. E., et al. "A Prospective Trial of the Effect of Vitamin D Supplementation on Metacarpal Bone Loss in Elderly Women," *American Journal of Clinical Nutrition* 42(3):470–474, 1985.
8. "Vitamin D for Elderly," *Medical Tribune*, April 22, 1987, p. 31.
9. Ensminger, Audrey H., et al. *Foods and Nutrition Encyclopedia.* Clovis, Calif.: Pegus Press, 1983, p. 2260.

15

Iodine Protects Against Goiter and Cancer

IODINE was the first nutrient to be recognized as essential for humans and animals. As early as 3000 B.C., the Chinese treated goiter by feeding seaweed and burnt sponge. Hippocrates used the same treatment for enlarged thyroid glands. Iodine gets its name from the Greek word *iodes*, which means violet color, from the color of the fumes of iodine.

French chemist Bernard Courtois discovered iodine in seaweed in 1811 and described some of its basic properties. Potassium hydriodate was introduced by Prout as a treatment for goiter five years later. However, goiter continued in much of the world for many years.

Then, in 1914, Edward C. Kendall isolated a crystalline compound containing 65 percent iodine from the thyroid gland and named it thyroxin. Based on research studies, the subsequent inclusion of iodine in the diets of man and animals brought a reduction of goiter in the United States and other developing countries. In 1950, Kendall and colleagues at the Mayo Clinic received the Nobel Prize for their work on thyroxin and other hormones of the adrenal cortex.

IODINE DEFICIENCY

In the absence of iodine, the thyroid gland attempts to compensate for the deficiency by increasing its secretory activity, causing the gland to enlarge. This is called simple, or endemic, goiter. Females are more apt to develop this disorder, since goiter often develops during periods when metabolic rate is high, such as puberty and pregnancy. Not all goiter is simple goiter and related to an iodine deficiency. Graves' disease (exophthalmic goiter) is due to overactivity of the thyroid gland, which is usually, but not always, enlarged.[1]

Iodine, an integral part of the thyroid hormones thyroxine and triiodothyronine, is present in food and water predominantly as iodide and, to a lesser degree, organically bound to amino acids. Iodide is rapidly and almost completely absorbed and transported to the thyroid gland for synthesis into the thyroid hormones, to salivary and gastric glands, and to the kidneys for excretion into the gastrointestinal tract and urine. Organically bound iodine is less well absorbed, and part of it is excreted in the feces.

Since all the iodide secreted into the gastrointestinal tract is reabsorbed, the main excretory route for the inorganic form of iodine is the urine. While losses in the milk of breast-feeding women and losses in sweat in hot climates can be considerable, urinary excretion is a reliable indicator of iodine status under most circumstances.

Iodine is not distributed evenly in the environment. In mountainous areas, environmental levels are inadequate for humans and animals. Deficiency can lead to a wide spectrum of diseases, ranging from severe cretinism with mental retardation to barely visible enlargement of the thyroid. Endemic goiter and the more severe forms of iodine deficiency disorders still can be seen around the globe. In 1983, there were an estimated 400 million iodine-deficient persons in the less developed regions of the world, and an estimated 112 million in the more developed areas.

Iodine deficiency disorders, including goiter, can be prevented (but not cured) by providing an adequate iodine intake. The incidence of endemic goiter in the United States fell sharply after the introduction of iodized salt in 1924. There are, however, residual cases of goiter remaining, mainly in women and children living in areas of California, Texas, Kentucky, Louisiana and South Carolina, and in the prairie regions of Canada. These are most probably not caused by iodine deficiency, because they bear no relation to urinary iodine excretion. Natural goitrogens, such as those found in cabbage or cassava, have been implicated in the pathogenesis of goiter in some parts of the world, but it is not known if they pose a problem in the United States.

Sources of Iodine

The environmental levels of iodine and their contribution to the daily intake of animals and humans vary widely in the U.S. In the coastal areas, for example, seafoods, water and iodine-containing mist from the ocean are important sources.

Further inland, the iodine content of plant and animal products is variable, depending on the geochemical environment and on fertilizing, feeding practices and food processing. In these areas, iodized table salt is a reliable source by providing 75 micrograms of iodine per gram of salt.

Iodates are still used as dough oxidizers in the continuous bread-making process, adding about 500 mcg/100 g of bread. Dairy products accumulate iodine because of the use of iodine-containing disinfectants on cows, milking machines and storage tanks, as well as by iodine-containing additives in the animals' feed.

In its Total Diet Study, the Food and Drug Administration found a tendency toward steadily declining iodine levels since 1982. Between 1985–1986, the typical intake for men and women was 250 mcg and 170 mcg/day respectively, excluding intakes from iodized salt.[2]

IODINE DEFICIENCY AND THE THYROID

As previously mentioned, members of the Brassica family—cabbage, kale, turnips, cauliflower, rapeseed and mustard seed—contain goitrogens, which interfere with the use of thyroxin and may produce goiter. However, goitrogenic action is usually prevented by cooking, and an adequate supply of iodine inhibits or prevents the problem. Deficiencies of iodine and vitamin A are said to cause a more severe thyroid disorder than lack of iodine alone.[3]

The thyroid gland is located in the middle of the neck and is formed like an H, with the bar of the H located one to two fingers beneath the Adams' apple, according to Niels Lauersen, M.D., and Steven Whitney in A Woman's Body. The gland's arms are located on each side of the bar of the H. Since this gland produces thyroid hormones, this is extremely important for metabolism.[4]

"One common function of the thyroid is regulation of weight," the authors continued. "If you have a low thyroid function, you might have a slow metabolic rate and will tend to be fat even with minimal food intake. On the other hand, if your thyroid is overactive, your metabolic rate will be high and you will be constantly hungry and able to eat without gaining weight. If that sounds too good to be true, it is; people with overactive thyroids also tend to feel hot and sweaty most of the time, whereas people with slow thyroid functions tend toward fatigue and are extremely sensitive to cold."

The thyroid gland is also closely associated with ovulation, since the gonadotrophic hormones, produced by the pituitary and regulating the ovarian function, are influenced by the thyroid hormones. A slow or fast thyroid function might interfere with ovulation through interaction with the pituitary hormone.

The thyroid gland can be checked by a blood test to examine the blood content of the thyroid hormone, the authors added, or it can be checked by a basal metabolism test. This test needs to be taken on an empty stomach, since food containing high amounts of iodine can upset the real values. They added that infertility has often been corrected just by giving small amounts of thyroid medication to the patient with a slow thyroid function.

Enlargement of the thyroid gland can occur from many causes, the authors said. It could be due to an overproduction of thyroid hormone by the glands, or it could be caused by a tumor or cancer of the thyroid gland. Insufficient intake of iodine will cause enlargement of the thyroid gland, since this causes the gland to enlarge in order to increase the production of thyroid hormone to keep pace with need.[4]

The late Broda O. Barnes, M.D. said that, of all the problems that can affect physical and mental health, none is more common than thyroid gland disturbance. He added that none is more easily corrected; none is more often untreated or detected.

Barnes, who at the time had been practicing medicine for over 25 years, and who had been studying the thyroid gland since he was in medical school, said that 40 percent of the American people (four of every 10 children and adults) today are suffering needlessly and many are dying for lack of an inexpensive, easily available ingredient.* The following cases, involving some of his patients, and which he and Lawrence Galton reported in *Hypothyroidism: The Unsuspected Illness*, show the magnitude of low thyroid function:

1. A sufferer from severe rheumatic pain and a potential heart attack victim.
2. A young housewife who feels rundown, tires easily, is sleepy much of the time, and strangely oversensitive to cold weather.
3. A middle-aged man who has fought a life-long battle against low energy reserves.
4. A victim of severe recurrent headaches.
5. A couple unable to have children.

---

*Although the "easily available ingredient" he is talking about is not iodine but thyroid therapy, I felt it important enough to include in this chapter.

6. A child or adult unusually prone to infections, especially respiratory ones, but not necessarily limited to them.
7. A woman whose skin is abnormally rough, scaly, almost fishlike and patients with other skin problems, such as eczema, psoriasis and acne.
8. A man or woman in a state of severe mental depression.
9. A woman with menstrual problems.

"These are a few of the people who will pass through my waiting room on almost any routine day," Barnes said. "There is one striking common fact about them: Varied as are their symptoms, the cause of their illness in every case is the same—low thyroid function."[5]

HYPOTHYROIDISM AND THE HEART

Barnes added that one of the great puzzles about heart attacks is the relationship between tuberculosis and coronary disease; the insight that heart attacks are occurring in a "new population" made up of those who have escaped earlier death from TB.

Thyroid deficiency can produce many changes in the body which encourage heart attacks. One of these is the deposition in abnormal amounts of mucopolysaccharides in the tissues. These are the compounds known to accumulate early in any injury or inflammation and in hardening of the arteries.

"In some cases," Barnes added, "blood pressure is elevated and thyroid therapy lowers the pressure in most of these, taking extra work off the heart. Swiss investigators many years ago demonstrated that in hypothyroidism, blood clotting is accelerated and heart attacks often occur when a clot blocks completely a narrowed, atherosclerotic artery. With thyroid therapy, blood clotting activity returns to normal."

Barnes said that another important factor is fatigue. "If overexertion can trigger a heart attack, what constitutes overexertion depends upon the condition of the individual," he said. "For a chronically tired person, an extra energy expenditure that could be taken in stride by a vigorous person may constitute overexertion. Thyroid deficiency is a common cause of undue fatigue."

Barnes and his wife, Charlotte W. Barnes, said in *Solved: The Riddle of Heart Attacks*:

Over the past 25 years, rarely has a patient on thyroid therapy had an initial heart attack. Many patients have been seen with a history of heart attack and hospitalization prior to seeing me. They have been put on small doses of thyroid, usually an initial dosage of one-half grain daily. After one or two months, the dosage has been increased one-half grain at a time, and in some cases, over a period of six months, has attained as much as two grains daily . . . The number treated with thyroid in the present study is too small for statistical analysis, but during the past 25 years a death among these patients has rarely occurred. Most of them are surviving the normal life span, and when a second attack does occur, it usually can be attributed to some exceptional stress. This rare occurrence among those on thyroid is in sharp contrast to a mortality of five to 10 percent annually among patients with a previous heart attack treated by conventional means.[5]

Barnes added that if we can learn to diagnose the susceptible people in child-hood and keep the thyroid hormone level near the normal requirement during the individual's lifetime, it would appear that a heart attack can be delayed until advanced age.

"The most susceptible patients," he said, "are the major problems at present. Since they represent only 27 percent of the total heart attacks, it seems reasonable that thyroid (replacement) therapy may be able to eliminate these untimely deaths."

Murray Israel, M.D., of New York, began treating cases of advanced hardening of the arteries with thyroid therapy long before Barnes entered the field. He found that the requirement for vitamin B is increased when the metabolism is raised. During periods of growth, pregnancy and any other condition with an elevation in thyroid secretion, more vitamin B must be ingested or symptoms of a deficiency appear.

With the usual therapeutic doses of desiccated thyroid, Israel added an excess of several vitamins. "To hasten the utilization of fat and lower the cholesterol, he has added another tablet containing choline, inositol and vitamin B6. As many as 30 of these tablets daily may be administered. In addition to the oral therapy, frequent intravenous injections of still another preparation composed of synthetic thyroxine, synthetic vitamin B12 and calcium gluconate were given.[6]

"Since Friedland's demonstration in 1927, repeatedly thyroid therapy has cor-rected the elevated serum fats and cholesterol in most cases," Barnes noted. "In hundreds of patients treated in the last 25 years, 95 percent of the cholesterol levels have returned to normal with only thyroid therapy. No premature heart attacks have occurred in the five percent whose elevated cholesterols persisted in spite of thyroid therapy . . . atherosclerosis results from the thyroid deficiency and not from the elevated serum fats that accompany it."

For those with a thyroid deficiency, a small quantity of the thyroid hormone must be supplied from the outside, just as extra insulin must be given to the diabetic. If too much thyroid is supplied, none is secreted by the patient's own gland; in this situation there is no way the patient can decrease the amount of hormone during periods when less is needed. The patient has a chronic case of hyperthyroidism, which brings on the symptoms of this disorder.[5]

In addition to its use in iodized salt, the mineral finds its way into animal feed, sanitizers and in food processing, according to Chris Lecos in *FDA Consumer*. This use, together with consumption of naturally occurring iodine, has led to concerns about excess amounts in the diet. In 1980, Lecos said, the Food and Nutrition Board reported that the amount of iodine consumed in the United States had risen "to levels well above the nutritional requirement, and concern has been expressed that certain population groups may be exposed to excessive levels of iodine.

"Although these higher intake levels were still viewed as safe, the board warned that any additional increases should be viewed with concern," Lecos added. "Already aware of the increased iodine in the food supply, FDA had identified likely sources and has been working with the American Medical Association and industry so that the amount of iodine in the food supply appears to be leveling off."[6]

IODINE DEFICIENCY DISEASES

While iodine deficiency seems to pose no health problems in the United States, it is a recurring problem in many countries, according to a World Bank report. Alan Berg, a nutritionist with the World Bank, was quoted as saying that deficiencies of vitamin A, iodine and iron cause blindness, goiter, anemia, retardation and death in more than one billion people, and that at least twice that many are at risk.

Berg added that vitamin A deficiency has blinded more than 13 million people, and that six of every 10 preschool children with the deficiency die; about one billion people lack adequate iodine, and that this deficiency kills five to 10 babies out of every 1,000 pregnancies, as well as leaving untold numbers retarded, deaf and mute; and that about one billion people suffer from iron-deficiency anemia.

"Micronutrient deficiencies aren't a major problem in most of the developed world," the World Bank report continued. "Americans, for instance, eat iodized salt, the easiest way to fight iodine deficiency. The bank is lending China $27 million in 1995 for its first salt iodization. But many developing countries don't have a centralized salt works, so the bank funded the world's first iodized water, in Mali. By simply rigging village wells so every bucket of water washes over an iodine pack, iodine deficiency among 500,000 people was lowered from 94 to 40 percent last year at a cost of 10 cents a person."

Berg added that millions spent on global nutrition every year are being wasted on obscure academic research and by programs that buy nutrients but cannot get them through local governments, or simply by overlooking simple behavior changes and education. As an example, he said, cassava is a root that is a staple in Africa, but people discard the nutrient-packed leaves.[7]

Although Denmark is hardly a Third World country, the government is considering introducing legislation making it compulsory to add iodine to salt after two studies found an extremely high rate of goiter, reported Margaret Dolley in the July 30, 1994 issue of the British Medical Journal. The World Health Organization recently estimated that 5 percent of Danish schoolchildren and 10 percent of adults had a goiter sufficient to raise their concentration of thyroid stimulating hormone. Another study, based on the town of Randers, found that 12 percent of the residents had a goiter.[8]

"The head of the National Food Committee's nutrition department, Lars Ovesen, said that 75 percent of adults could lack sufficient iodine, 50 percent could lack iron, 25 percent could be short on calcium and 10 percent be deficient in folic acid," Dolley added. "He believes that this is due to recent changes in Danish dietary habits, in particular a switch away from fish—which used to be an extremely important local staple—and green vegetables, towards more meat and dairy products."

Dolley went on to say that the Committee is also considering making it compulsory to add calcium, iron and folic acid, the B vitamin, to flour, even though European countries, and especially Denmark, have no tradition of adding minerals and other substances to food. Public opinion generally favors food as being as pure as possible. Phosphorus and calcium were once legally required to be added to flour and grain products, but this stipulation was withdrawn several years ago.

Ovesen said the level of deficiencies was unacceptable, but that the problem was too widespread to tackle with health information campaigns alone. That is because the authorities have been recommending that people cut their salt consumption.[8]

The mountains and plains of northern India, Nepal and Bhutan have long been infamous in medical circles as the "Himalayan goiter belt," reported Erik Eckholm in the April 2, 1985 issue of The New York Times. The soils and waters of the Himalayas are so lacking in natural iodine that even the goats develop goiter. In some mountain cultures, people with smooth necklines were once regarded as oddities.

"Outright cretinism remains shockingly commonplace in the Himalayas," the *Times* said. "Nepali officials thought they had found an unparalleled incidence in the mountain hamlet of Tulibesi, where 18 percent of 750 residents are cretins. Then a survey in the nearby kingdom of Bhutan revealed two villages in which one-third of the populace are cretins."

Robert Tyabji, who worked in Bhutan for UNICEF, told the *Times*: "Walking into these villages is absolutely mind-shattering. Daily tasks are carried on with an eerie lethargy. Mentally deficient, stunted and deaf and mute people, many moving with an awkward gait. Goiters deform every throat, sometimes reaching monstrous size."

The *Times* went on to say that teams of health workers, often traveling by foot over some of the world's most rugged terrain, are injecting millions of potential mothers with megadoses of iodine, hoping to prevent the birth of another generation of babies whose minds and bodies have been crippled for want of a few cents' worth of the mineral.[9]

In the January 23, 1992 issue of the *New England Journal of Medicine*, Rene Tonglet, M.D., et al., reported on a study to evaluate the use of low doses of iodized oil of 0.1 or 0.2 ml (47 and 118 mg of iodine respectively), and compared these amounts to placebo in a severely deficient area in Zaire. The researchers concluded that this amount of iodized oil is capable of correcting iodine deficiency for about a year and without any side effects.[10]

Relief for Fibrocystic Breasts

Iodine has been shown to relieve pain and soreness associated with fibrocystic breasts, according to Sheldon Saul Hendler, M.D., Ph.D., in *The Doctors' Vitamin and Mineral Encyclopedia*. Fibrocystic breasts are a very common condition in premenopausal women, as well as in postmenopausal women taking supplementary estrogens. He added that fibrocystic breasts are still referred to as fibrocystic disease in many medical textbooks and by many physicians. However, he said, fibrocystic breasts are not diseased breasts, even though they are frequently associated with pain and soreness.

"A Canadian physician reported in 1988 that a majority of women with fibrocystic breasts experienced complete relief from their symptoms after being treated with elemental iodine for four months," Hendler said. "When treatment was discontinued the symptoms returned. Other researchers have reported positive results with other iodine-containing compounds."[11]

Fibrocystic breast disease, also know as cystic mastitis, is a sometimes painful, but benign, cystic swelling of the breasts, according to Robert M. Giller, M.D., in *Natural Prescriptions*. Although this condition is an inconvenience and a discomfort, it is not a disease.

"Some 60 percent of all women suffer from fibrocystic breast disease, in which the breasts are sometimes cystic, or lumpy, and become swollen, typically before menstruation," Giller said. "Some women find that their breasts become so painful that they can't bear to touch them and have trouble sleeping at night. The condition is not medically dangerous, and is not a precursor of cancer, but it does complicate breast self-examination as it is difficult to identify a new lump among the existing ones. Consequently, regular mammograms are essential, particularly if there is a family history of breast cancer."

Giller added that the inflammatory processes of cystic mastitis appear to be aggravated by estrogen, both in its natural form and in birth control pills. The fluctuating levels of estrogen account for the cyclic nature of the inflammation and swelling. In his practice, he has noted that caffeine in coffee and colas, theophylline in tea and theobromine in chocolate have been shown to contribute to the inflammation and should be eliminated from the diet. Some asthma medications that contain caffeine can also aggravate the condition.

There is also evidence that what you eat and the regularity of your bowel movements have a direct bearing on cystic mastitis. Women having fewer than three bowel movements per week are 4.5 times more likely to have the condition than women who have at least one movement a day. A diet high in vegetables and fruits will regulate bowel function and help to reduce the serverity of the inflammation, Giller added.

In addition to the diet recommendations already mentioned, Giller said that women with fibrocystic breast disease should avoid animal fats and eat fish and other seafood rich in iodine. In addition to regular supplements, he recommends 400 IU/day of vitamin E; 10,000 to 20,000 IU/day of beta-carotene; and one or two capsules of evening primrose oil three times a day.

"There is experimental evidence linking iodine deficiency in animals with cystic mastitis," Giller said. "Some doctors have had good results prescribing kelp supplements for patients, but this isn't something you should do on your own. Your doctor will want to test you for thyroid activity before making a decision. If your intake of iodine is low because you are cutting back on iodized salt, you can compensate by eating seafood, which is rich in iodine, and by taking kelp daily."[12]

In 1979, T. B. Krouse, et al., reported that iodine-deficient rats developed lesions somewhat resembling human fibrocystic breast disease. This was generally more notable in the older rats.[13]

The April 24, 1976 issue of *Lancet* reported that the geographic distribution of cancer of the breast, ovary and uterus is inversely correlated with the distribution of iodine in the diet. In other words, geographical areas with low-dietary intake of iodine have significantly higher rates of cancer. The researchers conclude that low iodine levels may cause increased effectiveness of gonadotropins, thereby resulting in increased secretion of estrogen, along with a low ratio of estriol to estrone plus estradiol estrogen hormones. This ratio may be the reason for the increased incidence of these cancers, the researchers said.[14]

Bernard A. Eskin, M.D., chief of gynecologic endocrinology at the Albert Einstein Medical Center and the Medical College of Pennsylvania in Philadelphia, said that the highest breast cancer mortality rates in the United States are found in the "goiter belt" bordering the Great Lakes. Increased breast cancer rates are also found in specific goiter regions of Poland, Switzerland, Australia and the former Soviet Union. In addition, Mexico and Thailand have high incidences of goiter and breast cancer.

Eskin has shown that a dietary iodine deficiency in laboratory rats leads to abnormal breast tissue growth (dysplasia). He also showed that the female sex hormone estrogen hastens the development of dysplasia when iodine is lacking in the diet. In clinical trials with women, he discovered that iodine supplementation could prevent breast dysplasia and that the dysplasia process could be reversed by iodine supplements. However, the extension of dysplasia to cancer or linking thyroid disorders to breast cancer is controversial. Clinically, many physicians have found that using a simple, organic iodine preparation and painting the vagina relieves the symptoms of cystic breast disease, since iodine is rapidly absorbed through vaginal tissues.[15]

Radiation usually refers to high-energy radiation, such as X-rays or gamma rays that are capable of penetrating tissue and causing molecular disruption, according to Sheldon Saul Hendler, M.D., Ph.D., in *The Purification Prescription*. In a stricter sense, he added, this type of radiation is called ionizing radiation. Radiation of lower energy is nonionizing radiation and includes radio, TV, microwaves and radar emissions.[16]

All of the toxic effects of ionizing radiation are mediated through free radical mechanisms, Hendler said. Consequently, biological antioxidants can confer protection against these toxic effects. Radioactive pollutants produced following the meltdown of a nuclear reactor—for instance, Chernobyl—include isotopes of iodine, cesium, barium and strontium. And, he said, alginates, found in brown seaweed, protect against the toxicity of strontium, barium and possibly cesium as well. Nonradioactive iodine protects against the toxic effects of its radioactive isotope.

"Those at risk for radiation toxicity—those exposed to large doses of X-ray or radionuclides used for diagnostic and therapeutic purposes—should consider taking a vitamin and mineral supplement rich in biological antioxidant precursors," Hendler said. "Two to three ounces of edible brown seaweed weekly may confer significant protection against toxicity of radioactive strontium, barium, radium and cesium. A hundred milligrams of iodide daily for seven to 14 days helps protect against toxicity due to acute radioactive iodine exposure. It should be started right at the beginning of such exposure in order for it to be most effective."

Edible seaweed is a remarkable purifying and healing food, and we should include a liberal amount of it in our diets, Hendler continued. It is also a great cholesterol-lowering food.[16]

CANCER PREVENTION

In the March 1990 issue of the *East African Medical Journal*, Ruth K. Oniang'O and K. O. Rogo discussed the role of nutrition in preventing cancer. Factors which contribute to cancer, they said, include nutritional excesses and deficiencies; carcinogens naturally occurring in foods; contaminants and additives in foods; undetermined environmental factors; excesses of animal protein, refined sugar, fat and calories; and nutritional deficiencies, such as iodine, vitamin A, vitamin B2, vitamin B6; and contaminants such as DDT, nitrites, smoked or burned foods, aflatoxin, etc.[17]

In her classic book, *Let's Eat Right to Keep Fit*, Adelle Davis reported that a thyroid gland not adequately supplied with ordinary food iodine avidly absorbs the highly toxic radioactive iodine from fallout, leaving the gland particularly susceptible to cancer and precancerous nodules. Such cancers and particularly such nodules increased markedly in several Western states years after bomb testing in Nevada was discontinued, she added.[18]

"Some countries are still testing bombs, and because our Earth turns, the stratosphere over those countries is over ours before a day passes," she said. "Fallout, therefore, is still a problem. If the thyroid gland can obtain adequate iodine, none of the radioactive material is absorbed and no harm is done. Harvard physicians found that Massachusetts children absorbed radioactive iodine rapidly unless given a daily supplement of one or two milligrams of iodine. Their research indicates that adults would probably need at least three or four milligrams of iodine daily. In Japan, abnormalities of the thyroid do not exist; their per-day intake from iodine-rich seaweed averages three milligrams. It is difficult indeed for Americans to obtain this desirable amount."[18] (When Davis wrote the book in 1970, she could not have known about Chernobyl or the possibility of nuclear testing in some countries that still threatens us.)

Writing in the *International Journal of Clinical Nutrition* in July 1992, Benjamin H. S. Lau, M.D., Ph.D., discussed the potential anticarcinogenic and immune-potentiating properties of a green-food supplement, available in health food stores, which contains young barley leaves, wheat grass and two types of seaweed, chlorella (an algae) and laminaria (kelp). He added that the barley leaves and wheat grass are good sources of chlorophyll, calcium, magnesium, potassium, vitamins, enzymes and antioxidant enzymes. Kelp is a rich source of iodine, calcium, potassium, magnesium and vitamin C. Consequently, he said, the supplement may serve as a chemopreventive dietary agent as well as providing protection against cancer.[19]

Graves' disease is a condition that affects many parts of the body and is usually associated with overactivity of the thyroid gland (hyperthyroidism), according to Manfred Blum, M.D., in *Medical and Health Annual 1992.*[20]

"Descriptions of people with the typical manifestations of this disorder were recorded in antiquity," Blum said. "However, the modern awareness of its clinical characteristics come from three almost simultaneous descriptions in the medical literature of the first half of the 19th century."

These discoveries were made by Caleb H. Parry (1755–1822), an English physician and Robert J. Graves (1797–1853), an Irish physician, and Karl A. von Basedow (1799–1854), a German physician. In English-speaking countries, Blum said, Graves is given primary credit for identifying the condition, while much of Europe continues to honor Basedow, calling it Basedow's disease. It has been estimated that four out of every 1,000 people have Graves' disease, with more than one million of them in North America alone. Women are four to five times more likely to be afflicted than men.

"Typical symptoms include bulging of the eyes, anxiety, irritability, intolerance to heat, excessive sweating, sleeplessness, fatigue, palpitations (rapid heartbeat) with a rapid or irregular pulse, shortness of breath, weight loss in spite of a good appetite, frequent loose bowel movements, tremor, muscle weakness and clumsiness. Swelling of the neck may occur, but it is usually painless. Some patients develop a patchy loss of skin pigmentation (vitiligo). A rare complaint is swelling of the shin (pretibial myxedema)."

The course of the thyroid manifestations is highly variable, Blum added. Some people experience a single spurt of hyperthyroidism with no recurrence. Others have repeated cycles of thyroid overactivity that may be precipitated by emotional factors, physical trauma or infections. Hyperthyroidism may alternate with periods of hypothyroidism (deficient thyroid activity). Treatment usually includes drug therapy, sometimes the surgical removal of part of the thyroid gland (subtotal thyroidectomy) and radioactive iodine therapy.[20]

Among natural foods, the best sources of iodine are seafoods and vegetables grown on iodine-rich soils. In the United States, commercially iodized salt contains 0.01 percent of potassium iodide. Assuming that the average adult uses six to 6.5 grams of salt daily, his concurrent iodine intake from this source is 0.48 mg; this amount of iodine represents about twice the normal requirement and provides amply for a sufficient reserve. In Central America, iodates are used successfully instead of iodide; they have the advantage of greater stability in salt which is not highly refined.[21]

TABLE 15.1

RECOMMENDED DIETARY ALLOWANCES FOR IODINE

AGE AND CATEGORY	MICROGRAMS PER DAY
Infants, one to six months	40 mcg
Infants, six months to one year	50 mcg
Children, 1 to 3	70 mcg
Children, 4 to 6	90 mcg
Children, 7 to 10	120 mcg
Males, 11 and over	150 mcg
Females, 11 and over	150 mcg
Pregnant females	175 mcg
Lactating females	200 mcg

From *Recommended Dietary Allowances*, 10th Edition. Washington, D.C.: National Academy Press, 1989.

REFERENCES

1. Ensminger, Audrey H., et al. *Foods and Nutrition Encyclopedia*. Clovis, Calif.: Pegus Press, 1983, pp. 1242ff.
2. *Recommended Dietary Allowances*, 10th Edition. Washington, D.C.: National Academy Press, 1989, pp. 213ff.

3. *Foods and Nutrition Encyclopedia.* Ibid.

4. Lauersen, Niels, M.D., and Whitney, Steven. *A Woman's Body.* New York: Perigee Books, 1987, pp. 39ff.

5. Murray, Frank. *Program Your Heart for Health.* New York: Larchmont Books, 1978, pp. 254ff.

6. Lecos, Chris. "Tracking Trace Minerals," *FDA Consumer*, a reprint, July/August 1983, pp. 3–4.

7. "Nutrient Deficiency Causing Mass Ills," *The (Nashville) Tennessean*, December 16, 1994, p. 14A.

8. Dolley, Margaret. "Denmark to Tackle High Goitre Rate by Adding Iodine to Salt," *British Medical Journal* 309:294, July 30, 1994.

9. Eckholm, Erik. "Iodine Deficiency in Himalayas Is Believed to Disable Millions," *The New York Times*, April 2, 1985, pp. C1-C3.

10. Tonglet, Rene, M.D., et al. "Efficiency of Low Oral Doses of Iodized Oil in The Control of Iodine Deficiency in Zaire," *New England Journal of Medicine* 326(4):236–241, January 23, 1992.

11. Hendler, Sheldon Saul, M.D., Ph.D. *The Doctors' Vitamin and Mineral Encyclopedia.* New York: Simon and Schuster, 1990, pp. 144ff.

12. Giller, Robert M., M.D., and Matthews, Kathy. *Natural Prescriptions.* New York: Carol Southern Books, 1994, pp. 139ff.

13. Krouse, T. B., et al. "Age-Related Changes Resembling Fibrocystic Disease in Iodine-Blocked Rats," *Arch. Pathol. Lab. Med.* 103:631–634, 1979.

14. Stadel, B. V. "Dietary Iodine and Risk of Breast, Endometrial and Ovarian Cancer," *Lancet*, April 24, 1976, pp. 890–891.

15. Passwater, Richard A., Ph.D., and Cranton, Elmer M., M.D. *Trace Elements, Hair Analysis and Nutrition.* New Canaan, Conn.: Keats Publishing, Inc., 1983, pp. 170ff.

16. Hendler, Sheldon Saul, M.D., Ph.D. *The Purification Prescription.* New York: William Morrow and Co., Inc., 1991, pp. 229ff.

17. Oniang'O, Ruth K., and Rogo, K. O. "Nutrition and Cancer: A Review," *East African Medical Journal* 67(3):154–161, March 1990.

18. Davis, Adelle. *Let's Eat Right to Keep Fit.* New York: New American Library, 1970, pp. 181ff.

19. Lau, Benjamin H. S., M.D., Ph.D. "Edible Plant Extracts Modulate Macrophage Activity and Bacterial Mutagenesis," *International Journal of Clinical Nutrition* 12(3):147–155, July 1992.

20. Blum, Manfred, M.D. "Graves' Disease," *Medical and Health Annual.* Chicago: Encyclopedia Britannica, Inc., 1992, pp. 452ff.

21. Burton, Benjamin T., Ph.D. *The Heinz Handbook of Nutrition.* New York: McGraw-Hill Book Co., 1965, pp. 125–127.

16

Iron Deficiency Affects Many People

ELEMENTAL iron has been known since prehistoric times, and scientists are convinced that early, highly prized samples of iron came from meteors. References to "the metal of heaven" (thought to be iron) have been found in ancient writings. By about 1200 B.C., iron was being obtained from its ores, marking the beginning of the Iron Age.

The early Greeks were the first to consider this mineral a health tonic. In England in the 17th century, iron was found to be an effective treatment for anemia. The French chemist Boussingault proved iron's vital role in nutrition in 1867.

Although iron is the most common and cheapest of all metals, more deficiencies of iron (chiefly in the form of iron deficiency anemia) exist in the United States and in most other developed countries than of any other nutrient. It is estimated that between 10 and 25 percent of the population is affected. Lack of iron in the diet is attributed to the increased refining and processing of our food supply, and the decreased use of cast-iron cookware.

The greatest absorption of iron occurs in the upper part of the small intestine (in the duodenum and jejunum), although a small amount of absorption occurs from the stomach and throughout the whole of the small intestine. Only about 10 percent of the iron available in cereals, vegetables and legumes (excluding soybeans) is absorbed. But absorption from other foods is a little higher. As an example, 30 percent of the iron from meat is absorbed, as is 20 percent from soybeans and 15 percent from fish. It is believed that about 10 percent of the iron from mixed foods is absorbed.

There are two types of iron in food: heme or organic iron, and nonheme or inorganic iron. Heme iron is better absorbed from food than is nonheme iron and is independent of vitamin C or iron-binding agents. Although the proportion of heme iron in animal tissues varies, it amounts to about one-third of the total iron in all animal tissues, such as meat, liver, poultry and fish. The remaining two-thirds of the iron in animal tissues and all the iron of vegetables products are nonheme iron. Since animals eat vegetarian foodstuffs (grass, grains, etc.), meat contains both heme and nonheme iron.

Factors which increase the absorption of iron include:

1. Foods high in heme iron;
2. Body needs—increased by growth, menstruation and pregnancy;
3. The presence of vitamin C and gastric hydrochloric acid, which convert the iron from the ferric to the ferrous state;
4. Little iron being deposited in the intestinal mucosal ferritin curtain;
5. Increased hemoglobin synthesis—for example, following hemorrhages (bleeding), or as a result of anemia or hemopoetic abnormalities; and
6. The presence of calcium.

Iron absorption is impaired:

1. By foods high in nonheme iron;
2. When much iron is deposited in the intestinal mucosal ferritin curtain;
3. By excess phosphatges, phytates, oxalates and tannic acid (in tea), all of which form insoluble compounds that are not readily absorbed (hence, excesses of such substances should be avoided in individuals suffering from severe nutritional anemia); and
4. Following surgical removal of the stomach or when there are malabsorption disorders.

Mucosal ferritin delivers ferrous iron to the portal blood system, where iron is converted back to the ferric state by oxidation. Ferric iron combines with protein (transferrin) to form a combination known as transferritin. Iron is then transported to the bone marrow, where it can be incorporated into newly synthesized hemoglobin molecules. Or it can be stored in the liver, spleen and bone marrow, where it combines with a protein and is deposited as ferritin.

Absorbed iron is only lost by desquamation or the shedding or peeling off of cells from the alimentary, urinary and respiratory tracts as well as by skin and hair losses. Roughly 90 percent of the ingested iron is lost in the feces. Only small amounts of iron are excreted in the urine.

"The body conserves and reuses iron once it has been absorbed," according to *Foods and Nutrition Encyclopedia* noted. "The combined losses of iron by all routes are of the order of 1 mg/day for a healthy adult man, and about 1.5 mg/day for a woman during the reproductive period. Added losses of iron occur from blood donation and pathological bleeding (hookworm infections, bleeding ulcers, etc.), and in cases of kidney diseases, particularly nephrosis (degenerative disease of the kidneys, which involves edema, protein in the urine and an increase in cholesterol in the blood).

Iron combines with protein to make hemoglobin for red blood cells. Heme iron combines with protein (globin) to form hemoglobin, the iron-containing substance in red blood cells. Iron is involved in the transport of oxygen throughout the body, and the mineral is a component of enzymes which are involved in energy metabolism.[1]

Although the human body contains only about 0.004 percent iron (roughly three to four grams in an adult) it is one of the most significant elements in nutrition and consequently very necessary to life. Iron deficiency is said to be the second most common nutritional problem in the United States, following obesity. Several surveys have shown that women of child-bearing years have an iron intake that is only 61 percent of the Recommended Dietary Allowance.[2]

According to a survey by the United States Department of Agriculture in 1986, low-calorie diets are responsible for the prevalence of iron deficiency in women. The survey found that women of child-bearing years reported mean food energy intakes of 1,588 calories a day. However, the American diet averages only about seven milligrams of iron per 1,000 calories, meaning that the iron intake for women aged 19 to 50 or during their reproductive years is substantially below the RDA. (At the time of the study, the RDA for most women was 18 mg/day of iron. It is now 15 mg/day but still not sufficient.)

SYMPTOMS OF IRON DEFICIENCY

Without an adequate iron supply, people are at risk for developing a variety of symptoms, such as reduced work capacity; more rapid build-up of lactic acid in exercising muscles; irritability and apathy; lower resistance to infections; spoon-shaped, thin nails; and pale nail beds. It is difficult to get sufficient iron from the diet because all food sources are not all equal in value. For example, spinach is rich in iron, but the mineral is bound by chelates and takes it out of the body before it can be properly absorbed. Other chelates include tannins in tea; phytates in whole grains, brans and soybeans; polyphenols in coffee; and phosvitin in egg yolk.

Two dietary factors have been shown to enhance the absorption of nonheme iron—vitamin C and the Meat Factor in meat, fish and poultry, according to Elaine Monsen, Ph.D., R.D., professor of nutrition at the University of Washington in Seattle. Meat, fish and poultry play an important dual role in iron absorption because they provide both heme iron and the so-called Meat Factor, which helps the body absorb nonheme iron from other food sources, such as vegetables and grains.

Women and Anemia

"Women who have heavy or frequent menstrual flows are particularly prone to iron deficiency because of extensive menstrual blood loss," Monsen added. "In addition, concern has arisen in the dietary community regarding poorly selected vegetarian regimens. There are two reasons for this concern, the lack of heme iron and the lack of meat which increases the absorption of nonheme iron."[2]

Since women lose a great deal of iron in menstrual flow, it follows that those with menorrhagia (excessive menstrual flow) are in danger of becoming anemic. In fact, women with menorrhagia may be iron-deficient even though there are no overt signs of iron-deficiency anemia, reported the *British Medical Journal* in 1982.

In one study, serum ferritin (iron in the blood) levels for patients with excessive menstruation was significantly lower than it was in the controls, even though there wasn't much difference in hemoglobin concentrations or the amount of iron in corpuscular hemoglobin.[3]

Studies reported in the *Journal of the American Medical Association* in 1964 suggested that a chronic iron deficiency can cause menorrhagia. But patients often respond when given iron supplements. In one double-blind study, 75 percent of those given iron supplements improved, compared with 32.5 percent given a placebo. In another study, 74 patients with menorrhagia improved after taking iron supplements; nine patients didn't respond.[4]

In still another study, reported in a Scandinavian medical journal in 1981, 14 of 15 patients with excessive menstrual flow were able to retain more iron than they were losing after being given 100 mg/day of iron.[5]

Researchers at Lakehead University in Ontario, Canada, reported in *Medicine and Science in Sports* in 1993 that iron deficiency is common in women, and that the deficiency is often undetected unless serum iron levels are measured. In the study, blood samples for iron, copper, zinc, calcium and magnesium were taken from 111 healthy women, ranging in age from 18 to 40. While 39 percent of the volunteers were deficient in iron, only 3.6 percent were listed as anemic, suggesting that more accurate blood levels need to be administered. Iron supplements raised the blood ferritin level from 15.0 mcg to 36.5 mcg, without affecting the zinc and magnesium levels. Although the women were not deficient in magnesium and copper, 6.5 percent were low in zinc and 1.8 percent had low levels of calcium.[6]

In *New England Journal of Medicine*, Misha Pless, M.D., and Stuart A. Lipton, Ph.D., of the Harvard Medical School in Boston reported in the December 2, 1993 issue that some patients who were thought to have a brain tumor, when in effect they had swelling of the optic nerve, headaches, etc., related to iron deficiency anemia.

The authors discussed a 36-year-old woman who had been diagnosed with anemia, headaches and blurred vision. There was the presence of papilledema, which is a swelling of the optic nerve/disc due to increased intracranial pressure.

"Long-term treatment with iron led to resolution of the symptoms, return of serum iron concentrations to low normal levels and reversal of the papilledema," the authors said.

The patient subsequently did not comply with the treatment and her symptoms reappeared. Iron treatment again corrected the problem.

"Patients with iron-deficiency anemia and headache should undergo a careful examination of the optic fundi to rule out papilledema, since this can lead to visual loss if left untreated," the authors added.[7]

In the same issue of the *New England Journal of Medicine*, Martin H. Ellis, M.D., and James D. Levine, M.D., of New England Deaconess Hospital, said that they were surprised that pica was not mentioned in relationship to children with iron deficiency. This is an abnormal behavior in which people, especially children, chew ice, dirt, laundry starch, etc, and this is thought to be related to iron deficiency. "Pica may be associated with lead poisoning, which may cause iron deficiency and which is a serious health hazard to young children," they said.[8]

Routine iron supplementation to pregnant women is still being debated, according to the U.S. Preventive Services Task Force in the December 15, 1993 issue of the *Journal of the American Medical Association*. Anemia is present in about 20 to 40 percent of pregnant women, the task force reported. However, there have not been any extensive studies on the prevalence of iron deficiency in pregnant women. Low iron levels could also be passed on to the fetus.

Consequently, the task force does not advise against iron supplements, but leaves the decision up to the obstetrician as to whether the woman should be given iron supplements or should simply increase iron-rich foods in her diet. But all pregnant women should be tested for anemia and iron deficiency at their first prenatal visit and be given higher doses of iron if they are diagnosed with either condition.[9]

Commenting on the task force study in the January 6, 1994 issue of *Medical Tribune*, Laura Buterbaugh said: "A number of studies have found that anemic women who take iron supplements are less likely to have low birth-weight or premature babies than anemic women who do not take supplements. But the studies did not control for other potential influences, and some lacked statistical power to prove iron's effect, according to the government report."

Roy Pitkin, M. D., chairman of obstetrics and gynecology at the University of California at Los Angeles, said that he gives iron supplements to most of his pregnant patients. "There's no argument on the science here," he said. "It's basically a question of interpretation."

Buford Nichols, M.D., director emeritus of the Children's Nutrition Research Center at Baylor College of Medicine, added that he sees no reason for routine iron supplementation in the absence of anemia or iron deficiency. But it may be difficult to determine whether a patient needs the supplements, because there typically are no previous blood tests to use for comparison.

"It's probably better to give supplements when in doubt," Nichols added. "That's why a lot of physicians prescribe it routinely."

Nichols went on to say that studies have shown that, even for anemic women, iron supplements have no benefit unless they are initiated well before pregnancy. That is why it is important for women to receive proper nutrition in adolescence, not just as adults, he said.[10]

Although the prevalence of iron-deficiency anemia may not be easily recognized during a woman's pregnancy, it does pose ominous warning signs for both mother and infant, according to a study in the *American Journal of Clinical Nutrition*. In the study, completed at the University of Medicine and Dentistry of New Jersey and the Cooper Hospital/University Medical Center in Camden, 800 pregnant women, ranging in age from 12 to 29, were monitored during their pregnancy to determine how iron deficiency might impact on their pregnancy and the infant. The volunteers were mostly from inner city, minority families.

The New Jersey team reported that the women diagnosed with iron deficiency anemia had less energy and consumed less iron in their diet than the women who were not anemic. In addition, the anemic women were three times as likely to deliver infants with low birth weights and twice as likely to deliver prematurely than the women who did not have iron deficiency anemia. The researchers added that vaginal bleeding prior to or at entry into the prenatal care program increased the likelihood of premature delivery five-fold in anemic women, compared to two-fold for those women who were not anemic. They further revealed that the anemic women were likely not to gain sufficient weight during their pregnancy.[11]

Studies by a number of researchers have focused on the important relationships between feeding practices and iron intakes according to a newsletter, *Special Currents: Iron*, published by Ross Laboratories. It quoted John Dobbing, editor of *Brain, Behaviour and Iron in the Infant Diet*, as saying that iron deficiency anemia during the first year of life causes long-term deficits in mental and motor development, *even though* the deficiency is corrected with iron therapy. An infant is especially vulnerable during the second six months of life and any deficits may well be permanent.

Another chapter in *Brain, Behaviour and Iron in the Infant Diet* written by Betsy Lozoff, M.D., of Case Western Reserve University School of Medicine in Cleveland, and Hospital Nacional de Ninos, University of Costa Rica, in San Jose, reported that in every study that compared results on developmental tests in anemic and nonanemic infants, those with iron deficiency severe enough to cause anemia had lower scores. Studying Costa Rican children from a highly literate, healthy, lower-middle-class population, she found that, compared with appropriate controls, infants with moderate iron deficiency anemia had lower scores on both mental and motor tests, while infants with mild anemia had lower motor scores only. Behavioral disturbances were also noted in iron-deficient anemic infants, who seemed unduly fearful, unhappy, tired, tense and hesitant with the examiner.

A study by E. E. Ziegler, S. J. Foman, et al., maintained that prolonged feeding of cow's milk to infants is likely to lead to poor nutrition. ("Cow Milk Feeding in Infancy: Further Observations on Blood Loss From the Gastrointestinal Tract," *Journal of Pediatrics* 116:11–18, 1990.) They added that feeding of pasteurized cow's milk has been shown to induce gastrointestinal blood loss, which may be severe enough to cause anemia. Although the children do not experience major bleeding, even the loss of small amounts of blood may adversely affect iron status.

"Potentially important blood loss is associated with feedings of pasteurized cow's milk but not with milk-based commercial formulas," the newsletter continued. "In a study of 26 nonanemic infants fed cow's milk and 26 fed formula from days 168 through 252, the group fed cow's milk had significantly higher fecal hemoglobin losses. Of the infants fed cow's milk, only six of the 26 had no appreciable hemoglobin loss. Mean fecal hemoglobin in the 20 milk-fed infants who lost blood during the peak period (ages 175 to 196 days) was 4,773 mcg/g dry stool, representing an iron loss of 0.20 mg/day—a nutritionally significant quantity. Blood loss decreased with age and duration of cow's milk feeding."

The newsletter added that some physicians are reluctant to recommend iron-fortified formulas because they think they may induce behavioral problems, such as fussiness, or gastrointestinal complaints, such as constipation. But S. E. Nelson, et al. conducted a comprehensive cross-over study which compared iron-fortified with low-iron fortified formula and found no justification for this viewpoint.[12]

Writing in the *New England Journal of Medicine* in 1991, Betsy Lozoff, M.D., previously mentioned, and colleagues said that children who have iron-deficiency anemia in infancy are at risk for long-lasting developmental disadvantage as compared with their peers with better iron status.

In spite of a number of unresolved issues, the results of their study indicate that relatively severe and chronic iron deficiency in infancy may serve as a convenient marker for any associated factors that contribute to poor developmental outcome but are harder to identify during routine pediatric care.

"Our findings also call into question the adequacy of current therapeutic approaches," the researchers continued. "The possibility that earlier detection of iron deficiency or longer treatment in infancy might be effective in preventing developmental disadvantage needs to be assessed. Infants with severe and chronic iron deficiency may also require special intervention in addition to iron therapy. Such intervention—for example, enrichment programs—would ideally be targeted to the specific alternations in behavior observed in infants with iron deficiency and tailored to the special needs of their families. However, given the findings to date that lower test scores persist, a vigorous effort to prevent iron deficiency is the safest approach."[13]

In an Israeli study, Ami Ballin, M.D., of the E. Wolfson Hospital in Tel Aviv, reported that iron supplements may boost the mental and emotional status of teenage girls, according to *Medical Tribune* in 1992. Teenage girls are often deficient in iron because of poor dietary choices, losses during menstruation and periods of accelerated growth. During the two-month study, 29 girls, ages 16 and 17, received orally a 105-mg iron supplement each day. Thirty controls were given a placebo. All of the girls had complained of mood swings, inability to concentrate in school and lassitude. Those in the treatment group reported statistically significant improvements, Ballin said.[14]

In 1990, A. S. Ryan and colleagues reported that infants are born with only enough iron for the first four to six months. The researchers concluded that children fed breast milk and iron-fortified formulas are less likely to develop anemia.[15]

A study at the Children's Hospital in Helsinki, Finland, found that iron in human breast milk has a uniquely high bioavailability, reported *Current Prescribing* in 1979. Undertaken to find out whether breast-fed infants require supplemental iron, the study also compared iron status of breast-fed infants with that of bottle-fed infants.

The study involved 132 healthy newborns with similar birth weights and no significant hematologic differences—except slightly higher blood ferritin levels in the breast-fed group. Fifty-six received milk only from breast feedings until six months of age; 29 were given a non-iron-supplemented cow's milk formula; and 47 were fed a proprietary formula containing iron as ferrous gluconate. The latter two groups were also partially breast-fed an average of 2.5 and three months postpartum, respectively. All infants received cooked vegetables at 3.5 months; cereals with some iron supplementation at five months; and meat and eggs at six months. Daily vitamins were begun at two weeks.

Results showed that breast milk was superior to cow's milk for mean hematologic values. Differences were noted at four months in transferrin saturation and serum ferritin and at six months for most measurements. The mean values of the breast-fed and the iron-supplemented-formula group were similar to about age six months. But by nine months, lower values were seen in the breast-fed than in the formula group. Over half the breast-fed children had been weaned to cow's milk by nine months; the eight infants whose sole source of milk was still breast milk did not have better values than those weaned. The researchers concluded that nonfortified solid foods appear not to provide sufficient iron for infants breast-fed for prolonged periods. Therefore, supplemental iron should be considered for breast-fed infants after six months of age, and that infants weaned early need iron supplementation even sooner.[16]

In a 1991 screening of infants six- to 12-months-old in U.S. public health programs, about 216,000 were at risk of developing anemia because of low hemoglobin counts, reported the Centers for Disease Control and Prevention in Atlanta. The anemia was apparently due to a lack of iron in the children's diets. In addition to health problems caused by iron deficiency anemia, the deficiency can lead to reduced IQ scores five years later.

In 1992, the American Academy of Pediatrics reversed a long-standing policy by recommending only breast milk and iron-fortified infant formulas for children during their first year of life. Cow's milk is not recommended by the Academy for the first year of life, because the milk reportedly promotes loss of iron in the stools of susceptible infants. In addition to being a poor source of iron, cow's milk is also high in calcium and phosphorus, which may interfere with iron absorption, causing gastrointestinal bleeding and a loss of iron.[17]

In a study published in *Pediatrics* in 1989, Tomas Walter, M.D., and colleagues at the University of Chile in Santiago, reported that iron deficiency anemia affects the learning and development of infants. The double-blind, placebo-controlled study followed 196 infants from birth to 15 months of age.

"Developmental test performance in infancy has now been conclusively demonstrated to be impaired in children with anemia due to iron deficiency," the researchers said. "Among anemic infants, both severity and duration of anemia were associated with poorer performance. The selected areas most clearly affected were those of language acquisition and proficiency in body balance and coordination development leading to the erect position and walking."[18]

Low iron levels may increase the risk of severe menstrual symptoms, such as mood disturbances and greater pain, reported *Medical World News* in 1993. They discussed a meeting of the Federation of American Societies for Experimental Biology (FASEB) in New Orleans on March 31, 1993, in which James Penland, Ph.D., of the USDA's Human Nutrition Research Center in Grand Forks, North

Dakota, said that low iron levels were associated with behavioral changes, pain and autonomic sensations such as sweating and dizziness. The study involved 367 women, and those with clinically low levels of hemoglobin (red blood cells) experienced more behavioral changes prior to and during their periods. Symptoms included decreased efficiency, poor performance at work or school, increased daytime napping and avoidance of social activities.[19]

For a listing of the iron content of some common foods, refer to Table 16.2. Although heme and nonheme iron is available in a variety of foods, when you check the major sources of the mineral, it is easy to see why many Americans are deficient in iron.

TABLE 16.1

RECOMMENDED DIETARY ALLOWANCES FOR IRON

CATEGORY AND AGE	MILLIGRAMS OF IRON PER DAY
Infants, from birth to 6 months	6
Infants, 6 months to 1 year	10
Children, 1–3	10
Children, 4–6	10
Children, 7–10	10
Males, 11–14	12
Males, 15–18	12
Males, 19–24	10
Males, 25–50	10
Males, 51 and over	10
Females, 11–14	15
Females, 15–18	15
Females, 19–24	15
Females, 25–50	15
Females, 51 and over	10
Pregnant females	30
Lactating women, first 6 months	15
Lactating women, second 6 months	15

From *Recommended Dietary Allowances*, 10th Edition. National Academy Press, Washington, D.C., 1989.

TABLE 16.2

SOME COMMON FOODS HIGH IN IRON

FOOD	MILLIGRAMS OF IRON IN AN AVERAGE SERVING
Almonds, ½ cup	3.3
Beans, dried	4.6
Beans, lima	5.6
Beef	3
Blackstrap molasses, 1 tbsp.	2.3
Chicken	1.4
Clams	6
Collards, cooked	3
Dandelion greens	5.6
Eggs	1.1
Heart, beef	5.9
Liver, beef	4.4
Mushrooms	2
Mustard greens	4.1
Oysters, 1 cup	13.2
Peas	3
Pecans	2.6
Pork	2.2
Prunes, 1 cup	4.5
Raisins, 1 cup	5.6
Shrimp	2.6
Spinach	3.6
Walnuts, 1 cup	7.6
Wheat germ, 1 cup	5.5

From *Minerals: Kill or Cure?* by Ruth Adams and Frank Murray, Larchmont Books, New York, 1974.

REFERENCES

1. Ensminger, Audrey H., et al. *Foods and Nutrition Encyclopedia.* Clovis, Calif.: Pegus Press, 1983, pp. 1246ff.
2. McDermott, Tom. "Iron Deficiency—America's Second Greatest Nutrition Problem," Beef Industry Council, June 24, 1987.
3. Lewis, G. J. "Do Women with Menorrhagia Need Iron?" *British Medical Journal* 284:1158, 1982.
   4. Taymor, M. L., et al. "The Etiological Role of Chronic Iron Deficiency in Poduction of Menorrhagia," *The Journal of the American Medical Association* 187:323–327, 1964.
5. Arvidsson, B., et al. "Iron Prophylaxis in Menorrhagia," *Acta Obstetrics and Gynecology Scandinavia* 60:157–160, 1981.
6. Newhouse, I., et al. "Effects of Iron Supplementation and Discontinuation on Serum Copper, Zinc, Calcium and Magnesium Levels in Women," *Medicine and Science in Sports and Exercise* 25:562–571, 1993.
7. Pless, Misha, M.D., and Lipton, Stuart, M.D., Ph.D. "Iron Deficiency in Children," *New England Journal of Medicine* 329:1741–1742, December 2, 1993.
8. Ellis, Martin H., M.D., and Levine, James D., M.D. Ibid.
9. "Routine Iron Supplementation During Pregnancy," *The Journal of the American Medical Association* 270:2846–2854, December 15, 1993.
10. Buterbaugh, Laura. "Iron Supplements in Pregnancy Debated," *Medical Tribune*, January 6, 1994, pp. 1, 6.
11. Scholl, T., et al. "Anemia vs Iron Deficiency: Increased Risk of Preterm Delivery in a Prospective Study," *American Journal of Clinical Nutrition* 55:985–988, 1992.
12. *Special Currents: Iron*, March 1991, p. lff.
13. Lozoff, Betsy, M.D., et al. "Long-Term Developmental Outcome of Infants with Iron Deficiency," *New England Journal of Medicine* 325:687–694, September 5, 1991.
14. "Iron Slows Teen Mood Swings," *Medical Tribune*, September 10, 1992, p. 12.
15. Ryan, A. S., et al. "Changing Patterns of Infant Feeding in the United States: Evidence to Support Improved Iron Nutritional Status in Childhood." In Hercberg, S., et al. "Recent Knowledge on Iron and Folate Deficiencies in the World," *Colloque Inserm* 197:631–639, 1990.
16. "Iron Supplementation with Prolonged Breast Feeding?" *Current Prescribing*, January 1979, p. 74.
17. *Morbidity and Mortality Weekly Report*, Centers for Disease Control and Prevention, Atlanta, February 19, 1993, p. 1.
18. Walter, Tomas, M.D., et al. "Iron Deficiency Anemia: Adverse Effects on Infant Psychomotor Development," *Pediatrics* 84(1):7–17, July 1989.
19. "Low Iron Levels Linked to Menstrual Symptoms," *Medical World News*, April 1993, pp. 21–22.

17

Can You Get Too Much Iron?

ALTHOUGH iron deficiency is still a major health problem around the world, a Finnish study has implicated an excess of iron in some cases of heart disease.

Iron overload is referred to as hemochromatosis, a condition in which the body absorbs and stores too much iron. This is a common genetic error, according to the American Liver Foundation, Cedar Grove, New Jersey.

From studies in Europe, Australia and the United States, it is estimated that hemochromatosis affects about one in 300 to 400 people, the Foundation reported in their booklet, *Hemochromatosis: Not So Rare*.[1]

"Many people have no symptoms," the Foundation reported. "In advanced cases, injuries to the liver can slowly lead to cirrhosis if the illness is not treated. A bronze discoloration of the skin is often a sign that hemochromatosis is present. Damage to the pancreas can result in a severe form of diabetes mellitus. Damage to other organs may cause endocrine and heart problems, impotence and chronic fatigue. The wide range of symptoms, varying from individual to individual, makes diagnosis difficult."

Blood tests for serum iron and total iron binding capacity (TIBC) are the screening devices to detect iron overload. The normal blood iron level is about 100 and any level over 150 should be investigated further. The normal TIBC level is about 300. And the ratio of blood iron to the TIBC is normally about 0.30 or 30 percent. Figures above 50 percent (iron overload) or below 15 percent (iron deficiency) need more study. A reliable followup test is the serum ferritin level. If these tests are persistently high, a liver biopsy should be done to determine the amount of iron stored in the liver and to assess the damage (if any) to the liver.

Hemochromatosis is easily treated. One to two pints of blood (which is rich in iron) is removed each week until iron stores go down to a normal level. This can take from several months to several years, depending on the patient. When the iron stores are reduced to a normal level, the therapy needs to be continued every two to four months throughout life. The blood, of course, can be donated to a blood bank.

For those who follow these procedures, the prognosis is very good, so that the patient can usually lead a normal, active life. The situation becomes more serious if the illness has advanced to cirrhosis, in which the liver is marked by excessive formation of connective tissue and the eventual contraction of the organ. Liver cancers can occur in up to 25 percent of these patients. Ironically, since there are many forms of anemia, it is possible for a patient with iron overload to have both anemia and hemochromatosis.

"Hemochromatosis is most often diagnosed between the ages of 40 and 60, but it has been detected in younger and older people," the Foundation added. "The gene responsible for the disease is inherited from both parents. Women frequently develop symptoms at a later age than men, since women normally lose significant amounts of iron through menstruation, pregnancy and lactation. Anyone who has a blood relative with hemochromatosis should be tested with the various blood tests, even if there are no symptoms."

Hemochromatosis is an inherited disease that can develop in individuals eating a normal diet. It is rare for people to develop iron storage problems after taking heavy amounts of iron tonics and medications for a long time. However, these medications should be avoided by those with hemochromatosis. The same goes for consuming large amounts of iron-rich foods. The Foundation recommends that patients with hemochromatosis follow a normal, balanced diet, keeping in mind foods that are rich in iron. Megadoses of iron supplements should, of course, be monitored by a professional.[1]

Writing in the June 1990 issue of the *American Heart Journal*, Randall B. Lauffer, Ph.D., of the Massachusetts General Hospital in Boston, believes that iron's ability to stimulate the production of free radicals may accelerate cellular damage and increase the oxidation of low-density lipoprotein cholesterol (LDL, the harmful kind). He added that premenopausal, menstruating women, who are often deficient in iron, have a lower incidence of coronary artery disease than men. But as they reach menopause, their risk is virtually comparable to men. He further believes that the benefits of exercise may be due to iron depletion from the gastrointestinal serum loss and sweat, thereby inhibiting the production of free radicals. If this theory is correct, he continued, phlebotomy (donating blood) of 0.5 liter of blood two to three times a year (400 to 600 mg of iron annually) may prevent iron accumulation in both men and women and prove to be a preventive approach to ischemic heart disease. Iron fortification of foods and the monitoring of iron levels, along with screening for hemochromatosis, may be subjects that need to be discussed.[2]

"Most physicians were taught that hemochromatosis is a very rare inherited disease, but it's not so rare," stated H. Ralph Schumacher, Jr., M.D., of the University of Pennsylvania, reported the June 8, 1987 issue of *Medical World News*. His remarks came at the New York Academy of Sciences' first international conference on the iron overload disorder. He came to his conclusions after sending questionnaires to patients on the rolls of the Hemochromatosis Research Foundation in Albany, New York.

"Of 129 patients with the disorder who had arthritis-like symptoms, only 16 were correctly diagnosed as having 'the arthritis of hemochromatosis,'" Schumacher said. "Thirty-six others were diagnosed as having osteoarthritis. Regarding 13 patients who were told they had rheumatoid arthritis, that's extremely unlikely. Maybe one or two really did have rheumatoid."

As to why physicians are not recognizing hemochromatosis more often, Margaret A. Krikker, M.D., president and founder of the Hemochromatosis Research Foundation, Inc., said that "they're not aware of the new gene frequency figures." In addition, she added, the usual symptoms of iron-damaged organs are similar to symptoms of other chronic diseases such as diabetes, heart failure and thyroid deficiency. Symptoms are quite variable and joint pain is not always the first sign of a problem, she said. Initial symptoms have been as diverse as amenorrhea and the sudden onset of shortness of breath.

"Untreated hemochromatosis can lead to a severe form of diabetes, cardiac arrhythmias, arthritis, liver failure and death," *Medical World News* reported. "Among early symptoms are pseudogout, fatigue, premature menopause, loss of sex drive and impotence in men and an enlarged liver."[3]

Acquired hemochromatosis is secondary to a primary medical condition, according to the Hemochromatosis Research Foundation, Inc. These patients are usually under medical care, their physicians are aware of their iron-loading tendencies and their treatments are individualized and do not include phlebotomies. This form of hemochromatosis is not due to the inheritance of the iron-loading H gene, but is due to:

1. Many transfusions of blood (over 80) given to patients with chronic anemias (congenital or acquired types), so as to sustain their lives; and
2. Increased iron absorption secondary to chronic anemias and to chronic liver diseases, especially alcoholic cirrhosis;
3. Although secondary hemochromatosis may also occur when dietary iron intake is excessive, this is usually rare.

Since all foods except fats and oils contain iron, it is not practical or nutritionally advisable for patients with hemochromatosis to limit a diet to low-iron foods. However, a patient can reduce the amount of foods containing highly available iron, such as meats. So, instead of eating three ounces of meat, eat one ounce. And fish contains less available iron.[4]

Sean R. Lynch and colleagues reported in the November 1982 issue of the *American Journal of Clinical Nutrition*:

The ease with which iron intake can be increased markedly by the ingestion of pharmaceutical preparations makes a brief consideration of the possible hazards of excessive iron consumption necessary. Individuals who have a normal regulatory mechanism for absorption appear to be able to maintain iron stores in the physiological range despite high dietary iron or even iron supplementation. Failure of this homeostatic mechanism occurs in hereditary hemochromatosis, certain iron loading anemias such as thalassemia and sideroblastic anemia. Tissue iron deposition in these disorders is associated with significant morbidity and increased mortality that may be aggravated by a rise in dietary iron intake. They are relatively rare conditions and usually present before the age of 65, although the protective effect of menstrual blood loss may delay the onset of symptoms in some women with idiopathic hemochromatosis.

The researchers added that it has recently been demonstrated that idiopathic hemochromatosis is an autosomal recessive disorder genetically linked to the HLA locus and that the gene may be present in up to two to 10 percent of the population in some areas of the world, including the U.S.

"Male heterozygotes accumulate four to five grams of iron by the age of 40," the researchers continued. "Although most of them appear to stabilize at this level, it is not clear whether a high iron intake might lead to a progressive increase in body iron. These observations may have particular relevance to the elderly since studies carried out in the United States and Sweden suggest that some elderly people take large quantities of supplemental iron."[5]

Overdoses May Be Fatal

Although iron pills are entirely safe when prescribed by a physician or administered by a parent following label directions, these pills must be kept out of the reach of children, who mistake them for candy. During 1991, the most recent year tabulated, 5,144 children took accidental overdoses of iron pills, which resulted in 11 deaths. Those who died had accidentally ingested 30 iron tablets, reported the Centers for Disease Control and Prevention in Atlanta.[6]

For additional information about hemochromatosis, contact:

American Liver Foundation, 998 Pompton Ave., Cedar Grove, New Jersey 07009; telephone 201–256–2550.

The Hemochromatosis Research Foundation, Inc., P.O. Box 8569, Albany, New York 12208; telephone 518–475–2875.

REFERENCES

1. "Hemochromatosis: Not So Rare," American Liver Foundation, Cedar Grove, N.J., undated.
2. Lauffer, Randall B., Ph.D. "Iron Depletion in Coronary Disease," *American Heart Journal* 119(6):1448, June 1990.
3. "Iron Overload Diagnosis Missed," *Medical World News*, June 8, 1987, p. 110.
4. "Some Facts About Hemochromatosis," Hemochromatosis Research Foundation, Inc., 1984.
5. Lynch, Sean R., et al. "Iron Status of Elderly Americans," *The American Journal of Clinical Nutrition* 36:1032–1045, November 1982.
6. *Morbidity and Mortality Weekly Report*, February 19, 1993; Centers for Disease Control and Prevention, Atlanta.

18

Magnesium Keeps Your Heart Healthy

IN ancient times, the Romans believed that *magnesia alba* (white magnesium salts from the region of Magnesia in Greece) possessed unusual curative powers. However, it was not until 1808 that Sir Humphrey Davy (1778–1829), a British chemist, isolated a substance in the salts, which we now know as magnesium. Sir Davy also discovered the anesthetic properties of nitrous oxide, better known as "laughing gas."

Magnesium is an essential mineral that makes up about 0.05 percent of the body's weight, roughly 20 to 30 grams. An estimated 60 percent of this mineral is found in the bones in the form of phosphates and carbonates, with 28 percent of the mineral located in soft tissue. Another two percent is found in body fluids. The highest amount of the mineral in the soft tissues is in the liver and muscles (and remember that the heart is a muscle). Blood serum contains between one and three milligrams of the mineral per 100 milliliter (one thousandths of a liter). Most of the mineral is attached to proteins, with the rest in the form of ions, which are atoms with a positive or negative electrical charge.

MANY FACTORS INFLUENCE ABSORPTION

"From 30 to 50 percent of the average daily intake of magnesium is absorbed in the small intestine," the *Foods and Nutrition Encyclopedia* reported. "Almost all of the magnesium in the feces represents unabsorbed dietary magnesium. Its absorption is interfered with high intake of calcium, phosphate, oxalic acid (spinach, rhubarb), phytate (whole-grain cereals), and poorly digested fats (long-chain saturated fatty acids). Its absorption is enhanced by protein, lactose (milk sugar), vitamin D, growth hormone and antibiotics."[1]

147

Most of the mineral is excreted in the urine, and aldosterone, an adrenal gland hormone, regulates the amount of magnesium that is excreted through the kidneys. Diuretics, or water pills, which increase urination, and alcohol are known to deplete magnesium stores in the body.

Caffeine is responsible for increasing the excretion of magnesium, as well as calcium and sodium, according to researchers at Washington State University in Pullman. There was little effect on the excretion of potassium, phosphorus and chloride, according to the report in *Nutrition Reviews*.[2]

A study conducted by the University of Helsinki and the National Public Health Institute in Finland found that alcohol lowers the amount of magnesium and selenium in the blood. After analyzing data from the 48 male and 37 female volunteers, all alcoholics, it was determined that the increased alcohol intake was responsible for removing magnesium and selenium from the blood, since there was no indication that the people had overt dietary deficiencies.[3]

In a study reported in the *American Journal of Cardiology*, 20 percent of 45 consecutive patients with atrial fibrillation (irregular heartbeat) had a magnesium deficiency.[4] Another study, reported in *Critical Care Medicine*, found that, out of 102 consecutive patients admitted to a medical intensive care unit, 20 percent were deficient in magnesium.[5]

Magnesium and calcium are useful in reducing high blood pressure, according to Abram Hoffer, M.D., Ph.D., in *Orthomolecular Medicine for Physicians*. In fact, he said, 1,000 mg of calcium and 500 mg of magnesium each day will decrease the incidence of high blood pressure and, therefore, decrease the load on the heart.[6]

Sodium is apparently much less involved as a cause of hypertension, Hoffer believed. The chloride ion in sodium chloride (table salt) is still an important factor, he adds, but other sodium salts, such as sodium ascorbate, are not involved. (Sodium ascorbate was the late Dr. Linus Pauling's favorite form of vitamin C. He ingested 16 grams of sodium ascorbate daily, most of which he sprinkled on his food. He also kept one-gram capsules of vitamin C in his pocket.)

Hypertension Decreases Magnesium Stores

Hoffer reported:

> A series of hypertensive patients on antihypertensive medication were given one gram (1,000 mg) of calcium per day. After a few months half of them no longer required their antihypertensive medication. Since calcium and magnesium interre-

late, this means both ions are important . . . Magnesium is decreased in hypertension. The incidence of hypertension is high in areas where drinking water is soft or where there is little magnesium in the soil. It has been known since 1925 that magnesium salts lower blood pressure. Magnesium also plays an important role in regulating vasomotor tone. Low magnesium increases it.[6]

The earliest symptoms of a magnesium deficiency include: a loss of appetite, nausea, vomiting, diarrhea, mental changes and irritability. Spontaneous or induced muscle spasms are noted and seizures may occur. Since there are no syndromes specific to magnesium, a magnesium deficiency is often overlooked by attending physicians, Hoffer noted. And neurologic and cardiac symptoms may be associated with calcium and potassium deficiencies, as well as too little magnesium.

"Fouty (1978) maintains that magnesium deficiency should be suspected in any situations associated with potassium deficiency, even though serum levels are normal, as they are in half the subjects," Hoffer explained. "A few cases have been diagnosed with multiple sclerosis. A clinical background of diuretics, steroid treatment, hypercalcemia (excessive calcium in the blood), diarrhea, alcoholism, hypokalemia (potassium deficiency) and liquid protein diets should lead one to suspect magnesium deficiency."[6]

Most physicians do not realize that magnesium and calcium are intimately related. That is why a magnesium deficiency can cause calcium deposits in muscles and kidneys. This also results in kidney stones in susceptible people, and is probably related to the deficiencies that can result with the increasing use of modern foods.

Magnesium sulfate proved to be useful in reducing ventricular arrhythmias in eight patients at the Institute of Experimental and Clinical Oncology, Reggio Calabria University in Italy. No side effects were noted.[7]

H. Alexander Heggtveit, M.D., Professor of Pathology at the University of Ottawa in Canada, said that there is strong evidence that lack of magnesium plays a decisive role in human heart ailments. When he examined heart muscle from victims of fatal heart attacks, he found that certain portions contained up to 42 percent less magnesium than heart muscle from individuals who died of other causes. Such a magnesium deficiency may predispose the human heart to fatal arrhythmias, or disturbances in the heart's beating rhythm.

Mildred S. Seelig, M.D., believes that a magnesium deficiency accounts for the high incidence of heart disease in the United States and other Western countries. In 1964, Seelig reported on the magnesium levels of people in various parts of the world, including England and the U.S. She found that only the people living in the Orient—where hardening of the arteries is not common—have sufficient reserves of magnesium. She added that American diets are grossly deficient in the mineral, and that large amounts of vitamin D, calcium and protein interfere with the absorption and retention of magnesium. She added that magnesium has been declining in the American diet since 1900, largely because of food processing and changes in food preferences. Seelig pointed out that the milling of wheat strips away much of the magnesium, and that certain chemical additives used to keep frozen vegetables a bright shade of green pull out essential minerals, including magnesium.[8]

In his book, *Nutrigenetics*, R. O. Brennan, D.O., reported that 85 percent of the magnesium is removed from wheat during the milling process to make white flour. Other losses, he said, include: vitamin A (90 percent); vitamin B1 (77 percent); vitamin B2 (80 percent); vitamin B3 (81 percent); vitamin B6 (72 percent); vitamin B12 (77 percent); pantothenic acid (50 percent); vitamin D (90 percent); vitamin E (86 percent); folic acid, the B vitamin (67 percent); calcium (60 percent); chromium (40 percent); cobalt (89 percent); iron (76 percent); manganese (86 percent); phosphorus (71 percent); potassium (77 percent); selenium (16 percent); sodium (78 percent); zinc (78 percent).

"The flour industry did nothing to improve its product until it was pressured to do so in 1941 (when strong bodies were needed during World War II)," Brennan said. "The resulting 'enrichment,' however, meant replacement of thiamine (B1), riboflavin (B2), niacin (B3) and iron. That was all. Processing took out parts of 22 elements. The industry put back parts of four."[9]

When researchers at the University of Southern California at Los Angeles examined over 100 consecutive admissions to its coronary care unit, they found that 53 percent were short on magnesium, reported Rick McGuire in the August 27, 1986 issue of *Medical Tribune*.

McGuire reported that special tests revealed unexpectedly high rates of magnesium deficiency in heart patients, suggesting that serum testing for the mineral is inadequate. Since magnesium, like potassium, is primarily an intracellular cation (positively charged ion), blood levels may not accurately reflect total body balance. Robert Rude, M.D., one of the researchers, said that blood levels indicated that only five percent of the patients were hypomagnesemic (having low blood levels of magnesium), but a check of lymphocyte magnesium levels boosted the incidence to 53 percent.

"I think hypomagnesemia certainly could be a contributing factor [to cardiovascular disorders]," Rude said. "We know that magnesium depletion predisposes to hypertension and cardiac arrhythmias, and may predispose to coronary vasospasm and perhaps myocardial infarction."

In *Medical Tribune*, Jean Durlach, M.D., Hopital Cochin, Paris, president of the International Society for the Development of Magnesium Research, reported that his study "shows a consistent global pattern indicating that the higher the magnesium content of drinking water, the lower the morbidity and mortality rates for heart disease."[10]

A 1983 study from South Africa found a 10-percent reduction in coronary heart disease mortality for every 6 mg/1 increase in water magnesium levels. A 1960 study from Dartmouth University reported the same effect per 8 mg/1 increase. And in a study at Glostrup Hospital, University of Copenhagen, myocardial infarction patients were shown to have decreased levels of magnesium, when judged by a parenteral magnesium retention test.

Because of difficulties in accurately detecting magnesium deficiency, Robert Rude suspects that the problem is more common than originally thought, especially in seriously ill patients. In a sample of consecutive admissions to the Los Angeles County-USC Medical Center, Rude found low blood levels of magnesium in 10 percent of the general patients and 67 percent in the intensive care patients.

"If a patient has a complication that may be secondary to magnesium deficiency, such as cardiac arrhythmias which are especially resistant to antiarrhythmic therapy, perhaps the patient should receive magnesium therapy as a diagnostic/therapeutic trial," Rude said. "In patients with normal kidney function, you can give magnesium with a fair degree of safety. If renal function is not normal, then you do have to drop your dose and monitor daily."[10]

In 1982, doctors at the Veterans Administration Medical Center in Oklahoma City found that patients with low serum magnesium required more drugs to control their high blood pressure than those with normal levels of the mineral, according to *The Complete Book of Vitamins and Minerals for Health*. They also reported that low magnesium levels may be caused by the diuretics given for high blood pressure, which in turn may interfere with the effectiveness of the other blood pressure medications.

At University Hospital in Umea, Sweden, 20 patients receiving long-term diuretics (18 for high blood pressure, 2 for congestive heart failure) were given 365 mg/day of magnesium supplements for six months. Nineteen of the 20 showed a drop in blood pressure. In three patients, blood pressure dropped so low that the amount of magnesium was reduced. In three other patients, the amount of diuretic being used to treat the high blood pressure was reduced.

Burton M. Altura, Ph.D., and his wife, Bella T. Altura, Ph.D., of the Downstate Medical Center in Brooklyn, New York, believe that magnesium deficiencies are a likely factor in many diseases or conditions that involve constriction or spasm of the heart and circulatory system, the publication added. Their findings also indicate that an optimum intake of magnesium can go a long way toward preventing those diseases and alleviating their symptoms. They also believe that magnesium may control the "sodium-calcium pump," which is essential for the maintenance of normal coronary artery muscle tone. Too little magnesium permits calcium and sodium to flood the cells, and, since those two minerals are constricting agents, the muscle tissue turns to knots, the Alturas explained. This means that sufficient amounts of magnesium allow our hearts to beat smoothly and regularly and to withstand daily stress. The mineral also helps blood vessels to remain open, thereby lowering blood pressure.[11]

MANY AT RISK

A magnesium deficiency is thought to occur in between 20 and 80 percent of the population, according to M. A. Brodsky in the *Journal of the American College of Nutrition*. In acute ischemia and myocardial infarction, magnesium therapy has been shown to reduce life-threatening ventricular tachyarrhythmias. And in seven studies, he added, involving over 1,300 patients, magnesium therapy resulted in a 55 percent reduction in the odds of death in the volunteers given the mineral. It interacts with potassium ions and may help replete hypokalemia and thus reduce arrhythmias, he said. Magnesium is also helpful in treating the arrhythmias associated with digitalis toxicity and coronary artery spasm. The mineral is an important therapy in cardiovascular disease and will help to reduce morbidity and mortality with increased use, he added.[12]

"One recent study, by Honolulu Heart Program researchers, clearly shows magnesium's importance in blood pressure control," stated *Medical Care Yearbook* 1989. "The scientists examined 61 different factors in the diets of healthy older men. Magnesium came out on top, having the strongest link between high intake and low blood pressure. Many mineral researchers think an average-size man should be getting about 420 to 475 milligrams of magnesium a day to make up for what he loses—and to help protect him from developing high blood pressure as he ages. That's about 125 to 150 mg/day more than most men get."[13]

Since magnesium serves as a natural calcium channel blocker and calcium blockers relax vascular cells, R. Touyz, M.D., of the University of the Witwatersrand Medical School in Johannesburg, South Africa, suggests that the hypotensive therapeutic effect of synthetic calcium channel blockers, combined with magnesium supplements, would be very compatible, he reported in 1991. A magnesium deficiency inhibits vascular smooth muscle tone and leads to elevated blood pressure, he said. Magnesium has been referred to as "the endogenous calcium channel blocker," because it blocks calcium's entry into vascular smooth muscle;

it inhibits calcium's release within the cell; it competes with calcium for nonspecific binding sites on plasma membranes; and it blocks the slow calcium channels, Touyz reported.[14]

"Treating patients with magnesium in the acute phase of a heart attack will reduce early mortality, early complications and late mortality," reported researchers from Kent Woods Leicester Royal Infirmary, Leicester, England. The research was reported at the XVth Congress of the European Society of Cardiology in Nice, France.

The English trial, involving 2,000 patients, found a 20-percent reduction in mortality over four years in myocardial infarction patients treated with magnesium, compared with those not receiving the therapy. Volunteers were given the mineral intravenously over 24 hours following a suspected MI.

Earlier information from the study revealed a significant reduction in death rates 28 days after the victims' MIs occurred, from 10.3 percent not receiving magnesium, to 7.8 percent in the magnesium group, or a reduction of 24 percent.

Rory Collins, M.D., codirector of the Clinical trial Service Unit at the University of Oxford in England, said that magnesium is simple to give, it's cheap and well-tolerated. If the results are confirmed by a later study, he would consider magnesium's protective effect on the heart "to be as great as aspirin's."

Peter Elwood, M.D., of the Medical Research Council Epidemiology Unit in South Wales, told the French meeting about his observational Caerphilly Heart Disease Study that is tracking the magnesium intake of 2,182 men over 10 years. The 152 men who have died during the study had an average magnesium intake of 235 mg/day, compared to the survivors, who had intakes of 266 mg/day. Elwood's study, which involves healthy men ranging in age from 45 to 59, suggests that dietary magnesium can provide long-term heart protection.[15]

In the *Journal of the American College of Cardiology*, Stephen S. Gottlieb, M.D. of the University of Maryland School of Medicine in Baltimore reported that, out of 199 patients with chronic congestive heart failure, 19 percent were found to have below normal blood levels of magnesium; 67 percent were in the normal range; and 14 percent were above that. Those with low serum magnesium levels had a worse prognosis during long-term follow-up than normomagnesemic patients. He added that magnesium intervention needs further study to see if it can change the course of chronic congestive heart failure patients.[16]

Hiroo Miyagi, M.D., et al., of the Kumamoto University Medical School in Kumamoto City, Japan, reported in *Circulation* that intravenous magnesium may be useful for the treatment of coronary spasm and play an active role in the treatment of ischemic heart disease, unstable angina and myocardial infarction.[17]

In patients with myocardial infarction and/or cardiac arrhythmias, liberal amounts of magnesium should be given to them, unless they have kidney failure, heart block or severe respiratory complications, reported A. Sjogren, et al., of Varnamo Hospital in Sweden in the *Journal of Internal Medicine*. They added that digitalis intoxication can result in low serum magnesium levels, which may increase the likelihood of arrhythmias. And magnesium should be considered as an adjuvant treatment for cardiac arrhythmias, especially in conjunction with hypokalemia, digitalis intoxication, following coronary bypass surgery or in *torsades de pointes* ventricular tachycardia.[18]

A magnesium-rich diet lowered blood lipids in a group of patients at the Medical Hospital and Research Centre in Moradabad, India, according to R. Singh, et al., in *Biology and Trace Elements*. The researchers gave 200 volunteers a diet high in magnesium and potassium, while the control group ate a standard diet. Following six weeks of the study, serum cholesterol, low-density lipoprotein cholesterol (LDL) and triglycerides were lower in the group getting the minerals. There was a slight rise in high-density lipoprotein cholesterol (HDL, the good kind) in the treatment group, while HDL values decreased in the control group.[19]

Patients with labile (unstable) high blood pressure and poor magnesium status should supplement their diet with magnesium, reported H. Ruddel and colleagues at the University of Bonn in Berlin, Germany, in the *Journal of the American College of Nutrition*. The patients with initial low concentrations of magnesium in red blood cells improved on the mineral therapy, which brought a decrease in systolic blood pressure, especially during emotional stress. Symptoms did not improve in the volunteers with initial magnesium levels in the normal range.[20]

Magnesium is the second most abundant intracellular cation in the body, and is involved in more than 300 enzymatic reactions involving glucose, fat, protein, nucleic acid, adenosine triphosphate and muscle and membrane transport metabolism, according to Michael Shechter, M.D., et al., of the Heart Institute, Sheba Medical Center, Tel-Hashomer, Israel, in *Archives of Internal Medicine*. After reviewing a number of recent studies, they noted that magnesium improves myocardial performance by reducing systemic and pulmonary vascular resistance, bringing a concomitant decrease in blood pressure and a slight increase in cardiac index. They concluded that the current data available suggests that magnesium has significant potential for myocardial protection and enhanced survival in patients with acute myocardial infarction. The therapy is inexpensive, safe and simple.[21]

Magnesium may reduce hardening of the artery lesions by modulating cholesterol accumulation in the aortic wall, possibly by inhibiting the formation of foam cells, protecting the vascular endothelial cells, or possibly by some unknown effect that is related to the reduction in serum triglycerides, reported Y. Ouchi, et al. of the University of Tokyo in Japan in *Arteriosclerosis*. This was an animal study, in which rabbits were given a standard diet, a diet containing one percent cholesterol, a one percent cholesterol diet supplemented with either 300, 600 or 900 mg of magnesium as magnesium sulfate.[22]

Since magnesium is so important for keeping us healthy, how much should you be getting in your diet and/or supplements? The Recommended Dietary Allowances, which were designed to meet the needs of healthy people under the age of 51, follows.

TABLE 18.1

RECOMMENDED DIETARY ALLOWANCES FOR MAGNESIUM

AGE AND CATEGORY	MILLIGRAMS PER DAY
Infants, to six months	40
Children, six months to one year	60
Children, 1 to 3	80
Children, 4 to 6	120
Children, 7 to 10	170
Males, 11 to 14	270
Males, 15 to 18	400
Males, 19 and over	350
Females, 11 to 14	280
Females, 15 to 18	300
Females, 19 and over	280
Pregnant women	320
Breast-feeding women, first six months	355
Breast-feeding women, 2 to six months	340

From *Recommended Dietary Allowances*, 10th Edition. Washington, D.C.: National Academy Press, 1989.

References

1. Ensminger, Audrey H., et al. *Foods and Nutrition Encyclopedia*. Clovis, Calif.: Pegus Press, 1983, pp. 1338ff.
2. Massey, L., et al. "Acute Effects of Dietary Caffeine and Aspirin on Urinary Mineral Excretion in Pre- and Postmenopausal Women," *Nutrition Reviews*, Vol. 8, pp. 845–851, 1988.
3. Karkkainen, P., et al. "Alcohol Intake Correlated with Serum Trace Elements," *Alcohol and Alcoholism*, Vol. 23, pp. 279–282, 1988.
4. DeCarli, C., et al. "Serum Magnesium Levels in Symptomatic Atrial Fibrillation and Their Relation on Rhythm Control by Intravenous Digoxin," *American Journal of Cardiology*, Vol. 57, p. 956, 1986.
5. Reinhart, R., et al. "Hypomagnesemia in Patients Entering the ICU," *Critical Care Medicine* 13(6):506, 1985.
6. Hoffer, Abram, M.D., Ph.D. *Orthomolecular Medicine for Physicians*. New Canaan, Conn.: Keats Publishing, Inc., 1989, pp. 122–123.
7. Peticone, F., et al. "Protective Magnesium Treatment in Ischemic Dilated Cardiomyopathy," *Journal of the American College of Nutrition* 7:403, 1988.
8. Murray, Frank. *Program Your Heart for Health*. New York: Larchmont Books, 1978, pp. 328–329.
9. Brennan, R. O., D.O. *Nutrigenetics*. New York: M. Evans and Co., Inc., 1975, pp. 43ff.
10. McGuire, Rick. "How Come Hypomagnesemia in 50% of CCU Admittees?" *Medical Tribune*, August 27, 1986, p. 3, 23.
11. *The Complete Book of Vitamins and Minerals for Health*. Emmaus, Pa.: Rodale Press, 1988, pp. 195ff.
12. Brodsky, M. A. "Magnesium, Myocardial Infarction and Arrhythmias," *Journal of the American College of Nutrition* 11(5):607/Abstract 36, October 1992.
13. Ferguson, Sharon Stocker, editor. *Medical Care Yearbook*. Emmaus, Pa.: Rodale Press, 1989, p. 90.
14. Touzy, R. "Magnesium Supplementation as an Adjuvant to Synthetic Calcium Channel Antagonists in the Treatment of Hypertension," *Med. Hypo.* 36:140–141, 1991.
15. Phillips, Pat. "Magnesium May Extend Survival After Myocardial Infarctions," *Medical Tribune*, October 7, 1993, p. 8.
16. Gottlieb, Stephen S., M.D., et al. "Prognostic Importance of Serum Magnesium Concentration in Patients with Congestive Heart Failure," *Journal of the American College of Cardiology* 16(4):827–831, October 1990.
17. Miyagi, Hiroo, M.D., et al. "Effect of Magnesium on Anginal Attack Induced by Hyperventilation in Patients with Varying Angina," *Circulation* 79:597–602, 1989.
18. Sjogren, A., et al. "Magnesium Deficiency in Coronary Artery Disease and Cardiac Arrhythmias," *Journal of Internal Medicine* 229:213–222, 1989.

19. Singh, R., et al. "Does Dietary Magnesium Modulate Blood Lipids?" *Biology and Trace Elements* 30:59–64, 1991.
20. Ruddel, H., et al. "Effect of Magnesium Supplementation in Patients with Labile Hypertension," *Journal of the American College of Nutrition* 6:445, 1987.
21. Shechter, Michael, M.D., et al. "Rationale of Magnesium Supplementation in Acute Myocardial Infarction: A Review of the Literature," *Archives of Internal Medicine* 152:2189–2196, November 1992.
22. Ouchi, Y., et al. "Effect of Dietary Magnesium on Development of Atherosclerosis in Cholesterol-Fed Rabbits," *Arteriosclerosis* 10:732–737, 1990.

19

More Reasons Why You Need Magnesium

In addition to protecting us against cardiovascular disease and high blood pressure, magnesium is useful in treating premenstrual syndrome (PMS); it helps to prevent kidney stones; it helps to fight depression; it has proved to be effective in the treatment of convulsions in pregnant women and prevents premature labor; it aids in the treatment of neuromuscular and nervous disorders; it is effective in the treatment of diarrhea, vomiting and indigestion, among other things, according to Sheldon Saul Hendler, M.D., Ph.D., in *The Doctors' Vitamin and Mineral Encyclopedia*.

"A few studies report the beneficial effect of magnesium supplementation in the prevention of recurrent calcium-oxalate stones," Hendler said. "One study used 200 mg/day of magnesium oxide plus 10 mg/day of vitamin B6. In a second study, magnesium was used alone, in the amount of 300 mg/day of magnesium oxide. Magnesium hydroxide was used in a more recent study. The current evidence suggests that magnesium supplementation is effective in preventing calcium oxalate stones in people who have this recurrent problem. (It is presently estimated that about one million Americans now living will die from causes related to kidney stones.)"[1]

PREVENTS KIDNEY STONES

Hendler was referring to the work of Stanley F. Gershoff, Ph.D., and Edwin L. Prien, Sr., M.D., who reported in the *American Journal of Clinical Nutrition* in 1967, that habitual stone formers had a 90-percent reduction in stone formation with the magnesium-B6 therapy. Thirty of the 36 patients, who were followed for five years, experienced either no recurrence or a slightly decreased recurrence of the stones.[2]

Writing in the *Journal of Urology* in 1974, the two researchers discussed another study of 149 patients, who had at least one kidney stone annually for five years, for a total of 871 stones. Each patient received 100 mg of magnesium oxide three times a day, plus a daily dose of 10 mg of vitamin B6. During the following four and one-half to six years, only 17 patients (11 percent) developed stones, bringing an overall reduction of 92 percent in the occurrence of calcium-oxalate stones in this group.[3]

The pain brought on by kidney stones is caused by the passing of the stone as it blocks the flow of urine and causes stretching of the ureters and the kidney pelvis, explained Robert M. Giller, M.D., in *Natural Prescriptions*. The kidney pelvis is like a funnel that directs urine into the ureters, the tubes that lead to the bladder. Pain usually begins at the flank, then moves to the front and down toward the groin. It sometimes takes weeks or even months for a stone to pass, Giller said, with the pain coming in intense periodic waves. If there are complications, or the pain becomes too intense, a nonsurgical procedure, such as ultrasound, can shatter the stone, allowing it to pass. Kidney stones develop when calcium oxalate, or uric acid, in the urine is present in such high concentrations that it forms crystals.

"The most serious complication of kidney stones is infection caused by the blocked flow of urine," Giller said. "Chills, nausea and a high fever are all signs of infection, an emergency that requires immediate medical attention. Even when no infection is present, your doctor may prescribe medication to help manage the pain, and may order a urinalysis X-ray to support the diagnosis."

Giller added that kidney stones can be prevented by dietary modifications and by increasing fluid intake. For those susceptible to kidney stones, Giller recommends they:

- Drink at least eight glasses of water a day;
- Eat a low-protein diet (three ounces only at lunch and dinner);
- Avoid eating large meals late at night;
- Avoid sugar, salt, caffeine and alcohol, all of which increase the amount of calcium in the urine;
- Limit vitamin C intake to 2,000 mg/day if they are prone to stones; and
- See that they get enough magnesium, which is in such foods as barley, bran, corn, buckwheat, rye, oats, brown rice, potatoes and bananas.[4]

You can also see Table 19.1 which lists the magnesium content of some familiar foods.

At a roundtable briefing, "Magnesium: The Misunderstood Mineral," held May 19, 1994 at the New York Academy of Sciences, a team of renowned researchers discussed the importance of this mineral, which is involved in the activation of more than 300 enzymes and body chemicals. (Biochemists are still counting the number of involved enzymes.)

"Magnesium is both a versatile and a vital mineral," said Mildred Seelig, M.D., M.P.H., Adjunct Professor of Nutrition at the University of North Carolina School of Public Health in Chapel Hill. "The role of magnesium in human health is not fully understood or appreciated because the mineral has numerous functions. Among these is its importance in maintaining healthy bones. As in the case of calcium, its main function is accepted in the prevention of osteoporosis."

Almost three-quarters of Americans have magnesium intakes below the recommended amounts, the panelists agreed. On average, women are consuming only 296 mg/day of magnesium, while men are getting 376 mg/day. This contrasts with the recommended dietary intake of 400 mg/day.

When combined with other known risk factors, a magnesium deficiency can contribute to such health problems as osteoporosis, cardiovascular disease, kidney stones, diabetes, hypoglycemia, migraine headaches, morning sickness, menstrual cramps and premenstrual syndrome. A severe deficiency in the mineral is related to irregular heart rhythm and convulsions.[5]

In addition to insufficient amounts of magnesium in our diets, a deficiency of the mineral can be caused by such illnesses as diabetes and hyperthyroidism; medications such as antibiotics, diuretics, estrogen and oral contraceptives; alcoholism; diarrhea; excessive exercise; and prolonged stress, such as that caused by penetrating noise levels. As for the proper calcium-magnesium ratio, the panelists said that there is still controversy. Some are suggesting 3:1, 2:1 or 1:1.

"Preliminary research suggests that the shift in estrogen and progesterone balance that immediately precedes menstruation may reduce the level of magnesium in the blood," Seelig said. "Since magnesium insufficiency can cause tension and irritability, clinicians have shown that magnesium supplementation can ease similar symptoms of PMS."

She added that some doctors have been treating headache sufferers with magnesium supplementation to reduce the frequency of attacks. In fact, there is some evidence that magnesium can stop a migraine in its tracks, when given at the earliest stage, and good evidence that it mitigates the number of headaches a migraine sufferer gets. This is explained by the fact that migraine headaches are due to a constriction of blood vessels in the brain, and that the mineral helps to dilate or expand the blood vessels to allow more blood to flow.

"Millions of people in this country suffer from magnesium insufficiency, or hypomagnesemia," said Leo Galland, M.D., a New York City internist, another speaker. "But the symptoms of marginal hypomagnesemia are subtle and not easily diagnosed. Blood tests may be helpful, but they are not always conclusive. The symptoms are, for the most part, neuromuscular and include fatigue, headache, insomnia, irritability and muscle tension or cramps."

He added that the symptoms of low-level hypomagnesemia are reversible with over-the-counter magnesium supplements over a period of three to six months. For those who think they may be deficient n the mineral, Galland recommends that they confer with their physician, who can determine whether diet and/or supplementation are required.[5]

Magnesium Eases PMS

A number of studies have reported the beneficial effects of magnesium for premenstrual syndrome. For example, 192 PMS patients were given 4.5 to 6 grams of magnesium daily for one week premenstrually and for two days menstrually. Nervous tension subsided in 159 of 179 patients (89 percent), while 155 of 162 patients (96 percent) reported less painful breasts, according to *Endocrinology*.[6]

One of the most commonly cited causes of PMS cravings is magnesium deficiency, and yet blood tests on PMS patients seldom reveal this deficiency, according to Douglas Hunt, M.D., in *No More Fears*. Jeffrey Bland, Ph.D., has said that magnesium is often low in the cells, and when red blood cells are studied *instead* of the blood, the magnesium deficiency then becomes apparent.

"Magnesium has also been helpful in relieving cramping that comes with menstruation," Hunt added. "Two to four magnesium orotate tablets every time the cramping occurs has been reported effective. Those of us in preventive medicine have often used magnesium as a substitute for certain drugs. One of the drug groups that magnesium sometimes substitutes for are the calcium channel blockers."[7]

In her book, *Complementary Natural Prescriptions for Common Ailments*, Carolyn Dean, M.D., recommends that PMS patients avoid foods which retain salt and sugar and in turn retain fluid in the body. She advised against chips, sugar, desserts, alcohol, tea, coffee, soft drinks. Eat an optimum diet which contains whole grains, nuts, seeds, vegetables, legumes, fish and chicken.

The next step is to use vitamin B6 to decrease fluid build-up, 100 mg one to three times a day from midcycle to the period. Another supplement that is deficient in premenstrual syndrome is magnesium; 300 mg/day is a good amount to continue all month and can be taken with a calcium supplement of equal strength. This is especially important for those women who suffer painful periods. Evening primrose oil is used for many of the premenstrual symptoms, especially breast tenderness and can also be used for painful periods. This is taken four to six capsules per day. A good all-around vitamin and mineral is also an asset, especially for its B vitamin content to help balance the use of extra B6.[8]

APPLICATIONS IN AUTISM

Autism, the cause of which is unknown, is a child's inability from birth—or a loss of the ability within the first 30 months of life—to develop normal human relationships with anybody, even with parents, according to *The American Medical Association Family Medical Guide*. Although the symptoms of autism vary greatly, they follow a general pattern.[9]

"As a baby the autistic child will have difficulty with feeding and toilet training," the Guide reported. "He or she will not give, or will cease to give, smiling recognition to the parent's face. It will become increasingly apparent that the child lives in a world of his or her own. Speech, facial expressions, or any other form of communication are absent or unintelligible. In some cases a few words are spoken, but are repeated interminably for no apparent reason."

An autistic child makes no distinction among people, other living things, and inanimate objects, and treats them all in the same way. He or she cannot evaluate situations, and so reacts inappropriately to them. For example, the child may become fiercely agitated if the furniture is rearranged in the home or if he or she is taken into new but harmless surroundings, but the same child may also run across a dangerously busy road without any sign of fear.

"By not communicating," the Guide reported, "the autistic child remains isolated from other family members. Such children behave unpredictably. They may be violent one moment, and then sit completely still, in some strange position, for hours on end. Autistic children may adopt strange postures and mannerisms that can unsettle those around them. And although an autistic child may have normal intelligence, he or she may give the impression of being subnormal, or in some cases deaf."[9]

The dynamic duo of magnesium-vitamin B6 has been useful in treating some autistic children. For example, writing in *Developmental Medicine and Child Neu-*

rology, J. Martineau and colleagues in France discussed a study of 12 autistic children, ranging in age from four to 10. Six of them received 30 milligrams per kilogram of body weight per day of pyridoxine chlorhydrate and 10 mg/kg/day of magnesium lactate. The other six received the drug fenfluramine in a double-blind trial. Electrophysiologic evaluations were done on the children, and the researchers reported that the auditory evoked responses in those receiving B6-magnesium showed a significant increase. The research team noted that other studies have shown the two nutrients produce an overall improvement in autistic children. They concluded by saying that 15 percent of autistic children will respond to B6-magnesium therapy and that 30 percent may have mildly positive effects.[10]

In an earlier study, the same French researchers did another double-blind study, which consisted of giving 60 autistic children either vitamin B6 alone, magnesium alone, or the B6-magnesium combination. They recorded that behavioral improvement was observed only when the children got the B6-magnesium combination.[11]

Writing in the *Journal of Orthomolecular Psychiatry* in 1984, M. Marlow, et al., reported that hair analysis of 28 autistic children showed that magnesium levels were lower than those of 18 controls, including siblings, and that the mineral was the main element that statistically distinguished the two groups.[12]

Bernard Rimland, Ph.D., of the Autism Research Institute in San Diego, California, studied 4,000 questionnaires that were completed by parents of autistic children, beginning in 1967. He reported that the use of B6-magnesium was rated beneficial by 43 percent of 318 parents, although 5 percent said this therapy made the children worse. Twenty-nine percent of the children were helped with the drug deanol, while 16 percent were made worse, according to 121 parents. Twenty-nine percent of the parents said that the drug fenfluramine was effective, although 19 percent said it made their children worse. Rimland concluded that, while many practitioners overlook the possible benefits of B6-magnesium in treating autistic children, there is considerable support for recommending the two nutrients for reducing the severity of autistic symptoms.[13]

Although the case history is anecdotal, a letter to *Autism Research Review International* reported that B6-magnesium and dimethylglycine brought an improvement to an older patient who was nonverbal and who would flip the visors in parked cars as she walked by; she would move office desks; and she would throw items in inappropriate places. When this behavior was brought to her attention, she would scream, bite and stamp her feet. With the above therapy, she is accepting criticism more easily, and her speech pathologist has become very excited about her progress, both verbally and gesturally.[14]

At the University of Missouri's 22nd Annual Conference on Trace Substances in Environmental Health, held May 24–26, 1988 in St. Louis, Mildred S. Seelig, M.D., said that she is convinced that between 80 and 90 percent of the American population is deficient in magnesium. She added that the data suggest that many people are facing serious consequences from a preventable magnesium deficiency—including death—and that this deficiency is often "silent until it is severe." Those especially at risk of severe magnesium deficiency include alcoholics and those taking medications that interfere with the absorption of the mineral or speed up its excretion. These drugs include diuretics, digitalis and other heart drugs, antibiotics and some anticancer drugs. And stress of any kind, whether psychological or physical, tends to increase the requirements for magnesium.

Seelig went on to say that our diet rich in sugar, fat and phosphate increases our need for magnesium, and yet we often supplement our diet with calcemic agents such as vitamin D and calcium without realizing the impact this may have on an already magnesium-deficient intake. Many physicians are accustomed to giving magnesium as the "drug of choice" to correct convulsions near the end of a pregnancy. And the mineral is gaining recognition as a safe way of controlling irregular heartbeats. Either of these life-threatening conditions is often associated with a severe magnesium deficiency. The roles of magnesium in numerous enzyme systems have been spelled out by numerous researchers, and yet the clinical ramifications of a magnesium deficiency on metabolic processes dependent on magnesium-dependent enzymes are virtually unexplored. And this applies to disorders that are caused by dependencies on vitamins that require magnesium as a cofactor, Seelig said.

"Cardiovascular, kidney and bone lesions—to which a magnesium deficiency contributes—are recognized in experimental models," Seelig added. "Requiring further study is the possibility that a magnesium deficiency can contribute to such clinical diseases as high blood pressure, arteriosclerosis, myocardial infarction, kidney stones and possibly several bone diseases that resemble lesions caused by a magnesium deficiency alone or in combination with excesses of other nutrients."

DEFICIENCY DANGEROUS DURING PREGNANCY

Kenneth Weaver, an obstetrical researcher at East Tennessee State College of Medicine, Johnson City, another speaker, discussed his studies with sheep and human beings, which show that a deficiency in magnesium during pregnancy can bring on not only migraines and pregnancy-associated high blood pressure, but also babies with low birth weight, miscarriages and stillbirths. Conversely, "magnesium supplements can dramatically reduce the incidence of these events."

Although magnesium is available in a variety of foods, it is difficult to get the RDA from food alone. He added that, "If I were to name just one thing I'd supplement everybody with, it would probably be magnesium."

According to Weaver's data, a deficiency in magnesium can provoke spasms in blood vessels. With this, blood platelets can become a problem by plugging up some of the small blood vessels in the placenta and in the mother's body. Contributing to the problem is the fact that phosphates, widely available in soft drinks, bind magnesium in the bowel and prevent its absorption. A 12-ounce can of carbonated soft drink, he added, which might contain 30 milligrams of phosphate, might easily eliminate an equivalent amount of magnesium from the diet.

Another speaker, Ruth Schwartz, of Cornell University, Ithaca, New York, said that the effects of low magnesium levels include reduced bone growth and maturation, brittleness and reduced breaking strength, as well as interference with the removal of old bone tissue. She added that, "which abnormalities occur or predominate apparently depends on the length and severity of magnesium depletion, the age and species being depleted and other dietary constituents such as the level of calcium."

Burton M. Altura, Ph.D., and Bella T. Altura, Ph.D., from the State University of New York in Brooklyn, told the conference that considerable experimental and clinical evidence indicates that magnesium deficiencies have probably been overlooked as important causal factors in the development of high blood pressure, hardening of the arteries and disorders of the blood vessels.

"On the basis of epidemiologic and experimental findings," the Alturas said, "we and others have suggested that there is an association between the dietary intake of magnesium (and errors in the magnesium metabolism and distribution of magnesium in the body), the concentration of this element in the myocardium (heart muscle) and blood vessels, and the risk of development of cardiac arrhythmias, sudden death ischemic heart disease (caused by insufficient blood flow), high blood pressure, transient ischemic (TIAs) attacks or little strokes, strokes and pre-eclampsia (a serious disorder near the end of a pregnancy which threatens both the fetus and the mother). A deficiency in magnesium leads to the constriction of numerous blood vessels as well as reducing the amount of oxygen in the blood."[15]

AIDS IN ASTHMA TREATMENT

A deficiency in magnesium and vitamin B6 may be related to asthma, according to Gershon M. Lesser, M.D., a Los Angeles physician, in his book, *Growing Younger*.[16]

"While it is in no way a cure or even a total treatment for asthma," Lesser said, "testing to date confirms that elevated amounts of B6 intake can decrease the occurrence, duration and intensity of attacks in the asthmatics studied. Another current finding . . . is the role of magnesium in the onset and treatment of asthma. The study, reported in the *Journal of the American Medical Association*, said that, 'Lower magnesium uptake or a deficiency in this mineral may play a role in some types of asthma, and may therefore be useful as a supplementary therapy in controlling bronchial asthma.' "[16]

As "rejuvenation insurance," Lesser recommends 100 mg/day of vitamin B6, a B-complex supplement, and 500 mg of magnesium in the morning and 500 mg in the evening. He added that many people fail to realize that magnesium is dependent on calcium, vitamin C and protein for its absorption.[16]

Magnesium-aspartate hydrochloride and magnesium sulfate were given to a number of asthmatic patients in Switzerland and the United States, and the researchers concluded that magnesium therapy is a beneficial adjunctive treatment in severe asthma.[17,18]

In an article in the *Journal of the American Dietetic Association*, Jean Pennington, Ph.D., from the Food and Drug Administration in Washington, D.C., said that many Americans continue to consume inadequate diets. The Total Diet Study, which ran from 1982 to 1989, tabulated the intakes of various minerals among eight age-sex-matched groups, and compared these intakes with the Recommended Dietary Allowances. The results showed that most Americans consume too much sodium and not enough copper; teenage girls are getting inadequate amounts of calcium, magnesium, iron and manganese; adult women consume below level amounts of calcium, magnesium, iron and zinc; toddlers' diets were deficient in calcium and zinc; teenage boys and older men were not getting enough magnesium.[19]

Nocturnal leg cramps, which can be very painful, are often caused by your prescription drugs, according to Robert M. Giller, M.D., in *Natural Prescriptions*. As an example, diuretics taken for high blood pressure or heart disorders can cause an imbalance of your potassium and magnesium levels. However, the most common cause of nocturnal leg cramps is a calcium deficiency, he said. If neither calcium nor vitamin E gives you relief, Giller recommends magnesium, potassium or vitamin A.

"Because as it has been shown that sugar and caffeine reduce the absorption of vitamins and minerals, particularly calcium, I advise patients with cramping problems to eliminate as much sugar and caffeine from their diets as possible," Giller added.[20]

Research by Gustawa Stendig-Lindberg, Ph.D., of the Department of Physiology and Pharmacology in Tel Aviv University's Sackler School of Medicine and her colleagues has shown, in a sample of 19- to 50-year-old Israelis otherwise considered healthy, a clear magnesium deficiency in 25 percent of the women and eight percent of the men, and a marginal deficiency in the remainder. All of the 70 individuals showed a fluctuation in their magnesium levels, which the professor had only previously observed in ill patients in a study she conducted in Sweden. She believed that this phenomenon reflects the presence of intracellular magnesium deficiency, which is probably the result of living in Israel's hot climate, under the stress that its citizens have come to expect daily.

Working with Prof. Yair Shapira and other Israeli researchers, and Prof. Warren Worker at Harvard University, Stendig-Lindberg has found that strenuous exertion gives rise to persistent magnesium deficiency in young, highly trained, healthy young men eating an average Israeli diet. She added that almost everyone in Israel—especially those engaged in strenuous physical activity—would benefit from taking a magnesium supplement. A supplement is especially indicated for Israelis undergoing strenuous exertion with heat exposure. She added that sudden drops in the magnesium level can be dangerous, because of the risk of occurrences of life-threatening cardiac arrhythmias, or spasm of the coronary arteries.[21] (Although she did not go into this, one wonders if a magnesium deficiency might explain the sudden deaths of athletes while running marathons, playing basketball and football, etc.)

Mildred S. Seelig, M.D., made this observation in an article in the *Journal of the American College of Nutrition*. She reported that stress can release catecholamines and corticosteroids which, along with a magnesium deficiency, may increase the risk of sudden cardiac death. During stress, she added, free fatty acids, which are released by lipolytic effects of catecholamines, inactivate magnesium. These hormones step up the plasma calcium-magnesium ratio, which can increase the risk of intravascular coagulation and arrhythmias, as well as stimulate catecholamine secretion by the adrenal medulla and the myocardium. With marginal magnesium status, she added, athletes undergoing exhausting physical exertion can develop induced magnesium loss, which brings on muscle cramps and impaired performance and endurance. Younger athletes may be more at risk, she said, because they need magnesium for development and growth.[22]

In an article in *Clinical Nutrition*, I. B. Hessov, M.D., Ph.D., a Danish researcher, said that four out of nine patients with Crohn's disease that he studied were deficient in magnesium. And in evaluating 58 patients with ileal reactions from Crohn's disease, it was found that skeletal muscle deficiency was often found in spite of normal serum values.[23] (Crohn's disease, or regional ileitis, is a chronic inflammation of part of the digestive tract. If the disease continues for years, it can cause a gradual deterioration of bowel functioning, causing peritonitis and malabsorption of nutrients.)

Magnesium depletion was recorded in 21 of 25 patients with Crohn's disease, according to R. I. Russell in the *Journal of the American College of Nutrition*. Fifteen of the patients required intravenous nutrition. Following discharge from the hospital, five patients, who had received IV feedings, complained of muscle cramps, tetany and bone pain and were found to have low blood levels of magnesium over several months.[24]

A magnesium deficiency is prevalent in patients with diabetes mellitus, which can result in increased risk for cardiac arrhythmias, high blood pressure, myocardial infarction and altered glucose metabolism, according to Robert K. Rude, M.D., in *Postgraduate Medicine*. The association between low magnesium levels and diabetes has been documented as early as 1946. For diabetics with a magnesium deficiency, oral doses of 300 mg of elemental magnesium can be given, but doses gradually increased up to 600 mg/day may be required to achieve a therapeutic effect. To avoid diarrhea, divided doses are suggested. For those with impaired kidney function, magnesium therapy should be used with caution, he added.[25]

Researchers from the University of Naples, in Italy, reported in the *American Journal of Clinical Nutrition* that age-related depletion of magnesium from red blood cells might be responsible for impaired glucose tolerance in older people, and that correcting the magnesium deficiency could improve glucose handling. Magnesium supplementation increased the amount of the mineral in red blood cells and improved insulin response and action.[26]

A daily dose of magnesium may help to lower blood pressure in hypertensive people with Type II diabetes, the glucose-processing disorder that generally strikes after the age of 40 and is usually controlled without insulin, according to the September 22, 1990 issue of *Science News*.

Samuel A. Malayan of the University of Southern California in Los Angeles and colleagues stated that, compared to healthy nondiabetics, Type II diabetics with high blood pressure had lower magnesium levels in their red blood cells.

"In the new study, the California team gave seven hypertensive diabetics 260 mg/day of magnesium chloride," the publication reported. "After six weeks, blood pressure levels among these volunteers dropped from a starting average of 157/96 millimeters of mercury (mmHg) to just 128/77. Physicians consider a reading of less than 140/90 normal and a sign of healthy vessels."

Malayan added that the findings suggest that some non-insulin dependent diabetics may control their high blood pressure with magnesium supplements or a diet rich in the mineral. However, Jerry Nadler of the City of Hope Medical Center in Duarte, California, a coauthor of the study, added that people with diabetes can experience kidney failure, resulting in high blood levels of magnesium. He, therefore, suggests that diabetics should consult their physicians before taking magnesium supplements.[27]

CHRONIC FATIGUE SYNDROME

Researchers at the University of Southampton in England reported in *Lancet* in 1991 that patients with chronic fatigue syndrome often have low blood levels of magnesium and that they respond favorably to magnesium supplementation. The research team said that, in a case-controlled study, 20 patients with CFS had lower red blood cell levels of the mineral than did healthy, matched controls. And in a clinical trial involving 32 patients with CFS, intramuscular injections of magnesium sulfate or a placebo every six weeks revealed a marked improvement of symptoms in the magnesium-treated volunteers. They reported improved energy levels, better emotional states and less pain than did the controls. Other investigators have found that magnesium is often useful in treating anxiety, insomnia and organic mental disorders. A symptom of magnesium deficiency is psychiatric disturbance.[28]

OSTEOPOROSIS

At the 5th annual meeting of the American Society for Magnesium Research, which was held September 25–26, 1989 in Norfolk, Virginia, in conjunction with the 30th annual meeting of the American College of Nutrition, 40 papers were read dealing with the importance of magnesium to human and animal health. Mildred S. Seelig, M.D., told the conference that postmenopausal women and alcoholics are especially prone to osteoporosis because of a magnesium deficiency that is due to either poor absorption of the mineral or excess urinary losses. She added that women who are at risk in developing osteoporosis, who are being given estrogen and calcium supplements, should have blood magnesium and coagulation monitored, especially since calcium and magnesium can be antagonists.

"Estrogen causes a shift of magnesium from serum to soft and hard tissues, including bone, with the result that it lowers serum magnesium, especially in those with poor magnesium intake," she said. "Postmenopausal women treated with replacement estrogens to prevent or arrest progression of bone wasting, who also take excess calcium, may be at risk of thromboembolic events. Increasing magnesium intake—which is needed for formation of bone matrix—is a safe means of reducing the risk of intravascular coagulation."[29]

MUSCLE HEALTH AND SPORTS

Patricia A. Deuster, Ph.D., of the Human Performance Laboratory, University of the Health Sciences, Bethesda, Maryland, reported that, since magnesium is the second most abundant intracellular cation in the body, it plays an essential role in muscle metabolism, muscle cell permeability and muscle contractibility. These critical functions, she added, indicate the importance of magnesium in sports medicine and also suggest that either a dietary deficiency of magnesium or supplemental magnesium may influence exercise performance.

Another speaker, Howard S. Friedman, M.D., Professor of Medicine at the Medical School of SUNY Downstate, and Chief of Cardiology at Brooklyn Hospital in New York, said that potent diuretics, which are sometimes given to patients with advanced congestive heart failure, can cause a magnesium deficiency with the resulting ominous consequences. He added that magnesium is also useful as adjunct therapy when vasodilators are administered to heart patients. Vasodilators are drugs that cause blood vessels to dilate, thus increasing the flow of blood. He added that, "the significance of magnesium deficiency states in congestive heart failure has not only become increasingly evident, but a role for magnesium as a pharmacological agent in the treatment of this disorder has begun to emerge."

Added Lloyd T. Iseri, M.D., Emeritus Professor of Medicine, University of California at Irvine, magnesium should be considered in the treatment and prevention of most tachyarrhythmias (irregular heartbeats).

Magnesium is used to offset the side effects of sodium fluoride in the treatment of osteoporosis, according to K. J. Muenzenberg, M.D., and colleagues at the Orthopedics University Clinic in Bonn, Germany. For the past 20 years, they have been giving 20 mg of sodium fluoride daily to patients being treated with osteoporosis. A common side effect is arthralgia or severe joint pain. During the past 15 years, they have added magnesium, in doses of 400 to 600 mg/day to the fluoride treatment and have observed fewer adverse affects.

X. Y. Yang, M.D., and colleagues at the National Institutes of Health, Bethesda, Maryland, have observed that Type I (insulin dependent) diabetics have significantly lower blood levels of magnesium, while Type II patients had a significantly increased excretion of the mineral in the urine when compared to controls.[29]

TABLE 19.1

MAGNESIUM IN ONE SERVING OF FOODS
100 GRAMS OR ABOUT ¼ POUND

	MILLIGRAMS		MILLIGRAMS
Almonds	270	Molasses (blackstrap)	50
Apricots, raw	62	Oats, whole grain	169
Asparagus, raw	20	Peanuts	206
Banana, raw	33	Peanut butter (⅓ cup)	82
Barley, whole grain	124	Peanut flour	360
Beans, lima	67	Peas	35
Beets	25	Pecans	142
Beet greens	106	Pistachios	158
Brazil nuts	225	Rice, brown	88
Brussels sprouts	29	Rye flour	73
Cashew nuts	267	Sesame seeds	181
Chard, Swiss	65	Soybeans	265
Corn, fresh	147	Soybean flour, defatted	310
Cottonseed flour	650	Walnuts	190
Cowpeas (blackeyed)	55	Wheat bran	490
Dandelion greens	36	Wheat germ	336
Filberts	184	Whey, dried	130
Lentils	80	Yeast, brewer's	231
Millet	162		

From *Minerals: Kill or Cure?* by Ruth Adams and Frank Murray. New York: Larchmont Books, 1974.

REFERENCES

1. Hendler, Sheldon Saul, M.D., Ph.D. *The Doctors' Vitamin and Mineral Encyclopedia.* New York: Simon and Schuster, 1990, pp. 157ff.
2. Gershoff, S. F., and Prien, E. L. "Effect of Daily Magnesium Oxide and Vitamin B6 Administration to Patients with Recurring Calcium Oxalate Kidney Stones," *American Journal of Clinical Nutrition* 20(5):393–399, May 1967.
3. Prien, E. L., and Gershoff, S. F. "Magnesium Oxide-Pyridoxine Therapy for Recurrent Calcium Oxalate Calculi," *Journal of Urology* 112(16):509–512, October 1974.
4. Giller, Robert M., M.D., and Matthews, Kathy. *Natural Prescriptions.* New York: Carol Southern Books, 1994, pp. 227ff.
5. "Magnesium: The Misunderstood Mineral." Seminar held May 19, 1994 at the New York Academy of Sciences, New York City.
6. Mahaffee, D., et al. "Magnesium Promotes Both Parathyroid Hormone Secretion and Adenosine 3',5'-monophosphate Production in Rat Parathyroid Tissues and Reverses the Inhibitory Effects of Calcium on Adenylate Cyclase," *Endocrinology* 110:487–495, 1982.
7. Hunt, Douglas, M.D. *No More Fears.* New York: Warner Books, 1988, p. 149.
8. Dean, Carolyn, M.D. *Dr. Carolyn Dean's Complementary Natural Prescriptions for Common Ailments.* New Canaan, Conn.: Keats Publishing Inc., 1994, p. 135.
9. Kunz, Jeffrey R. M., M.D., editor-in-chief. *The American Medical Association Family Medical Guide.* New York: Random House, 1982, p. 672.
10. Martineau, J., et al. "Electrophysiological Effects of Fenfluramine or Combined Vitamin B6 and Magnesium on Children with Autistic Behavior," *Developmental Medicine and Child Neurology* 31:721–727, 1989.
11. Martineau, J., et al. "Vitamin B6, Magnesium, and Combined B6-Magnesium Therapeutic Effects in Childhood Autism," *Biol. Psychiat.* 20:467–478, 1985.
12. Marlow, M., et al. "Decreased Magnesium in the Hair of Autistic Children," *J. Orthomol. Psychiat.* 13(2):117–122, 1984.
13. Rimland, B. "Controversies in the Treatment of Autistic Children: Vitamin and Drug Therapy," *J. Child Nev.* 3:568–572, 1988.
14. Campbell, Stephanie. "Vitamin B6," *Autism Research Review International* 5(4):7, 1991.
15. Abstracts from the University of Missouri's 22nd Annual Conference on Trace Substances in Environmental Health, May 24–26, 1988, Clarion Hotel, St. Louis, Missouri.
16. Lesser, Gershon M., M.D. *Growing Younger.* Los Angeles: Jeremy P. Tarcher, Inc., 1987, pp. 130ff.
17. Hauser, S. P. "Intravenous Magnesium for Bronchial Asthma," *Schweiz. Med. Wschr.* 119(46):1633–1635, 1989.
18. Skobeloff, Emil M., et al. "Intravenous Magnesium Sulfate for the Treatment of Acute

Asthma in the Emergency Department," *Journal of the American Medical Association* 262(9):1210–1213, September 1, 1989.

19. Pennington, J., and Young, B. "Total Diet Study Nutritional Elements," *Journal of the American Dietetic Association* 91:179–183, 1991.

20. Giller, Robert M., and Matthews, Kathy. *Natural Prescriptions*. New York: Carol Southern Books, 1994, pp. 234–235.

21. Cook, Carol. "Magnesium Deficiency May Be Giving Israelis a Headache," *Tel Aviv University Press Release*, September 1, 1987.

22. Seelig, M. S., M.D. "Adverse Stress Reactions and Magnesium Deficiency: Preventive and Therapeutic Implications," *Journal of the American College of Nutrition* 11(5):609/ Abstract 40, October 1992.

23. Hessov, I. B., M.D., Ph.D. "Magnesium Deficiency in Crohn's Disease," *Clinical Nutrition* 9:297–298, 1990.

24. Russell, R. I. "Magnesium Requirements in Patients with Chronic Inflammatory Disease Receiving Intravenous Nutrition," *Journal of the American College of Nutrition* 4(5):553–558, 1985.

25. Rude, Robert K., M.D. "Magnesium Deficiency and Diabetes Mellitus: Causes and Effects," *Postgraduate Medicine* 92(5):217–223, October 1992.

26. Paolisso, G., et al. "Daily Magnesium Supplements Improve Glucose Handling in Elderly Subjects," *American Journal of Clinical Nutrition* 55: 1161–1167, 1992.

27. "Magnesium Eases Diabetic Blood Pressure," *Science News*, September 22, 1990, p. 189.

28. Cox, I., et al. "Red Blood Cell Magnesium and Chronic Fatigue Syndrome," *Lancet* 337:757–760, 1991.

29. Abstracts from papers read at the 5th Annual Meeting of the American Society for Magnesium Research, and 30th Annual Meeting of the American College of Nutrition, September 25–26, 1989, Norfolk, Virginia.

20

Phosphorus Helps Keep Calcium Honest

ALTHOUGH phosphorus is an important mineral for keeping us healthy, we generally pay about as much attention to it as Einstein's Theory of Relativity. That is because phosphorus is available in so many foods. It is especially important for combining with calcium to produce healthy, strong bones and teeth.

Phosphorus, a nonmetallic element, was initially identified in urine by Hennig Brand, a German alchemist, in 1669. It created quite a stir because, in its unnatural free form, it glowed in the dark and took fire spontaneously upon exposure to the air. As white phosphorus, it is the flame of incendiary bombs, and as red phosphorus, it's the heart of the common match. As organic phosphate, it's nerve gas and insecticides; as organic combinations, it's a constituent of every cell and fluid of the body. Without this mineral, no cell can divide, the heart cannot beat and a baby cannot grow.

LINKED TO CALCIUM

Phosphorus and calcium are so closely related that a deficiency or an overabundance of one may interfere with the utilization of the other. Both minerals are found in the same major food source—milk. In addition to building bones and teeth, the two minerals are related to vitamin D in the absorption process; they are regulated metabolically by the parathyroid hormone and calcitonin; they exist in the blood serum in a definite ratio to each other; and both, as the main components of bone ash, were used in many ancient medieval remedies.

"Phosphorus comprises about one percent or 1.4 pound (650 grams) of the adult body weight," the *Foods and Nutrition Encyclopedia* said. "That's about one-fourth the total mineral matter in the body. Eighty percent of the phosphorus is in the skeleton (including the teeth) in inorganic combination with calcium, where the proportion of calcium to phosphorus is about 2:1. The remaining 20 percent is distributed in the soft tissues, in organic combination, where the amount of phosphorus is much higher than calcium."[1]

In the soft tissues, phosphorus is found in every living cell, where it is an essential component in interrelationships with proteins, fats and carbohydrates to produce energy, to build and repair tissues and to serve as a buffer. Whole blood contains between 35 to 45 milligrams of phosphorus per 100 milliliters. Of this amount, about one-half is found in red cells. In adults, 2.5 to 4.5 mg/100 ml is in the serum. But in children, the blood phosphorus level is a little higher, ranging from 4 to 7 mg/100 ml. Between 4 to 9 milligrams of the whole blood phosphorus is inorganic phosphorus, which is affected by dietary intake and is in constant exchange with the organic phosphate of the blood. According to the encyclopedia:

> Since much of the phosphorus in foods occurs as a phosphate compound, the first step—prior to absorption—is the splitting off of phosphorus for absorption as the free mineral. The phosphorus is then absorbed as inorganic salts. Phosphorus is absorbed chiefly in the upper small intestine, the duodenum. The amount absorbed is dependent on several factors, such as source, calcium-phosphorus ratio, intestinal pH, lactose intake and dietary levels of calcium, phosphorus, vitamin D, iron, aluminum, manganese, potassium and fat. As is the case for most nutrients, the greater the need, the more efficient the absorption. Absorption increases, although not proportionally, with increased intake.[1]

About 70 percent of the phosphorus ingested in foods is generally absorbed, reported *The Heinz Handbook of Nutrition*. It is believed that intestinal phosphatases liberate simple phosphorus compounds from the ingesta before absorption takes place. As with calcium, absorption takes place in an acid medium. Excesses of iron, aluminum and magnesium interfere with phosphorus absorption through the formation of insoluble phosphates. For optimum absorption of calcium and phosphorus, both minerals should be supplied by the food in about equal amounts. But an abnormal calcium-phosphorus ratio in food interferes with the absorption of both and may result in a calcium deficiency. As is the case with calcium, the absorption of phosphorus is enhanced when vitamin D is available.[2] (The calcium-phosphorus ratio is still being debated by nutritionists. It is variously reported as 1:1, 1:1.5, 1:2, etc.)

"Phosphorus in the feces represents both the unabsorbed mineral and phosphorus secreted into the intestinal tract," the handbook reported. "Urinary phosphorus is principally inorganic phosphate; the amount fluctuates with the quantity absorbed from foods. Catabolism of body tissues during starvation releases much phosphorus into the urine. In individuals with a constant phosphorus intake, intense carbohydrate metabolism, which requires phosphorus, tends to decrease urinary phosphorus temporarily."[2]

The daily intake of phosphorus in the American diet, mainly in the form of phosphate, ranges between 800 and 1,500 milligrams, according to Sheldon Saul Hendler, M.D., Ph.D., in *The Doctors' Vitamin and Mineral Encyclopedia*. Milk and its products are the richest sources of dietary phosphorus, but phosphorus is also available in other foods, such as fish, meat, poultry, vegetables, eggs, etc. The major dietary form of phosphorus is inorganic phosphate, but phosphorus is also found in organic, that is, bound to carbon, forms such as lecithin.[3] (For the calcium and phosphorus content of some common foods, refer to Table 20.2.)

"Phosphorus deficiency can and does occur," Hendler said. "One can predict that the symptoms of such deficiency would affect all of the body's systems, since even mild phosphate deficiency leads to a decrease in the production of energy. Feeling easily fatigued, weak and having a decreased attention span could be symptoms of mild phosphate deficiency. Severe phosphate deficiency could produce seizures, coma, even death. Phosphate deficiency typically requires intensive medical management."

WHO IS AT RISK?

Hendler added that those at risk for phosphate depletion include:

- Patients being treated for diabetic ketoacidosis;
- Patients with urinary losses of phosphate due to malfunction of certain kidney structures;
- Those with gastrointestinal malabsorption syndromes, such as Crohn's disease, celiac disease, short bowel syndrome and radiation damage of the small intestine;
- Those who are starving; and
- Those with acute and chronic alcoholism, along with alcoholics admitted to the hospital for treatment of acute alcoholism or alcohol withdrawal and given intravenous fluids which don't contain phosphate.

"Many antacids, which are widely used for treatment of peptic ulcer disease, gastritis (heartburn) and acid reflux, contain magnesium and aluminum, both of which bind to phosphate, preventing its absorption into the body," Hendler added. "Several cases have been reported which describe severe phosphate depletion in people who have used these antacids between two and 12 years. An alcoholic who uses such antacids would certainly increase his or her vulnerability to phosphate deficiency."

Those with a mild phosphate deficiency may profit by taking one gram daily of supplementary phosphate, but this should be done under a physician's supervision, Hendler continued. Although there are several vitamin-mineral formulations on the market which contain phosphate, calcium, iron and other minerals and vitamins, Hendler does not recommend them since, he said, calcium phosphate may impair the absorption of other minerals, such as iron.[3]

While on the subject of antacids, in a study of 11 patients at the Veterans Administration Hospital in Hines, Illinois, Herta Spencer, M.D., reported that antacids caused a 75-percent loss of phosphorus in the patients' stools compared to the normal level of 25 percent, reported Mark Bricklin in *The Practical Encyclopedia of Natural Healing*. The patients also absorbed up to 20 times less fluoride.[4]

In addition, Spencer reported, long-term consumption of antacids may seriously deplete calcium stores, resulting in thinning of the bones and possible bone pain. In laboratory experiments, she found that relatively small amounts of one widely sold antacid caused a loss of about 130 mg/day of calcium. Another product caused twice this level of calcium loss.

"Adding weight to these findings," Bricklin said, "was the case of a 48-year-old man who had 'marked demineralization of the skeleton, probably a mixture of osteoporosis and osteomalacia,' but who had 'none of the usual causes of osteoporosis.' What he did have was a history of having taken aluminum-containing antacids for 10 to 12 years."[4]

Writing in *Psychosomatics* in 1981, W. L. Webb and M. Gehi reported that low levels of phosphorus are associated with irritability, apprehension, numbness, tingling sensations and weakness.[5]

Carlton Fredericks, Ph.D., and Herbert Bailey reported in *Food Facts and Fallacies*

It has long been known by biochemists that vitamin E is involved in the processes—almost miraculous as they are—by which the heart derives energy from food. The actual chemistry has been set up at least on a hypothetical basis. The body produces a substance called adenylic acid, which has an affinity for phosphorus. The body then proceeds to form from adenylic acid three phosphorus compounds. These compounds are somewhat analogous to the phosphorus compounds formerly used in the manufacture of matches. Like the head of a match, they carry within them potential energy. The heart, by breaking down these phosphorus compounds, releases this latent energy, obtains the fuel it needs and proceeds to rebuild the compound. Some biochemists theorize that it is impossible for these phosphorus compounds to be manufactured from the adenylic acid unless two vitamins are present. One of these is vitamin E; the other is inositol, a B-complex substance.[6]

Many enzymes and the B vitamins are activated only in the presence of phosphorus, according to Robert H. Garrison, Jr., M.A., R.Ph., and Elizabeth Somer, M.A., R.D., in *The Nutrition Desk Reference*. Therefore, the oxidation of carbohydrates, proteins and fats leading to the formation of adenosine triphosphate (ATP) requires phosphorus. (ATP is the energy that activates heartbeat, muscle contraction, the activity of the nervous system among other things.)

"The phospholipids (such as lecithin) contain phosphorus in their structure," Garrison and Somer continued. "These lipids carry fats in watery mediums and form the part of cell membranes responsible for transporting nutrients in and out of the cell."[7]

In an article in *Nutrition Reviews* in 1984, M. Parrot-Garcia and D. A. McCarron reported that low dietary calcium to phosphorus ratios are associated with high blood pressure.[8]

Evelyn P. Whitlock, M.D., who is in private practice in Portland, Oregon, said in *Health News and Review* that childhood and teenage years are the most critical in building a healthy skeletal mass. She said that diet surveys show that many teenage girls are favoring soft drinks (high in phosphorus) over milk, thus paving the way for virtually all of the women of the next generation to develop osteoporosis. As we have learned, a high-phosphorus diet depletes calcium stores.[9]

Researchers reported in *Nutrition Reports International* in 1986 that the treatment of osteoporosis may be fruitless as long as the calcium-to-phosphorus ratios are greater than 1:1.25. The study involved 158 females, ranging in age from 20 to 75, whose average calcium intake was only 600 mg/day.[10]

Jennifer Jowsey, M.D., of the Mayo Clinic, told a meeting of the California Dairy Council in 1976 that the average American diet, high in phosphorus and low in calcium, almost guarantees osteoporosis later in life.

"Americans in general tend to decrease their intake of calcium as they get older," Jowsey said. "However, the shift from big meals to snack foods has caused phosphorus intake to go up and calcium intake to go down in the United States."

Jowsey went on to say that when there is an abnormal absorption of calcium in the stomach and intestines, or when too much calcium is lost in the kidneys, the skeleton provides the only source of calcium. Bone tissue is therefore borrowed (resorbed) to put more calcium in the blood. And the same thing happens when the diet is too high in phosphorus without enough calcium to balance it.

Michael B. Miller, M.D. said that immobilization, such as in patients in rest homes and nursing homes, results in losses of calcium, phosphorus, potassium and other minerals in urine and feces.

It is well known that circulatory troubles also increase during bed rest, for the simple reason that the valves in the legs do not function properly unless one is up and about. Walking purposefully and briskly is the best way to keep these valves pumping blood along the blood vessels in the leg so that it does not accumulate, become sluggish and clot. The additional loss of so many minerals from bones compounds the health problems.

Prolonged immobilization affects the personality and social outlook of the bedridden patient, Miller pointed out. He discussed the cases of six elderly women who were put to bed in a nursing home because of broken hips, heart disorders, infections, amputations and so forth. After four weeks of immobilization, the women had apparently decided they were dying and began to behave appropriately. Although there was no measurable evidence of any damage to legs or nerves, they began to act irrationally, refusing to eat, to stand, etc. Fortunately, this syndrome is reversible, Miller said, and the old people can be rehabilitated.[11]

Sugar Interferes with Bone Formation

Marshall Ringsdorf, M.D., of the University of Alabama said that, for at least two hours after you have eaten two to four ounces of sugar, the phosphorus in your blood decreases from about three and one-half or four milligrams percent down to about one and one-half milligrams percent. This means that for about two hours after this much sugar is eaten, there is often so little phosphorus in the blood that calcification or bone formation cannot take place. Bone is constantly being replaced and reformed, so that in those whose sugar consumption creates a negative balance of phosphorus, destruction of bone may exceed bone formation for two to five hours every day. This is part of the problem of osteoporosis, both in the mouth and in the rest of the body, Ringsdorf said.[11] (The first signs of osteoporosis often appear when the jawbone begins to lose calcium and teeth begin to loosen and fall out.)

In the U.S. Department of Agriculture longitudinal surveys, which were conducted between 1971 and 1979, it was reported that, beyond the ages of 19 to 22, the daily calcium intake of 3,438 women fell from 800 to 500 mg/day, while the consumption of phosphorus remained at about 1,000 mg/day. This resulted in a calcium-to-phosphorus ratio of 1:1.4 to 1:1.8.[12]

As we know, excess phosphorus in the diet (meat, grains, soft drinks, etc.) results in impaired calcium absorption. In several studies, it has been suggested that periodontal disease is a result of a decreased calcium-phosphorus ratio, which causes secondary hyper-parathyroidism in order to maintain normal blood calcium levels.[13]

TABLE 20.1

THE RECOMMENDED DIETARY ALLOWANCES FOR PHOSPHORUS

AGE AND CATEGORY	MILLIGRAMS OF PHOSPHORUS, DAILY
Infants, to six months	300 mg
Infants, six months to one year	500 mg
Children, 1 to 10	800 mg
Males, 11 to 24	1,200 mg
Males, 25 and over	800 mg
Females, 11 to 24	1,200 mg
Females, 25 and over	800 mg
Pregnant women	1,200 mg
Breast-feeding women	1,200 mg

From *Recommended Dietary Allowances*, 10th Edition. Washington, D.C.: National Academy Press, 1989.

Table 20.2

CALCIUM AND PHOSPHORUS CONTENT
OF SOME COMMON FOODS

Food	Milligrams of Calcium in One Serving	Milligrams of Phosphorus in One Serving
Whole liquid milk	285 in 1 cup	230 in 1 cup
Milk, powdered, skim	520 in ½ cup	850 in ½ cup
American cheese	133 in 1-inch cube	130 in 1-inch cube
Yogurt	294 in 1 cup	230 in 1 cup
1 egg, whole	27	112
1 serving lean beef	10	214
1 serving chicken	10	232
1 serving haddock	15	197
10 almonds	25	45
20 cashew nuts	16	160
18 peanuts	15	73
1 serving peas	28	127
1 serving potatoes	9	52
whole-grain bread	20 in 1 slice	102 in 1 slice
wheat germ	70 in ½ cup	1050 in ½ cup
brewer's yeast	49 in 1 heaping tablespoon	945 in 1 heaping tablespoon

From *Minerals: Kill or Cure?* by Ruth Adams and Frank Murray. New York: Larchmont Books, 1974.

References

1. Ensminger, Audrey H., et al. *Foods and Nutrition Encyclopedia.* Clovis, Calif.: Pegus Press, 1983, pp. 1749ff.
2. Burton, Benjamin T., Ph.D. *The Heinz Handbook of Nutrition.* New York: McGraw-Hill Book Co., 1965, pp. 119–120.

3. Hendler, Sheldon Saul, M.D., Ph.D. *The Doctors' Vitamin and Mineral Encyclopedia.* New York: Simon and Schuster, 1990, pp. 172ff.
4. Bricklin, Mark. *The Practical Encyclopedia of Natural Healing.* New York: Penguin Books, 1990, pp. 200–201.
5. Webb, W. L., and Gehi, H. "Electrolyte and Fluid Imbalance: Neuropsychiatric Manifestations," *Psychosomatics* 22(3):199–203, 1981.
6. Fredericks, Carlton, Ph.D., and Bailey, Herbert. *Food Facts and Fallacies.* New York: ARC Books, Inc., 1971, pp. 33–34.
7. Garrison, Robert H., Jr., M.A., R.Ph., and Somer, Elizabeth, M.A., R.D. *The Nutrition Desk Reference.* New Canaan, Conn.: Keats Publishing, Inc., 1990, pp. 71–72.
8. Parrot-Garcia, M., and McCarron, D. A. *Nutrition Reviews* 42:205–213, 1984.
9. Mitchell, John. "Osteoporosis: It Takes More Than Calcium to Preserve Bone Health," *Health News and Review*, January/February 1988, pp. 1, 10.
10. *Nutrition Reports International* 33(6):879–891, 1986.
11. Adams, Ruth, and Murray, Frank. *Improving Your Health with Calcium and Phosphorus.* New York: Larchmont Books, 1978, pp. 16–17, 20, 60ff.
12. Chinn, H. I. "Effects of Dietary Factors on Skeletal Integrity in Adults: Calcium, Phosphorus, Vitamin D and Protein." Life Sciences Research Office, Federation of American Societies for Experimental Biology, Bethesda, Maryland, 1981.
13. Wical, K. E., et al. *J. Prosthet. Den.*, January 1979.
14. *Recommended Dietary Allowances*, 10th Edition. Washington, D.C.: National Academy Press, 1989.

21

Selenium: The Neglected Antioxidant

ALTHOUGH selenium was discovered in 1817 by Jöns Jacob Berzelius (1779–1848), a Swedish scientist, it was not until the 1950s that the mineral was determined to be an important fighter against disease. At that time, Klaus Schwarz, M.D., then at the National Institutes of Health in Washington, D.C., reported that the mineral could prevent a serious nutritional deficiency disease in laboratory animals. Since then, researchers around the world have found that the mineral protects against heart disease and stroke; strengthens the immune system; reduces the risk of many forms of cancer; enhances longevity; detoxifies environmental pollutants; and helps to defend against arthritis, Crohn's disease, respiratory infections, a variety of skin diseases and infertility, among other things.

In his introduction to *Selenium As Food and Medicine* by Richard A. Passwater, Ph.D., Julian E. Spallholz, Ph.D., of Texas Tech University at Lubbock, said that, "Selenium was named for the goddess of the moon, Seléne; but for nutrition it has been a shining star of the last decade. Not since the recognition of the mineral cobalt as part of vitamin B12 in the mid-1950s has a mineral been recognized as having a precisely definable function in human or animal nutrition as has happened with selenium. In 1973, Dr. J. T. Rotruck (then at the University of Wisconsin) and his associates identified selenium as a necessary component of an enzyme, glutathione peroxidase."

Spallholz added that, as a component of that enzyme, and perhaps other as yet undiscovered functions, selenium is thought to:

- Protect cell membranes
- Prevent cardiovascular disease

183

- Reduce the incidence of cancer
- Suppress arthritis
- Reduce aging
- Contribute generally to better health.[1]

Discussing the Third International Symposium on Selenium in Biology and Medicine, which was held May 28–June 1, 1984 in Beijing, China, S. P. Yang, Ph.D., of the Food and Nutrition Department at Texas Tech University, said that, until recently, clinical symptoms of selenium deficiency in humans, even in low selenium regions, had not been reported. But, he added, recent studies in China have identified a fatal cardiomyopathy (Keshan disease) and an arthritic disease (Kaschin-Beck disease) as being associated with severe selenium deficiency.

"In a long geographical belt in China where the soil is deficient in selenium, Keshan disease is reported to affect about one percent of infants and children with a fatality rate approaching 80 percent," Yang said.

At the time of the conference, Yang and Spallholz were working with two Chinese scientists, Dr. X. M. Luo and Dr. H. J. Wei, to determine the extent of selenium deficiency in parts of China.

Spallholz, who has been researching selenium for almost 30 years, said that, "Marco Polo described selenium toxicity in horses about the year 1265, and selenosis among horses and other livestock has long been known in the western United States where it is known to cause loss of hooves and hair from manes and tails. Some even claim too much loco weed might have contributed to Custer's defeat at Little Big Horn because of selenium in the plant, which affects the animals' central nervous systems."[2]

Elaborating on the Chinese problem, Passwater reported that, since 1976, all children in the affected region of China have been given selenium supplements. In the first year, there were only four cases of Keshan disease out of 12,579 children who were studied. By 1977, there were no new fresh cases out of 12,747 children who were given selenium supplements. At the time, the Chinese were considering putting the mineral in table salt as a preventive measure.[3]

Writing in *Nature* in 1985, Thomas H. Jukes, M.D., of the University of California at Berkeley, was alarmed that officials in Monterey, California, were concerned that selenium was discovered in the Kesterson reservoir and refused to allow the "toxic fluid" to be released into the Pacific Ocean. Apparently the town officials were unaware that selenium is an essential dietary supplement.

Jukes pointed out that geological variations in the Earth's crust, flaciation during the Ice Age, the effects of vulcanism and the results of erosion and leaching are some of the factors that decide which parts of the Earth's surface are either deficient or oversupplied with trace minerals.

> In some parts of the world, most conspicuously in Australia, the soil is so deficient in certain trace minerals such as zinc and copper that plants will not grow. Elsewhere, soil contains a toxic excess of some minerals. One of these is selenium, which was known for many years only as being poisonous, even carcinogenic. It came into prominence because certain plants such as Astragalus (loco weed) concentrate it from high-selenium soils so that horses that eat Astragalus may become poisoned, or locoed ("blind staggers"). In the 1930s, Franke and his coworkers reported effects of "toxic wheat" grown in South Dakota on high-selenium soil. Feeding toxic wheat or selenium to hens produced deformed embryos in their eggs with eyes and beaks missing, and with distorted wings and feet. No such injuries were detected in human beings; the only bad effects were dental caries.[4]

"Toxin" Found Essential

Jukes added that the bad reputation of selenium was abruptly changed in 1957, when it was found in laboratory studies to be a nutritionally essential trace element for rats, chickens and pigs. This news was followed with startling rapidity by reports of selenium deficiency in farm animals all over the world, especially in New Zealand. He added that selenium provided one of the most dramatic illustrations of the rule of Paracelsus that "the dose alone determines the poison," a rule that seems to have been forgotten by most of us.

"Among the many studies of the toxicity of selenium were some carried out by the Food and Drug Administration, which led to the conclusion that high levels of selenium are carcinogenic," Jukes said. "Since official thinking does not permit the extension of Paracelsus' rule to carcinogens, FDA agonized for 15 years before it allowed selenium to be added to the diet of farm animals. Ironically, selenium had meanwhile emerged as an anticarcinogen and as a component of an important enzyme, glutathione peroxidase, an enzyme important in the metabolism of injurious hydroperoxides."

Meanwhile, officials in Monterey were concerned about the "contaminated" water supply and were predicting "another year's crop of what may very well be contaminated produce." In reality, Jukes maintained, "the contaminated produce is probably helping to protect consumers against cancer." While the objective of the town officials seemed to be to treat selenium as a toxicant that must be sequestered, much of the land in California and more in Oregon is deficient in selenium, he said.

"Until FDA gave approval for selenium as an animal feed additive, farmers literally had to return to the ocean, the original source of selenium for animals, to obtain selenium for their livestock," Jukes continued. "This was done by feeding fish meal, the selenium in which was natural and therefore legal. Selenium has another role in ocean fish; it prevents the injurious action of mercury that is naturally present in seawater and is added to the ocean by volcanic discharge and run-off from coastal soils."[4]

In the United States, Ray Shamberger, M.D., and Charles Willis, M.D., of the Cleveland Clinic in Ohio, reported in 1976 that people who live in low-selenium areas had three times more heart disease than those living in areas where the soil and water are rich in the mineral, according to Richard A. Passwater, Ph.D., in *Selenium Update.*[5]

Low-selenium areas were also found by Shamberger and colleagues to contribute to cancer deaths, as Ruth Adams and I reported in *Minerals: Kill or Cure?* Their study involved an analysis of cancer incidences in 34 American cities (*Medical Tribune*, June 27, 1973), where they found that cancer incidence is not nearly so great where there is plenty of selenium in the soil. A low-selenium area was said to be where grass which forage animals eat contains up to 0.05 ppm of the mineral; a medium selenium area has concentrations up to 0.10 ppm, while a high area has up to 0.11 ppm of selenium. (See Table 21.1.)[6]

Shamberger said that antioxidants, such as selenium, prevent cancer by decreasing peroxidation that may enhance the attachment of the carcinogen to desoxyribonucleic acid. In other words, the antioxidant prevents oxygen from reacting with other substances, thereby preventing the cancer-causing substances from attaching themselves to an extremely important substance in the cell called DNA. Such antioxidants as selenium, vitamin E, vitamin C and BHT (a food preservative) seem to behave in this way.

The selenium content of soils/crops is naturally of interest to farmers and ranchers, whose animals in low-selenium areas are subject to white muscle disease, which is caused by a selenium deficiency. The antidote, of course, is to give the animals a selenium supplement. The subject was reviewed in the May/June 1967 issue of *Agricultural and Food Chemistry* by J. Kubota, et al. in which a map of the U.S. reveals the amount of selenium in soils. They reported that in the Pacific Northwest, Northeastern United States and the Southeastern Seaboard states, there are extensive areas where crops are generally low in selenium. Selenium-responsive diseases in livestock are most likely to occur in these areas.

TABLE 21.1

SELENIUM PATTERNS ACROSS THE U.S.

LOW SELENIUM AREA	HIGH SELENIUM AREA
Chicago, Ill.	Los Angeles, Calif.
Bridgeport, Conn.	Atlanta, Ga.
Cincinnati, Ohio	San Diego, Calif.
Fall River, Mass.	Fort Worth, Texas
Providence, R.I.	Dallas, Texas
Youngstown, Ohio	Oklahoma City, Okla.
Dayton, Ohio	Phoenix, Ariz.
Albany, N.Y.	Denver, Colo.
Worcester, Mass.	Houston, Texas
Rochester, N.Y.	New Orleans, La.
Allentown, Pa.	San Antonio, Texas
Brockton, Mass.	Salt Lake City, Utah
Gary, Ind.	Tulsa, Okla.
Utica, N.Y.	Birmingham, Ala.
Toledo, Ohio	Omaha, Nebr.
Wilmington, Del.	Wichita, Kansas

From *Minerals: Kill or Cure?* by Ruth Adams and Frank Murray. Larchmont Books, 1974.

The researchers, from the U.S. Department of Agriculture in Ithaca, New York, and Twin Falls, Idaho, added that in a very extensive area in the west-central U.S., the selenium contents of crops are predominantly in the protective, but nontoxic, range of selenium concentrations. Therefore, animal feeds in this area may be valuable additions to animal diets in the low-selenium areas, they said.[7]

A more complete analysis of the selenium content of forage and hay crops in the Pacific Northwest was given by D. L. Carter and colleagues in the September/October 1968 issue of *Agronomy Journal.*[8]

SELENIUM LEVELS AND CANCER RISK

An estimated 200 scientific studies involving human volunteers have shown an association between relatively low selenium levels and an increased risk of developing cancer, according to Larry Clark, M.D., of the University of Arizona School of Medicine. Before going to Arizona, Clark researched the mineral at Cornell University in Ithaca, New York. Clark and Gerald Combs, Jr., Ph.D., a professor of nutrition at Cornell, reported that a sampling of patients with gastrointestinal disorders, who had lower than mean selenium blood levels of the mineral, were three and one-half times more likely to have neoplastic polyps—a precursor to colorectal cancer—than patients with higher plasma selenium levels.

"We do not think that selenium causes or prevents cancer," Combs said, "but many human and animal studies suggest that selenium may modify the effects of other cancer-causing agents."

How effective selenium is in reducing the cancer risk may depend on a person's nutritional status, especially relating to the other antioxidants, Combs continued. In addition to selenium, other major antioxidants are vitamin A/beta-carotene, vitamin C, vitamin E, zinc, copper and manganese.

In earlier studies, Clark and Combs have found that high blood levels of selenium may offer protection against nonmelanoma skin cancer. Recognizing that skin cancer patients tend to be of the age of greatest risk to colorectal cancer, the researchers became interested in a possible link between selenium stores and colonic polyps. They enlisted the aid of Lee Hixon of the Arizona university, who evaluated the selenium status and polyp incidence in a sampling of 100 patients undergoing rectal exams at the Tucson VA Hospital. The study revealed that patients who ranked below the mean in blood selenium concentration had a much higher prevalence of neoplastic polyps of the colon.[9]

Researchers at the University of Wisconsin in Madison, and the Roswell Park Memorial Institute in Buffalo, New York, have documented the ability of some selenium compounds to reduce by half the incidence of breast cancer in laboratory animals treated with a powerful cancer-causing chemical.

On a per-weight basis, the anti-carcinogenic properties of the stronger selenium compounds are 50 to 100 times more powerful than other known anti-carcinogens such as the retinoids (vitamin A-like compounds), according to Howard Ganther, Ph.D., of Wisconsin. In addition, the selenium substances are 1,000 times stronger in this instance than conjugated linoleic acid, a cancer preventive unsaturated fatty acid in meat and dairy products.

Ganther, who is working with Clement Ip, Ph.D., and his colleagues in New

York, said that other researchers have found selenium to be effective against a broad spectrum of chemicals and viruses that result in cancer in many types of tissues.

"The latest studies provide strong, new evidence that the chemical form of selenium is an important determinant of its anticarcinogenic activity," Ganther explained.

In 1949, Carl Baumann and a graduate student at the Wisconsin university found that selenium lessened the incidence of cancer in experimental animals. Since selenium in very large doses can be toxic, it had been assumed that selenium might increase cancer risk.

The Wisconsin-New York researchers now know that people need selenium to make an enzyme that protects the body from peroxides, which are severe oxidizing molecules that can damage cells. Selenium is actually a key component for at least two essential enzymes, and it provides antioxidant protection in collaboration with vitamin E.[10]

In an article in the *International Journal of Cancer* in 1988, researchers at Finland's Social Insurance Institution and other facilities reported that selenium and vitamin E may offer protection from gastrointestinal cancer, especially among men, but not for colorectal cancer. The longitudinal study was based on 36,365 men and women, ranging in age from 15 to 99, who initially did not have cancer. The research team made their observations after analyzing blood samples of 150 people who developed gastrointestinal cancer six to 10 years afterwards, compared with 276 controls.[11]

Cancer Preventive

Selenium has gained attention as an important nutrient in cancer prevention, according to Ronald Ross Watson, Ph.D., of the University of Arizona College of Medicine in Tucson, in *Food and Nutrition News*, May/June 1989. It enhances the immune response and functions as an antioxidant to help prevent free radical formation, which damages cell membranes and can initiate the cancer process, he added. Selenium appears to act synergistically with vitamin E and possibly with vitamin A in exerting its protective effect. Unfortunately, he said, selenium intake is unpredictable. Although dietary sources include lean meats, seafood and vegetables, intake is dependent upon the amount of the mineral in the soil where the food (if from a plant source) is grown. Watson continued:

Many studies in both animals and humans have shown an inverse correlation between cancer incidence and selenium intake. Research on animals supplemented with selenium revealed that tumor incidence was approximately one-half that of control animals. In humans, epidemiological evidence from 27 countries indicated that individuals with higher dietary selenium intakes and higher blood selenium levels had lower cancer mortality rates. However, selenium compounds are toxic in large amounts, and excesses have been linked with an enhancement of the cancer process in animals. Thus, while significant data are available suggesting that selenium acts as an anticarcinogenic agent, further studies are required to determine optimal levels of selenium to be used in cancer prevention in humans.[12]

Writing in *Food and Nutrition News*, May/June 1986, Watson said that data such as the geographic distribution of types of tumors in man and experimental animal studies point toward dietary components such as vitamin A and its precursors or selenium as important factors in prevention of some cancers. For example, certain subgroups of the American population, such as members of the Church of Jesus Christ of Latter-Day Saints (Mormons), demonstrate significantly lower cancer rates, which in part reflect different dietary patterns.

He added that nutrients that act as anticarcinogens to prevent cancer initiation or growth may function by:

1. Picking up active forms of cancer-initiating compounds (carcinogens) and preventing them from functioning to initiate cancer cell growths;
2. Alteration of the body's defense systems;
3. Inhibition of tumor initiation via alteration of cell metabolism;
4. Prevention of gene activation and cellular proliferation by tumor promoters;
5. Inhibition of cancer progression once it has been initiated by the alteration of cell differentation.

"Selenium has the ability to affect both initiation and promotion stages of chemically induced cancers, as well as development of nonchemically induced tumors," Watson continued. "LeBoeuf and Hoekstra suggested that selenium at concentrations shown to reduce cancer initiation delays the process by decreasing cell proliferation. One explanation is that selenium alters the metabolism of glutathione, an enzyme. Selenium protects membranes from damage by oxygen compounds through the action of selenium-dependent glutathione peroxidase, which breaks down peroxides before they can attack cell membranes."[13]

Decreased protein synthesis may be involved in the antiproliferative effects of selenium on cancer cells, he said. Selenium causes increased levels of enzymes that reduce protein synthesis when isolated from cells for study. And selenium deficiency can lead to hyperkeratosis of the skin and metablastic changes in gastrointestinal, respiratory and urogenital tract epithelium.

Watson added that the very low dietary selenium intake in areas with Keshan disease is less than half the minimum daily selenium requirement of 24 mcg/day suggested by balance studies in New Zealand women. Daily intakes of 116 mcg/day in the selenium-adequate area falls in the U.S. National Research Council's "safe/adequate range"—50 to 200 mcg/day. In the high-selenium areas without selenosis, he added, intakes of 750 mcg/day are somewhat greater than the tentative maximum acceptable intake of 500 mcg/day, calculated on the basis of fish-eating populations in Japan. Recent evidence suggests a role for selenium, at least at supranutritional levels, in reducing tumor formation in animals. In the majority of studies that demonstrate a protective effect of selenium against cancer, he said, dietary selenium concentrations of 20 to 60 times the nutritional requirement have been used.[13]

In a study reported in the *Journal of Trace Elements, Electrolytes and Health Disease*, Z. Pawlowicz and colleagues studied 29 women, 34 to 74, who had breast cancer; 28 volunteers, 49 to 74, with gastrointestinal cancer; and 36 patients, 22 to 74, with colorectal cancer, who were admitted to a hospital in Poland for an operation. The controls were 35 healthy people, 20 to 74, who served as controls for the gastric and colorectal cancer patients, and 18 women, 31 to 66, who were controls for the breast cancer study. The research team found that, in all the cancer patients studied, there were significantly lower whole blood and plasma selenium concentrations, and significantly lower red cell and plasma glutathione peroxidase activity.[14]

Researchers from the Research Institute for Nutritional Diseases in Tygerberg, South Africa, and three other South African facilities, reported in *Cancer* in 1988 that selenium levels were significantly lower in rural blacks who lived in areas with moderate to high incidences of esophageal cancer, compared to people in rural and urban areas where there is a low incidence of the disorder.[15]

Chinese researchers reported in *Biological Trace Element Research* in 1990 that supplemental selenium reduces the risk of developing lung cancer in high-risk populations. The study, conducted at the Beijing Food Industrial Institute in China, concerned workers at the Yunnan Tin Corporation, where the miners have a very high incidence of lung cancer. During the study, 40 healthy miners were given 300 mcg of selenium in selenium-containing malt cakes or a placebo for one year. Prior to the study, low concentrations of the mineral in plasma and hair were documented. Following selenium supplementation, selenium status was increased in the blood by 178 percent and in the hair by 194.8 percent.

Glutathione peroxidase activity went up 155.7 percent, while lipid peroxide levels were reduced 74.5 percent when compared with placebo. The researchers concluded that a daily intake of 300 mcg of selenium, which is slightly above the recommended amount, is a safe and effective way for humans to possibly prevent lung cancer, especially among these tin miners who have an incidence of lung cancer of greater than one percent per year.[16]

At a meeting of the Federation of American Societies for Experimental Biology in New Orleans in 1993, Larry Clark, Ph.D., of the University of Arizona, reported that those with low blood levels of selenium appear to be at greater risk for developing adenomatous colon polyps than those with "median" or higher selenium levels, according to the April 8, 1993 issue of *Medical Tribune*. One-third of the people in the lowest quartile of blood selenium levels had colon polyps, which can progress to colon cancer. But Clark said that only nine percent in the highest quartile had these lesions.[17]

Writing in *Cancer Detection and Prevention* in 1990, Sir Richard Doll, of Radcliffe Infirmary, Oxford, England, said that it is estimated that lifestyle changes may be able to reduce the risk of cancer by 70 to 80 percent in adult life. This might be achieved, he added, by modifying the diet, eliminating tobacco and alcohol, reducing calories, by increasing the intake of fruits and vegetables (especially members of the Brassica family), vitamin C, vitamin E, beta-carotene, fiber and selenium.[18]

Blood levels of selenium and lycopene (a carotenoid) were lower among the people with pancreatic cancer, according to P. Burney, et al. in the *American Journal of Clinical Nutrition* in 1989. Vitamin E was also shown to provide a lesser but protective effect. The researchers, from the Johns Hopkins School of Hygiene and the University of Missouri, collected and stored blood samples in 1974. Blood samples of those who subsequently developed cancer between 1975 and 1986 were then examined.[19]

HOW SELENIUM HELPS

Selenium, which was first recommended for cancer therapy more than 70 years ago, may offer protection because it is a component of the antioxidant enzyme glutathione peroxidase, and because it may also help repair DNA, reduce DNA binding of carcinogens, inhibit neoplastic transformation and suppress gene mutations, according to Karen Burke, M.D., Ph.D., of the Cabrini Medical Center in New York City. She added that a study of 240 skin cancer patients in general good health demonstrated significantly lower mean plasma selenium concentrations than control volunteers without skin cancer. A recent study, she continued, in the October 1992 issue of *The Nutrition Report*, used both oral and topical L-selenomethionine supplementation, which showed a reduction in the incidence of acute and chronic damage to the skin induced by ultraviolet radiation and with no signs of toxicity. The study, which involved mice, reported that there was less damage to the skin of the animals from UV radiation when they were treated with selenium. None of the animals given either oral or topical selenium developed any blistering sunburn, as did the animals not treated with selenium.[20]

Burke pointed out that UV radiation-induced skin cancer is a cumulative process that begins with the initial exposure. It is thought that one blistering sunburn in a child doubles the potential for developing skin cancer later in life. She added that regular use of a sunscreen with a sun-protection factor of 15, during the first 18 years of life, may reduce 78 percent of the lifetime incidence of nonmelanoma skin cancer. The potential importance of topically or orally given selenomethionine may be significant with regards to skin cancer prevention, because of the reduction in the ozone layer and an increase in UV irradiation. Skin cancer deaths have increased more than any other form of cancer except for lung cancer. She suggested that every adult take 100 mcg/day of selenomethionine, especially during the summer months. But for those who have a family history of cancer, she recommended 200 mcg/day.[20] Writing in *Nutrition and Cancer* in 1992, Burke and colleagues at the Scripps Clinic and Research Foundation in La Jolla, California, reiterated their belief that the topical application of selenium might lessen the damaging effects of UV radiation on the skin and help to prevent skin cancer and other disorders induced by too much exposure to the sun.[21]

In a meeting abstract reported in *FASEB Journal* in 1993, researchers at Texas Tech University Health Sciences Center in Lubbock, said that increasing the selenium content of the diet does not eliminate, but it does significantly reduce, the risk of developing UV-induced skin cancer.[22]

Against Heart Disease

Using laboratory animals, researchers at Meharry Medical College in Nashville reported that vitamin E and selenium may be useful in preventing heart disease. Their study was published in *Annals of Nutrition and Metabolism* in 1986. The research team, consisting of William L. Stone, M.D., director of pediatric research, M. E. Stewart and Nicholas S. Pavulur, said that when the animals were fed a diet deficient in vitamin E and selenium, they developed high levels of low-density lipoprotein cholesterol (LDL), the damaging kind that is associated with hardening of the arteries and heart attacks. Since vitamin E and selenium are antioxidants, and since they are known to protect fatty substances from unwanted chemical changes, the Tennessee team hypothesized that a diet short on these nutrients "might permit chemical changes in LDLs that would hinder their normal passage from the bloodstream into body cells. If this were the case, elevated levels of LDL and its cholesterol cargo would be found in the blood."

In one experiment, the researchers compared the amount of LDL-cholesterol in rats fed a diet short on vitamin E and selenium and another group fed the same diet but with vitamin E and selenium supplements added. After 20 weeks on this regimen, the cholesterol levels were 68-percent higher in the group not getting the supplements than in the supplemented group. The researchers then reversed the procedure, giving rats from the deficiency group vitamin E and selenium supplements, while the other group was deprived of the supplements.

"In the course of 55 additional weeks, a complete reversal occurred in LDL-cholesterol," the scientists said. "The rats that were shifted to a deficiency diet at week 20 ended up with LDL-cholesterol levels more than three times as high as that of the animals switched to vitamin E and selenium supplements."[23]

In another experiment, the Tennessee team compared four groups of laboratory animals: 1) Those fed a basic diet deficient in selenium and vitamin E; 2) those fed the basic diet with a selenium supplement; 3) those fed the diet with a vitamin E supplement; and 4) those fed the same diet with supplements of vitamin E and selenium.

"After 13 weeks," said the researchers, "the No. 4 group had less than half the blood level of LDL-cholesterol than the No. 1 group had. Interestingly, the group fed the vitamin E supplement also had a high level, while the group fed the selenium supplement had the second lowest. This suggests that selenium is the more important of the two nutrients in keeping LDL-cholesterol levels down but that vitamin E appears to play a role in the process."

The results also suggest that the impact of vitamin E and selenium on LDL-cholesterol levels is probably not rapid but cumulative over an extended period, they said. But this is understandable. Vitamins and minerals do not work over-night, as is often the case with drugs. It takes time for the body to utilize the nutrients, whose absence in the body may have triggered the health problem to begin with.[23]

Annals of Clinical Research (18:1, 1986) devotes its entire issue to selenium.

Although this research is confined to the Scandinavian countries, it shows that selenium deficiencies can cause a variety of health problems in man and animals.[24]

A team of researchers from the University of Kuopio and the National Public Health Institute in Finland reported in *Atherosclerosis* in 1988 that low selenium levels were associated with an increase in platelet aggregability and lower high-density lipoprotein cholesterol (HDL), the beneficial kind. These two factors are associated with an increased risk for developing ischemic heart disease. The study involved 1,132 men, all 54 years of age.[25]

Prescription to Prevent Angina

As a protection against angina, Robert M. Giller, M.D., writing in his book, *Natural Prescriptions*, recommends that his patients:

- Take 50 mcg/day of selenium
- Eliminate alcohol
- Adopt an exercise and stress-management program
- In addition to your daily supplements, take Coenzyme Q10 (30 to 60 mg three times a day)
- Beta-carotene (five one-half cup servings of fruits and vegetables rich in this nutrient and 10,000 IU/day as a supplement)
- Vitamin E (400 IU/day)
- Vitamin C (1,000 mg/day)
- Magnesium (250 mg three times a day)
- DL-carnitine (250 mg three times a day)
- Max EPA, fish oil (1,000 mg three times a day)
- One baby aspirin (60 mg) daily (unless you suffer from aspirin sensitivity, high blood pressure or bleeding or peptic ulcer).

Although the research is preliminary, he added that there is some fascinating research supporting the effectiveness of L-lysine, the amino acid, in conjunction with vitamin C. This should be tried for a few weeks to see if it gives any relief.[26]

In a study involving 106 hospitalized patients who were to undergo coronary arteriography (100 men and six women), Julie Anne Moore, Ph.D., of the Creighton University School of Medicine in Omaha, Nebraska, and colleagues reported a significant inverse correlation between the blood levels of selenium and the severity of coronary atherosclerosis. The low levels of the mineral in the blood may be due to a dietary deficiency or by the use of alcohol and tobacco, which might further deplete the mineral's availability. They added that Keshan disease, the congestive cardiomyopathy affecting mostly children and young women living in selenium-deficient areas of China, is principally attributed to the low dietary intake of selenium.[27]

In a review of selenium's role against cardiovascular disease, O. Oster and W. Prellwitz of the University of Hospital Mainz in Germany, reported in *Biological Trace Elements* in 1990, that patients' serum selenium and whole blood selenium levels in patients with coronary heart disease were found to be lower than in healthy controls. This is also seen in patients with acute myocardial infarction. Selenium's protective mechanism includes its role in the enzyme glutathione peroxidase, which helps to remove hydrogen peroxide and lipid peroxides. Lipid peroxidation is known to damage cell membranes, causing impaired calcium transport and an accumulation of calcium in the cell. They added that selenium can activate the liberation of arachidonic acid from phospholipids, which can lead to metabolites that may inhibit prostacyclin, a substance which prevents blood clots, thereby increasing the risk to thrombogenesis, platelet aggregation and vasoconstriction. Selenium is also antagonistic to cadmium, mercury and lead, which have been related to high blood pressure. And selenium has a cardioprotective effect against drugs and other xenobiotics that are cardiotoxic, such as Adriamycin. Selenium may also protect the heart against such things as Coxsackie B4 viruses.[28]

ASTHMA LINK

Researchers at Karolinska Hospital in Stockholm, Sweden, reported in *Allergy* in 1990, that patients with asthma have low levels of selenium and glutathione peroxidase. The enzyme was significantly lower during acute asthmatic attacks, possibly due to the added oxidative stress brought on by the condition. The research team suggests that an insufficient supply of selenium and other antioxidants, as indicated by the lowered glutathione peroxidase activity, might initiate a vicious cycle. In other words, the oxidative stress results in enhanced abnormal arachidonic acid metabolism, which generates more reactive free radicals. But an adequate supply of selenium might prevent this process.[29]

In the same medical journal in 1993, some of the same Swedish researchers again suggested that selenium supplements increase serum selenium levels and platelet glutathione peroxidase activity, thus improving asthmatic symptoms.[30]

Amber Flatt, M.D., and colleagues from the Wellington School of Medicine in

New Zealand, came to a similar conclusion in *Thorax* in 1990, when they reported that low selenium levels may increase the risk to the inflammatory processes in asthma. The country has a low dietary intake of selenium and a high incidence of the disease. There was a 5.8-fold increase in the risk of asthma among subjects with low glutathione peroxidase levels and 1.9 for low whole blood levels. They concluded that their results support the hypothesis that lowered selenium and glutathione peroxidase levels may contribute to the incidence of asthma in New Zealand.[31]

CROHN'S DISEASE

Terje Rannem, M.D., et al. of Copenhagen, Denmark, reported in the *American Journal of Clinical Nutrition* in 1992, that 27 out of 66 patients with Crohn's disease, an inflammation of the digestive tract, had reduced levels of selenium and glutathione peroxidase in the plasma and erythrocytes (red blood cells). The authors concluded that patients with small bowel resections greater than 200 centimeters, and who have had Crohn's disease, are at risk for developing selenium deficiency.[32]

Writing in the *Journal of Clinical Pathology* in 1988, L. Hinks, et al., of the University of Southampton, England, studied whole blood, plasma and leukocyte levels of selenium, zinc and copper in 20 patients with a mild case of Crohn's disease. The researchers remarked that their study shows that selenium status might be impaired in Crohn's disease patients, and that satisfactory test results of zinc and copper do not necessarily guarantee that other minerals are within normal concentrations in those with any inflammatory condition or malabsorptive state that alters trace mineral digestion and absorption.[33]

Because some formula-fed and some breast-fed infants received inadequate selenium, consideration should be given to supplementing infant formulas with selenium, and perhaps also the diets of pregnant and/or breastfeeding mothers, especially in areas such as New Zealand where the soil is deficient in the mineral, according to Barbara Dolamore, Ph.D., and colleagues at the Christchurch School of Medicine, New Zealand, in the April 22, 1992 issue of the *New Zealand Medical Journal.*[34]

SIDS AND SELENIUM DEFICIENCY?

In infants who succumb to sudden infant death syndrome (SIDS), there is a nonspecific cardiac muscle necrosis similar to that seen in sudden death in calves and lambs, in Keshan's disease and in acute cardiomyopathy, reported John Fitzherbert, M.D., of New South Wales, in the February 3, 1992 issue of *The Medical Journal of Australia*. In a review of 1,700 cases of Keshan's disease, there were lesions of the pancreas described as being typical of cystic fibrosis in 35 percent of the cases. The lesions were found only in fetuses and preschool children. He added that, while Keshan's disease may be due to a selenium deficiency specifically related to low antioxidant status of the infant—due to an inadequate supply of the mineral from breast milk—cystic fibrosis may be due to a sudden lowering of serum selenium levels between 22 and 24 weeks of pregnancy. While in the U.S. there has been an attempt to achieve a daily minimum intake of selenium for infants between 10 and 45 mcg/day, in New South Wales, where selenium status is a problem, investigations of milk formulas and breast milk have revealed intakes as low as two mcg/day; sometimes in the range of 12 to 15 mcg/day. Most frequent intakes have been 10 mcg/day or less. He noted that, for an infant to receive a daily selenium intake of 20 to 26 mcg/day, the selenium intake of the nursing mother needs to be doubled, which can only be done with supplements. He concluded by saying that SIDs is only the tip of the iceberg with regards to selenium deficiency problems.[35]

Researchers at the University of Illinois in Urbana reported in *FASEB Journal* in 1991 that the amount of selenium in a breastfeeding mother's diet is linked to the quantity of the mineral secreted in breast milk and the quantities of various fatty acids.[36]

Blood levels of selenium decrease in older people, which might subject seniors to an increased susceptibility to oxidative stress, according to Claudine Berr, M.D., Ph.D., and colleagues from Epidemiological Research in Neuroepidemiology and Psychopathology at INSERM in Villejuif, France. They stated in the *Journal of the American Geriatric Society* in 1993 that those who are 65 and older are at greater risk for low blood levels of selenium than younger people, and that this translates into reduced glutathione peroxidase activity and lowered antioxidant defenses.[37]

When 16 women and four men switched from a mixed diet to a lacto-ovo vegetarian diet for one year, magnesium and zinc concentrations remained the same but selenium decreased by 40 percent, according to T. S. Srikumar, et al., of the University of Lund in Sweden, in the *American Journal of Clinical Nutrition* in 1992. Although the mineral status changed from time to time, the researchers concluded that changing to a lacto-ovo vegetarian diet for one year indicates that this would be less optimal than a mixed diet with regards to zinc, selenium and probably copper, but adequate for magnesium. The vegetarian diet did reduce concentrations of mercury, cadmium and lead in hair.[38]

An analysis of 20 sickle-cell anemia patients was compared to 14 nonanemic controls, revealing that levels of selenium and glutathione peroxidase were significantly lower in the plasma and whole blood of sickle-cell patients, reported C. L. Natta, et al., in *ACTA Hematologica* in 1990. This is consistent with the belief of increased oxidative stress in these patients, and low levels of the two antioxidants suggest that a weak antioxidant potential may be associated with sickle-cell anemia patients. Previous reports have also suggested that these patients may also be deficient in vitamin C, vitamin E, carotenoids and zinc.[39]

In a study reported in the *Journal of Clinical Biochemical Nutrition* in 1992, Tadotoshi Yamaguchi, et al., analyzed selenium and the activity of glutathione peroxidase in the plasma and erythrocytes of 72 healthy male controls, seven to 52, and compared to 32 hospitalized patients with Duchenne-type muscular dystrophy, ranging in age from nine to 24. In the healthy volunteers, selenium concentrations in the red blood cells showed a steep rise with age and ascending gradually in the plasma. Glutathione peroxidase activity in both plasma and erythrocytes increased with aging. But in the DMD patients, the selenium concentrations in the red blood cells decreased sharply with aging and decreased gradually in the plasma. The Japanese team also revealed that the glutathione peroxidase activity in both plasma and erythrocytes apparently increased as in the healthy men with aging, but the level was some 80 percent that of healthy men. The researchers said that a lower glutathione peroxidase activity is present in DMD patients, which may explain why the disease may intensify with age.[40]

ACTION IN AIDS CASES

In a review article in the Spring 1992 issue of the *Journal of Advancement in Medicine*, Raymond J. Shamberger, Ph.D., of Westlake, Ohio, said that states with high selenium forage crop content (i.e., Colorado, North and South Dakota and Utah) had significantly lower human death rates than states with a low forage selenium. He added that it has been suggested that careful selection of diets and antioxidant supplementation may add five to 10 more years to the average life span. Selenium deficiency is common in AIDS (Acquired Immunodeficiency Syndrome) patients, he added, and low red cell selenium and glutathione activity has been found in AIDS and ARC (AIDS-related complex) patients. Selenium supplementation, at 400 mcg/day in a selenium yeast, returned the selenium blood levels to normal in 20 patients in 70 days. Two of the 20 patients felt worse, four reported no change and 14 showed a subjective improvement in health status. Those given selenium showed improvement in gastrointestinal function, improved appetite, in neurologic and psychological function, etc. Low selenium concentrations have also been noted in patients suffering from rheumatoid arthritis and juvenile chronic arthritis. He added that patients with asthma, Down's syndrome and psoriasis have low blood levels of selenium.[41]

Writing in *Environmental Research* in 1987, Lidia Kiremidjian-Schumacher, M.D., and G. Stotzky, M.D., of the New York University College of Dentistry in New York City, suggest that selenium not only may offer protection against some forms of cancer, but also that the mineral may stimulate the immune system. They reported that selenium aids in the production of antibodies, which are necessary for fighting viruses, bacteria, etc., and that they boost the immune system in other ways, such as increasing T- and B-lymphocytes, which are also involved in the fight against disease.[42]

Researchers at the Georgia College of Pharmacy, a division of the University of Georgia at Athens, have published a hypothesis that the AIDS virus slowly depletes the body of selenium, which it uses to erupt into uninfected cells, reported the August 21, 1994 issue of *The New York Times*.

Will Taylor and his colleagues, whose paper originally appeared in the August 19 issue of the *Journal of Medicinal Chemistry*, and whose study was funded by a grant from the National Institute of Allergy and Infectious Disease, said that the human immune-deficiency virus (HIV), which can develop into full-blown AIDS, gradually depletes selenium stores. The theory bolsters the notion that selenium supplements could help combat the disease, the *Times* added. The theory also supports the belief that HIV produces proteins that consume the body's supply of the mineral.

"According to the theory," the *Times* continued, "the virus needs selenium, which preserves the elasticity of body tissue and slows the aging process, to trigger its growth. Once the virus exhausts the selenium in the infected cell, it breaks out in search of more, spreading the infection to new cells."[43]

Taylor added that selenium biochemistry may be the key to understanding the control of the life cycle of HIV and also in the pathology of AIDS. For example, the length of time it takes to deplete the body's stores of selenium could explain HIV's latency period, which can often last for years. And selenium supplements might help to keep the virus in check, he added.[43]

Brad M. Dworkin, M.D., and colleagues at the New York Medical College in Valhalla, stated in the *Journal of Parenteral and Enteral Nutrition* in 1989, that the congestive heart failure found in AIDS patients may be due to a selenium deficiency. The researchers added that this heart condition (cardiomyopathy) has been described in patients on long-term parenteral (fed through a tube) nutrition who have become selenium deficient. In six of eight patients with AIDS, there was improvement in left ventricular function after selenium supplements were given by mouth.[44]

Protein and calorie malnutrition, as well as zinc and selenium deficiencies, are sometimes responsible for the wasting syndrome and significant weight loss in AIDS patients, reported Pierre Singer, M.D., and colleagues at Montefiore Medical Center, Bronx, New York, in the March 1992 issue of the *American Journal of Gastroenterology*. The researchers said that a malnourished AIDS patient shows a profound reduction in the proportion of T4 helper cells and a moderately reduced proportion of T8 cytotoxic or suppressor cells, which are needed to fight the disease. They added that zinc deficiency has been associated with severe cell-mediated immune deficiency and T-cell lymphocyte dysfunction. Reduced T-helper-cell lymphocyte function during total parenteral nutrition has been noted in selenium deficiency, they said.[45]

In the *Journal of Nutritional Medicine* in 1992, Chris M. Reading, M.B., of New South Wales, Australia, discussed two AIDS patients who improved with nutritional therapy. The first patient was a 45-year-old, HIV-positive patient, who had been taking 100 mg of AZT, the AIDS drug, three times daily since 1986. His symptoms included emaciation, pallor, soft and flat nails, hemorrhoids, coated tongue, monilia, diarrhea, dry skin, glare intolerance, leg-feet cramps, painful stiff shoulders and painful hips. He was instructed to avoid foods that might produce adverse reactions, and he was supplemented with B1, B2, B6, phosphate and selenium. Before treatment, the patient could swim only one length of the pool. Now he can swim 40 lengths and his arm muscles have doubled in size. He has gained weight, has more energy and his mental state has also improved.

The second case was a 33-year-old male who was positive for HIV 16 months prior to therapy. He had been taking 100 mg of AZT three times a day and two daily packets of DDI. The patient complained of chronic sinusitis, itching, numbness in the feet, painful feet, depression, lassitude, poor memory, headaches, insomnia, anxiety, muscle weakness, cracked lips, hemorrhoids, constipation, cold intolerance and other health problems. He was placed on an allergy-free program and given B1, B6, magnesium, selenium, zinc. This resulted in a dramatic improvement, with relief from most of his symptoms, weight gain and a clearer mentation, Reading said.[46]

In a review article published in the March 1992 issue of *The Nutrition Report*, Gerhard N. Schrauzer, D.Sc., of the University of California at San Diego, discussed some of the studies reported here and added that selenium-mediated enhancement of antibody production may result from the mineral's ability to accelerate their assembly by speeding up the formation of -S-S-bonds from sulfhydryl precursors. He believes that the recommended dosages of 70 and 55 mcg/day for adult males and females may not be enough to stimulate the most optimum immune response. He hopes that future requirements for nutrients will be determined by assessing the resistance to pathogenic or environmental stress.[47]

SOURCES OF SELENIUM

Brazil nuts are one of the richest sources of selenium. Other reliable sources include wheat germ, brewer's yeast, fish, flour, butter, lobster, smelt, blackstrap molasses, beer, clams, crab, eggs, cider vinegar, lamb, mushrooms, oysters, pork, Swiss chard, turnips, whole grains, mushrooms, spices (garlic, nutmeg, cinnamon, chili powder), most nuts and a few other vegetables. That's assuming the foods were grown in selenium-rich soils and that the animals were eating selenium-rich foods.

REFERENCES

1. Passwater, Richard A., Ph.D. *Selenium As Food and Medicine*. New Canaan, Conn.: Keats Publishing, Inc., 1980.
2. Zeeck, B. *Texas Tech News*, August 3, 1984.
3. Passwater, Richard A., Ph.D. *Selenium As Food and Medicine*. New Canaan. Conn.: Keats Publishing, Inc., 1980, pp. 56–57.
4. Jukes, Thomas H., M.D. "Selenium Not for Dumping," *Nature* 316(22):673, August 1985.
5. Passwater, Richard A., Ph.D. *Selenium Update*. New Canaan, Conn.: Keats Publishing, Inc., 1987, p. 18.
6. Adams, Ruth, and Murray, Frank. *Minerals: Kill or Cure?* New York: Larchmont Books, 1974, pp. 182ff.
7. Kubota, J., et al. "Selenium in Crops in the United States in Relation to Selenium-Responsive Disease of Animals," *Agricultural and Food Chemistry* 15(3):448–453, May/June 1967.
8. Carter, D. L., et al. "Selenium Content of Forage and Hay Crops in the Pacific Northwest," *Agronomy Journal* 60:532–534, September/October 1968.
9. Lang, Susan. "Study Links Low Selenium with Increased Cancer Precursors in Colon," *Cornell University News*, June 27, 1991.
10. Ganther, Howard. "Selenium Shows Promise in Preventing Cancer," *Science Report*, University of Wisconsin-Madison, June 21, 1991.

11. Kneckt, P., et al. "Serum Vitamin E, Serum Selenium and the Risk of Gastrointestinal Cancer," *International Journal of Cancer* 12:816–850, 1988.

12. Watson, Ronald Ross, Ph.D. "B-Complex Vitamins and Trace Elements: A Role in Immunomodulation and Cancer Prevention?" *Food and Nutrition News* 61(3):15–18, May/June 1989.

13. Watson, Ronald Ross, Ph.D. "The Role of Selenium and Retinoids in Immunomodulation and Cancer Prevention," *Food and Nutrition News* 58(3):15–17, May/June 1986.

14. Pawlowicz, Z., et al. "Blood Selenium Concentrations and Glutathione Peroxide Activities in Patients with Breast Cancer and with Advanced Gastrointestinal Cancer," *Journal of Trace Elements, Electrolytes and Health Disease* 5(4):275–277, 1991.

15. Jaskiewicz, K., et al. "Selenium and Other Mineral Elements in Populations at Risk for Esophageal Cancer," *Cancer* 62:2635–2639, 1988.

16. Yu, Shu-Yu, et al. "Intervention Trial in Selenium for the Prevention of Lung Cancer Among Tin Miners in Yunnan, China," *Biological Trace Element Research* 24:105–108, 1990.

17. Skerrett, P. J. "Selenium Fights Colon Cancer," *Medical Tribune*, April 8, 1993, pp. 1, 8.

18. Doll, Sir Richard, M.D. "Lifestyle: An Overview," *Cancer Detection and Prevention* 14(6):589–594, 1990.

19. Burney, P., et al. "Serologic Precursors of Cancer: Serum Micronutrients and the Subsequent Risk of Pancreatic Cancer," *American Journal of Clinical Nutrition* 49:895–900, 1989.

20. Burke, Karen, M.D., Ph.D. "Skin Cancer Protection with L-Selenomethionine," *The Nutrition Report* 10(10):73–80, October 1992.

21. Burke, Karen, M.D., Ph.D., et al. "The Effects of Topical and Oral L-selenomethionine on Pigmentation and Skin Cancer Incidence by Ultraviolet Irradiation," *Nutrition and Cancer* 17:123–137, 1992.

22. Delver, E., and Pence, B. "Effects of Dietary Selenium Level on UV-Induced Skin Cancer and Epidermal Antioxidant Status," *FASEB Journal* 7:A290, 1993.

23. Haimowitz, Ben. "Vitamin E and Selenium May Help Prevent Heart Disease, Study Suggests," *Meharry Medical College News*, December 3, 1986.

24. *Annals of Clinical Research* 18(1), 1986.

25. Salonen, J., et al. "Relationship of Serum Selenium and Antioxidants to Plasma Lipoprotein, Platelet Aggregability and Prevalent Ischemic Heart Disease in Eastern Finnish Men," *Atherosclerosis* 70:155–160, 1988.

26. Giller, Robert M., M.D., and Matthews, Kathy. *Natural Prescriptions*. New York: Carol Southern Books, 1994, pp. 15ff.

27. Moore, Julie Anne, et al. "Selenium Concentrations in Plasma of Patients with Arteriographically Defined Coronary Atherosclerosis," *Clinical Chemistry* 30(7): 1171–1173, 1984.

28. Oster, O., and Prellwitz, W. "Selenium in Cardiovascular Disease," *Biological Trace Elements* 24:91–103, 1990.

29. Hasselmark, L., et al. "Lowered Platelet Glutathione Peroxidase Activity in Patients with Intrinsic Asthma," *Allergy* 45:523–527, 1990.
30. Hasselmark, L., et al. "Selenium Supplementation in Intrinsic Asthma," *Allergy* 48:30–36, 1993.
31. Flatt, Amber, et al. "Reduced Selenium in Asthmatic Subjects in New Zealand," *Thorax* 45:95–99, 1990.
32. Rannem, Terje, et al. "Selenium Status in Patients with Crohn's Disease," *American Journal of Clinical Nutrition* 56:933–937, 1992.
33. Hinks, L., et al. "Reduced Concentrations of Selenium in Mild Crohn's Disease," *Journal of Clinical Pathology* 41:198–201, 1988.
34. Dolamore, Barbara, Ph.D., et al. "Selenium Status of Christchurch Infants and the Effect of Diet," *New Zealand Medical Journal* 105(932):139–142, April 22, 1992.
35. Fitzherbert, John, M.D. "SIDS and Selenium," *The Medical Journal of Australia* 156:220, February 3, 1992.
36. Dotson, K., et al. "Maternal Selenium Nutrition Affects Both Milk Selenium and Lipid Patterns," *FASEB Journal* 5:917A, 1991.
37. Berr, Claudine, M.D., Ph.D., et al. "Selenium and Oxygen-Metabolizing Enzymes in Elderly Community Residents. A Pilot Epidemiologic Study," *Journal of the American Geriatrics Society* 41:143–148, 1993.
38. Srikumar, T. S., et al. "Trace Element Status in Healthy Subjects Switching from a Mixed to a Lacto-Ovovegetarian Diet for 12 Months," *American Journal of Clinical Nutrition* 15:885–890, 1992.
39. Natta, C. L., et al. "Selenium and Glutathione Peroxidase Levels in Sickle Cell Anemia," *ACTA Hematologica* 83:130–132, 1990.
40. Yamaguchi, Tadotoshi, et al. "Selenium Concentrations and Glutathione Peroxidase Activity in Plasma and Erythrocytes from Human Blood," *Journal of Clinical Biochemical Nutrition* 12:41–50, 1992.
41. Shamberger, Raymond J., Ph.D. "Selenium and the Antioxidant Defense System," *Journal of Advancement in Medicine* 5(1):7–19, Spring 1992.
42. Kiremidjian-Schumacher, L., and Stotzky, G. "Selenium and Immune Response," *Environmental Research* 42:277–303, 1987.
43. "New Theory Links H.I.V. to Depletion of Mineral," *The New York Times*, August 21, 1994, p. 42.
44. Dworkin, Brad M., M.D., et al. "Reduced Cardiac Selenium Content in Acquired Immunodeficiency Syndrome," *Journal of Parenteral and Enteral Nutrition* 13(6):644–647, November/December 1989.
45. Singer, Pierre, M.D., et al. "Nutritional Aspects of the Acquired Immunodeficiency Syndrome," *American Journal of Gastroenterology* 87(3):265–273, March 1992.
46. Reading, Chris M., M.B. "Nutritional Intervention for AIDS Patients," *Journal of Nutritional Medicine* 3:145–148, 1992.
47. Schrauzer, Gerhard N., D.Sc. "Selenium and the Immune Response," *The Nutrition Report* 10(3):17–24, March 1992.

22

Always Think Zinc!

ALTHOUGH many people think of zinc as only necessary for covering pipes, coating wire fences and making galvanized buckets, the mineral is essential for human health. It is widely distributed throughout the body, with the highest concentrations found in the skin, hair, nails, eyes and prostate gland. Traces are also found in the liver, bones and blood. The human body contains about 2.2 grams of zinc, more than any other trace element except iron.

Zinc is poorly absorbed, with less than 10 percent of dietary zinc taken into the body, primarily in the duodenum, the first section of the small intestine. Metallic zinc and its carbonate, sulfate and oxide forms are absorbed equally well, although large amounts of calcium, phytic acid or copper can inhibit zinc absorption.

"After zinc is absorbed in the small intestine, it combines with plasma proteins for transport to the tissues," the *Foods and Nutrition Encyclopedia* said. "Relatively large amounts of zinc are deposited in bones, but these stores do not move into rapid equilibrium with the rest of the organism. The body pool of biologically available zinc appears to be small and to have a rapid turnover, as evidenced by the prompt appearance of deficiency signs in experimental animals."[1]

Zinc is necessary for healthy skin, bones and hair (it imparts "bloom" to the hair), and it is a component of several enzyme systems which are involved in digestion and respiration. In addition, zinc is necessary for the transfer of carbon dioxide in red blood cells; for proper calcification of bones; for the synthesis and metabolism of proteins and nucleic acids; for the development and functioning of reproductive organs; for wound and burn healing; for the functioning of insulin; and for normal taste acuity (the ability to taste accurately). According to the *Foods and Nutrition Encyclopedia*:

The most common cause of zinc deficiency is an unbalanced diet, although other factors may be responsible. For example, the consumption of alcohol may precipitate a zinc deficiency by flushing stored zinc out of the liver and into the urine. Lack of zinc in the human diet has been studied in detail in Egypt and Iran, where the major constituent of the diet is an unleavened bread prepared from low-extraction wheat flour. The phytate present in the flour limits the availability of zinc in these diets, with the result that the requirements for the element are not satisfied. Zinc-response has also been observed in young children in the United States who consume less than an ounce (28 grams) of meat per day.[1]

A zinc deficiency is characterized by loss of appetite, stunted growth in children, skin changes, small sex glands in boys, loss of taste sensitivity, dull hair, white spots on fingernails and delayed healing of wounds.

In reviewing the dietary status of various nutrients in all age groups, Constance Kies, Ph.D., professor of Human Nutrition at the University of Nebraska in Lincoln, reported in *Food and Nutrition News* that the average zinc, copper and manganese contents of diets may be less than optimal. As an example, zinc intakes were low in all age-sex groups except for men 25 to 30 years old, she said.

"Although these minerals are required in small amounts, many Americans are eating less than optimal amounts of them," she added. "Many dietary constituents have adverse effects on the absorption of these nutrients from the intestinal tract."

Thus, she said, deficiencies of zinc, copper and manganese may influence normal bone, brain and blood vessel characteristics. And adequate amounts of these trace minerals may have a role in prevention or control of brittle bone disease (osteoporosis), heart disease and stroke.[2]

VITAL FOR IMMUNE SYSTEM FUNCTION

In addition to its role in metabolism and cell growth, zinc is also profoundly important for the functioning of the immune system, said Ronald Ross Watson, Ph.D., of the University of Arizona College of Medicine in Tucson, in an issue of *Food and Nutrition News.*

Zinc deficiencies result in decreased numbers of antibodies and lymphocytes, leading to impaired body fluids and cell-mediated immunity, as well as an increased susceptibility to a variety of infections, Watson said. In experimental animals, zinc has been shown to both enhance and inhibit cancer growth. In one study, zinc supplementation at 10 mg/kg body weight decreased tumor incidence by two-thirds as compared with controls.[3]

Writing in the *Journal of the American Dietetic Association*, Jean Pennington, Ph.D., R.D., of the Food and Drug Administration in Washington, said that adult women consume insufficient amounts of zinc, calcium, magnesium and iron. Toddlers' diets were also low in zinc and calcium. As for teenage girls, they were getting inadequate amounts of calcium, magnesium, iron and manganese, while teenage boys and older men were not getting enough magnesium. Most Americans were ingesting too much sodium and not enough copper, she said.

"The results of this national survey support previous nutrition surveys showing that American diets are inadequate in essential vitamins and minerals," Pennington said. "It is not surprising that the minerals typically low in female diets are those nutrients most closely associated with anemia and osteoporosis. For males, the low levels of certain nutrients place them at risk in developing heart disease and high blood pressure."[4]

Reduced dietary intake is the most common reason for a zinc deficiency, and this is frequently found in patients with acquired immunodeficiency syndrome (AIDS), especially in the advanced stages of the disease, according to Majed Odeh, M.D., of Haifa, Israel, in the *Journal of Internal Medicine* in 1992. AIDS is associated with acute and chronic infections caused by various viral, bacterial, fungal and parasite pathogens, and these infections are thought to cause a significant decrease in blood zinc levels. These patients also have increased serum tumor necrosis factor, and the extent of the disease may be related to a zinc deficiency. Odeh added that zinc supplementation may play a vital therapeutic role in the prevention or correction of immune disorders that are found in the course of HIV infection. Since zinc stimulates T-cell differentiation and maturation, stabilizes cell membranes and increases the number of circulating T-lymphocytes, it may diminish some of the immune defects in AIDS, inhibit the progression of the disease and increase resistance against opportunistic infections.[5]

In the January 1990 issue of *Better Nutrition*, I reported that 30 AIDS/ARC patients studied by John D. Bogden, Ph.D., and his colleagues at the New Jersey Medical School in Newark were deficient in a number of nutrients. For example, 30 percent had below normal levels of zinc; 27 percent were deficient in calcium; 30 percent had low magnesium levels; 31 percent were deficient in beta-carotene; 50 percent had low choline levels; and 27 percent had below-normal levels of vitamin C. Ninety-three percent were deficient in at least one nutrient, even though all of them were taking megadoses of supplements.[6]

I also quoted Professor N. N. Klemparsky of the Institute of Biophysics in Moscow, Russia, as saying that therapeutic doses of zinc, which should exceed the normal RDA amount of 15 milligrams by five to 10-fold, can be beneficial in treating AIDS. The necessary amount of zinc varies with the severity of the symptoms, and for those patients with a less severe illness, oral zinc supplements may be sufficient. He added that zinc is necessary for normal immunological reactivity, especially for the function of T-lymphocytes which are destroyed by the HIV virus.

"Excellent results were obtained when treating a lethal children's disease, acrodermatitis enteropathica, with zinc," Klemparsky said. "The clinical manifestations of this disease are very similar to those of AIDS: malnutrition, dyspepsia and injury of the skin, eyes and lungs. After injections of large doses of zinc, these symptoms disappeared within 10 days. However, it is necessary to use the oral zinc treatment for three months."

Added Susanna Cunningham-Rundles, Ph.D., associate professor of immunology at New York Hospital-Cornell Medical Center, "AIDS patients typically have enormous gastrointestinal problems, leading to decreased ability to absorb nutrients from the diet. Zinc deficiency occurs very early in HIV disease and may play a more direct role, such as depleting T-cell function."[6]

Gerhard Schrauzer, Ph.D., of the University of California at San Diego, said that selenium should be part of any AIDS/ARC therapy. He added that many AIDS patients are often deficient in the mineral, particularly those residing in New York state, where selenium levels are low in the soils. He went on to say that some impressive work with selenium and AIDS patients has been reported in Australia and France. In the later stages of the disease, patients often experience heart problems. Although researchers are unsure whether these problems are caused by AIDS or a selenium deficiency, French doctors apparently have been able to stabilize the heart condition in some patients with 1,000 mcg of selenium.

"Selenium cannot provide a cure for AIDS, but it does improve the quality of life," Schrauzer said. "We have prescribed 150 mcg/day of selenium to AIDS/ARC patients and find that the amount is well tolerated and absorbed. In fact, 400 mcg may be equally well tolerated."[6]

Gregg Coodley, M.D., of the Oregon Health Sciences Center University in Portland, reported in the November 15, 1990 issue of *Annals of Internal Medicine* that low levels of zinc have been suggested as a marker for progression of the HIV infection. Where there is a deficiency of vitamin B6, a supplement may raise CD4 levels. There are sometimes borderline deficiencies of B6, B12, B1 and vitamin A. One study reported that 25 percent of HIV-infected patients were deficient in vitamin C, carotenes, choline or zinc, with over 10 percent having deficiencies in vitamin A, vitamin B6 and vitamin E.[7]

Writing in the October 1992 issue of the *Journal of the American College of Nutrition*, A. M. De Gordon reported that 17 of 37 patients with HIV infection were placed on zinc therapy. Development of Kaposi's sarcoma and other opportunistic infections were markedly reduced in those getting zinc therapy. A subset of the zinc therapy group was placed on maintenance zinc therapy by mouth, intravenously and with low-dose inferferon therapy, which brought a remarkable improvement in their two-year mortality.[8]

AIDS patients often develop a wasting syndrome and significant weight loss, according to Pierre Singer, M.D., et al. in a comprehensive review article in the March 1992 issue of the *American Journal of Gastroenterology*. Protein and calorie malnutrition, along with zinc and selenium deficiencies, have been documented. Nutritional support has been beneficial in reversing the wasting of AIDS, but specific recommendations for enteral and parenteral nutrition have not yet been clearly defined. In checking the records of 50 AIDS patients admitted to New York hospitals, 60 percent were underweight upon admission, but only 34 percent received any form of nutritional supplementation. Prior to their death, these patients had sustained an average weight loss of 16 percent of their pre-illness weight. Singer, who is with the Montefiore Medical Center, Bronx, New York, added that generally a weight loss of about 10 percent is considered to have a significant impact on a patient's functional status.[9]

TROUBLED BY TINNITUS?

Patients with tinnitus (ringing in the ears) may require six times more zinc than the Recommended Dietary Allowance, according to Hansel M. Debartolo, Jr., M.D., of Sugar Grove, Illinois. Those who take calcium supplements but not zinc supplements often have decreased levels of zinc. Vitamin A, in conjunction with zinc, is often useful because there are high concentrations of the vitamin in the cochlea and sensory receptor cells of the ear. A reduction in fat, cholesterol and caffeine, and a balance of electrolytes, may also benefit these patients. Potassium iodide supplementation has resolved tinnitus symptoms, and an imbalance in magnesium may also contribute to the disorder. Salicylate-free diets have also been beneficial.[10]

BOOSTS ACTION OF ACNE DRUGS

When 66 patients with inflammatory acne were given 30 mg/day of zinc gluconate in a double-blind trial, they showed a significant improvement over the controls. It is believed that the mineral's effectiveness may be attributed to its actions on inflammatory cells.[11]

In a study reported in the *Journal of the American Academy of Dermatology* in March, 1990, 103 patients with acne vulgaris received either erythromycin, an acne drug, or zinc, or a topical solution of one percent clindamycin phosphate. The medication was applied twice daily, and patients were examined at three, six, nine and 12 weeks after beginning the therapy. At six weeks there was considerable improvement in the zinc-treated group when compared to the clindamycin-treated group. Of the 92 patients who completed the study, there were no reported side effects. Lawrence Schachner, M.D., and colleagues at the University of Miami School of Medicine, concluded that the zinc-drug combination provides a better therapeutic benefit in a shorter amount of time.[12]

Researchers at the Hopital Bichat in Paris, France, reported in the *American Journal of Clinical Nutrition* in 1993 that low-dose supplements of zinc (20 mg/day) improve food intake, blood albumin levels and other indicators of nutritional status in the elderly. Zinc status was compromised at the beginning of the study, but increased about 20 percent after the zinc supplements were given.[13]

CROHN'S AND CELIAC DISEASES

Crohn's disease is a chronic inflammation of part of the digestive tract. The final section of the small intestine is most commonly involved, although patchy inflammation can be found anywhere along the intestines. It begins with inflammation in the intestinal wall, which can spread to other parts of the digestive system. Although some of the lesions heal, they can leave scar tissue that thickens the intestinal walls and narrows the passageways.[14]

Some patients with Crohn's disease might have a tissue depletion of zinc, researchers at the University Hospital in Lund, Sweden, reported in the *Journal of the American College of Nutrition* in 1988. The research team found that blood concentrations of zinc were low in five of the patients, and muscle zinc levels were low in six of the 30 patients.[15]

Researchers from Spain reported in the *American Journal of Gastroenterology* in December 1990, that 29 patients with inflammatory bowel disease were evaluated for zinc, copper, selenium and alkaline phosphatase levels. Blood zinc levels were lower and serum copper levels were higher in those with active ulcerative colitis than the controls. More than 50 percent of the patients with active colonic or small bowel disease had zinc levels of less than 15 percent of the controls.[16]

Celiac disease is a disorder in which the lining of the small intestine reacts adversely to gluten, a protein found in wheat, rye, oat and barley. Writing in the *American Journal of Clinical Nutrition* in 1990, Richard W. Crofton, et al., of Law Hospital in Scotland, evaluated the zinc status of eight patients with celiac disease. In mild cases of untreated celiac patients, increased zinc turnover and endogenous loss was found, although the absorption of zinc from normal zinc intake remained unchanged. The increased turnover and zinc loss were decreased when the patients were put on a gluten-free diet.[17]

A zinc deficiency is a common feature of untreated celiac disease, and zinc normalization can be expected when patients are placed on a gluten-free diet, according to M. Statter, of the Hadassah Hebrew University Hospital in Jerusalem, Israel, in *Trace Elements in Medicine* in 1990. The study involved 27 children with celiac disease, who were compared to 14 healthy controls for zinc and copper status. There was a significant reduction in blood zinc concentrations in the gluten-containing diet group and the gluten-free or normal controls. Copper levels were normal in both groups. The researchers suggested that there is a decreased zinc/copper ratio in untreated celiac disease, which may be a useful tool in the assessment of celiac disease.[18]

HOPE FOR THOSE WITH EATING DISORDERS

Anorexia nervosa and bulimia nervosa are two serious health problems in which the patients (usually, but not always, females) do not eat, or they vomit and take laxatives after eating, for fear of gaining weight. The illness usually begins with normal dieting to lose weight, but the patient gradually eats less every day, according to the *American Medical Association Family Medical Guide*. The patients give false reasons for not eating, suggesting, for example, that their legs or arms are too fat. The less she eats, the less she wants and, in some cases, she goes on binges in which she gobbles up large amounts of a particular food and then vomits. To counteract family concern, the patient may take food and throw it away, claiming it was eaten. When her weight drops to about 26 pounds below normal, she may stop having periods (amenorrhea) and her body may become more hairy.

"A girl who has anorexia nervosa is often abnormally energetic," the Guide explained. "She may cook large meals for others while starving herself, and she will insist that she feels fine. But her skin may begin to look sallow and thin and she eventually will become obviously ill. Whether or not she is constipated, she may take large doses of a laxative in the belief that by hurrying food through her system she will keep from growing fat. In later stages of the illness, she may lapse into severe depressive illness."[19]

Anorexia nervosa and zinc deficiency have a number of symptoms in common, according to Rita Bakan, Ph.D., of the British Columbia Institute of Technology in Burnaby, Canada, and colleagues at various facilities. These include weight loss, alterations in taste, smell and appetite, depression and amenorrhea.[20]

The researchers reported in the *International Journal of Eating Disorders* in 1993 that their study involved nine outpatient vegetarians with anorexia nervosa and 11 outpatients with the disorder who were not vegetarians. It was found that the vegetarians had significantly lower intakes of zinc, fat and protein and significantly higher amounts of calories from carbohydrates than the non-vegetarians. There were no significant differences between the two groups for calories, calcium, copper, iron or magnesium. Approximately 50 percent of patients with anorexia nervosa are vegetarians, the researchers reported. This may be because of the phytates in the vegetarian diet, which interfere with zinc absorption, and because vegetarians do not usually eat meat, which is a rich source of zinc, and they usually avoid high-fat foods.[20]

"Young women who use vegetarian diets to reduce weight should be informed of the need to compensate for the potential adverse effects of a meatless diet on their zinc status," the researchers said. "Zinc supplementation, and nutritional management to improve the quantity and bioavailability of zinc intake, may serve as an effective adjuvant therapy for this subgroup."[20]

Writing in *Lancet* in 1984, researchers reported that a 13-year-old girl with anorexia nervosa was believed to have a zinc deficiency because she was unable to taste a zinc sulphate solution she was given. Following two weeks of zinc supplementation (15 mg/day at first and then 50 mg three times a day) her appetite and mood began to improve. After four months of zinc supplementation, the girl had gained 13 kg, her depression had cleared, and she was able to taste the zinc solution. Ten months after discontinuing the zinc therapy, she had returned to her initial state, but again improved after zinc supplements were given.[21]

In a study reported in the December 1989 issue of the *Journal of Clinical Psychiatry*, Laurie Humphries, M.D., of the University of Kentucky Medical Center in Lexington, and colleagues at various facilities, studied 62 patients with bulimia and 24 patients with anorexia nervosa.[22]

"Forty percent of the patients with bulimia and 54 percent of those with anorexia nervosa had biochemical evidence of zinc deficiency," the researchers reported. "For a variety of reasons, such as lower dietary intake of zinc, impaired zinc absorption, vomiting, diarrhea and bingeing on low-zinc foods, patients with eating disorders may develop zinc deficiency. The acquired zinc deficiency could then add to the chronic nature of altered eating behavior in those patients."[22]

Researchers at the University of Surrey in England reported in the *Journal of Nutritional Medicine* in 1990 that 15 female patients with anorexia nervosa had lower levels of zinc than the 15 controls. This was determined after examining the zinc content of whole blood, serum, plasma, urine and scalp hair. During the study, the volunteers were given either a placebo, 15 mg of zinc sulfate, 15 mg of zinc gluconate, 15 mg of zinc orotate or 15 mg of zinc citrate twice a day. All of the zinc supplements increased in the just-named parameters in the anorexic patients, with subjective improvement in appetite and taste sensitivity.[23]

In *Pediatric Dermatology* in 1992, Abby S. Van Voorhees and Michelle Riba, M.D., discuss the case of a 35-year-old female who developed a zinc deficiency due to anorexia nervosa. She had lost 30 pounds, was depressed and had lost her appetite. For 10 years she had suffered from amenorrhea. While in the hospital, the researchers noted that she had thinning hair, low zinc levels and skin lesions. During the previous 10 years, she had abused laxatives. After her diet was supplemented with 45 mg/day of zinc, the lesions were completely resolved in 10 days. But her appetite did not improve and she remained depressed. The researchers concluded that zinc levels should be monitored in any patient with anorexia nervosa, especially if there are skin changes compatible with acrodermatitis enteropathica.[24]

Researchers in Sweden are convinced that zinc therapy should be given along with conventional treatment for patients with anorexia nervosa. Their conclusions came after studying 20 patients, ranging in age from 14 to 26, who had the disorder. Each patient was given from 45 to 90 mg/day of zinc sulfate. Seventeen of the patients increased their weight by more than 15 percent during the eight to 56-month follow-up. One patient achieved a weight gain of 57 percent after 24 months of zinc treatment. Another patient had a 24-percent increase in weight after three months of zinc therapy. Menstruation returned in 13 patients between one and 17 months after the therapy began. The researchers suggest that anorexia nervosa may be related to a zinc deficiency, especially in teenagers who have poor diets, who have increased zinc demands due to rapid growth, and especially those who are athletic, who can lose zinc in urine and sweat. Excess fiber in the diet can also contribute to a zinc deficiency, they said.[25]

MALE INFERTILITY HELPED

A zinc deficiency is related to male infertility, according to researchers at the U. S. Department of Agriculture's Human Nutrition Research Center in Grand Forks, North Dakota. During the study, reported in the *American Journal of Clinical Nutrition* in 1992, 11 volunteers were evaluated while living in a metabolic ward. They were given conventional foods along with a semisynthetic formula supplemented with zinc sulfate. During the 28-day pretreatment evaluation, the men consumed 10.4 mg/day of zinc. In the subsequent 35-day treatment period, their zinc intake was either 1.4 mg, 2.5 mg, 3.4 mg, 4.4 mg or 10.4 mg each day. The men who consumed the smallest amount of zinc (1.4 mg/day) showed significant decreases in semen volumes as well as serum testosterone levels when compared to when they were getting 10.4 mg/day. The researchers also found that total semen zinc loss per ejaculate was reduced in the men consuming 1.4 mg to 3.4 mg of zinc each day. They concluded that serum testosterone levels, seminal volume and seminal zinc loss per ejaculate are affected by short-term zinc intake, which might contribute to male infertility.[26]

Writing in *Biological Trace Element Research* in 1992, Alain-Emile Favier, a French researcher, reviewed the association between zinc intake and reproduction. He noted that zinc is necessary for the formation and maturation of sperm, for ovulation and for fertilization. A zinc deficiency during pregnancy is associated with spontaneous abortions, pregnancy-related toxemia, extended pregnancy or prematuring, malformation and growth retardation. Zinc's role in reproduction is explained by its multiple action on the metabolism of the androgen hormones, estrogen and progesterone as well as with prostaglandins, he said. The amounts of zinc given in the various studies he reviewed ranged between 10 and 60 mg/day.[27]

In studying a group of pregnant smokers and nonsmokers, researchers at Case Western Reserve University, Cleveland, Ohio, found that an increased number of pregnancies is associated with elevated levels of cadmium and decreased levels of zinc in the placenta of smokers. The research team reported in *Obstetrics and Gynecology* in 1988 that smoking depletes placenta zinc concentrations while elevating placental cadmium levels, especially in older women. As we know, zinc plays an active role in growth and development, while cadmium can be harmful to the developing fetus. The researchers suggest that the alterations in the concentrations of zinc and cadmium (found in cigarette smoke) might help to explain the increased incidence of low birth-weight infants born to smoking women.[28]

In a letter to the editor in the *British Medical Journal* in 1990, Patrick A. Riley and Robin L. Willson commented on the discovery of a high association of leukemia in children whose fathers have been exposed to external radiation before conception at the Sellafield Nuclear facility in the United Kingdom. They suggested that the possibility of internal contamination by a radionucleotide might be the explanation. Zinc is found in large amounts in semen and it is crucially important for proper functioning of DNA and protein synthesis. Therefore, the authors said, a substitution of zinc by other metals could lead to DNA damage by the generation of free radicals that are known to be produced by radiation. They added that short-lived radionucleotides might bind to thiols at these zinc sites, which could be a source of radiation-induced metagenesis.[29]

In reviewing the importance of zinc, Henri Faure, DPharm.Sci., et al., reported in *The Journal of Nutritional Medicine* in 1992 that the mineral is involved in over 200 different enzyme pathways. It plays a significant role in DNA and RNA replication, which is required for cell division and protein synthesis. The French researchers were focusing on the beneficial role in surgery, indicating that stress caused by major surgical procedures can result in a serum zinc drop of about 46 percent of the pre-operative value. For major surgery, the researchers said, there is a need for zinc supplementation before the intervention, in order to restore zinc supplies to the peripheral tissue, which requires more zinc after surgery. The mineral plays a significant role in cellular and humoral immunity, and it is necessary for the production of serum thymic factor, produced by the thymus, which stimulates T-cell markers and functions in immature cells. The authors added that, in major surgery, parenteral supplementation with 30 mg/day of zinc, begun before the operation, can significantly reduce postoperative zinc depletion and facilitate wound healing.[30]

ALZHEIMER'S DISEASE

There is a considerable controversy concerning whether or not zinc prevents and/or contributes to Alzheimer's disease or senile dementia. *Family Practice News* reported in 1990 that a zinc deficiency may be a factor in the development of the neurofibrillary tangles in Alzheimer's disease. That is because zinc levels have been shown to be decreased in the hippocampus of Alzheimer's disease patients. Zinc is useful in preventing the deposition of certain metals, such as lead, which can contribute to neurofibrillary tangles. The publication also reported that a zinc deficiency might cause abnormal functioning of certain enzymes, resulting in abnormal DNA production leading to abnormal protein synthesis and the formation of neurofibrillary tangles. Zinc might also help to prevent neurofibrillary tangles by slowing the accumulation of amyloid, a protein. In a preliminary study of six presenile dementia patients, zinc aspartate has shown some promise.[31]

A report in Gerontology in 1989, evaluated lipid peroxidation products and free-radical scavengers in 55 patients with senile Alzheimer's disease and compared with 24 matched controls. The French research team reported that there was a significant decrease in the levels of glutathione peroxidase, vitamin A, vitamin C, vitamin E, zinc, transferrin and albumin in the Alzheimer's group. Most of the deficiencies turned up in the malnourished subgroup of the Alzheimer's patients. The researchers concluded that more research is needed as to whether or not Alzheimer's patients should be supplemented with these nutrients.[32]

Test-tube experiments have demonstrated a link between zinc and the formation of plaque on brain cells that is associated with Alzheimer's disease, according to the September 6, 1994 issue of The New York Times. The research team, headed by Rudolph Tanzi, M.D., director of the laboratory of genetics and aging at Massachusetts General Hospital, which is affiliated with Harvard University, said that zinc ions can cause certain peptides, or proteins, to convert into an insoluble form that is believed to kill brain cells. These can also accumulate into clumps known as plaque, which has been found in the brains of Alzheimer's patients.

"Slight increases of zinc in certain areas of the brain could presumably convert the amyloid peptide from its normal, safe form into this more dangerous type," Tanzi told the Times.

Tanzi and other researchers were quick to point out that people should not become concerned about ordinary dietary intake of zinc, which plays a fundamental role in learning and memory, the immune system and many other body processes, the Times added. "The amount of zinc you get in your food or in a one-a-day vitamin is not going to hurt you," Tanzi added. "As far as megadoses of zinc go, most people would warn against taking megadoses of anything."

Scientists are deeply divided over what triggers Alzheimer's disease, for which there is no cure, the Times continued. "While many believe that the conversion of the beta-amyloid protein plays a central role, others argue that it is merely a byproduct of another, more important process that has not yet been definitely identified."

The researchers, whose initial study appeared in Science, found that in low concentrations, zinc bound to beta-amyloid without causing it to clump. However, when the zinc was elevated slightly, the amyloid clumped rapidly. The research team, which calls its findings "highly preliminary," will now compare levels of zinc in the brains of Alzheimer's patients with those who do not have the disease.[33]

Commenting on the research in the September 13, 1994 issue of *The New York Times*, Richard D. Levere, M.D., of the New York University School of Medicine, said that, although the Massachusetts researchers were not concerned about the amount of zinc we get from foods and supplements, "this neglects to consider the possible effect on amyloid protein formation from the zinc in hair shampoos."[34]

"Zinc in the form of pyrithione zinc, is used to control dandruff, and sales of dandruff shampoos containing zinc amount to more than $200 million a year," Levere said. "This means that many risk absorbing large amounts of zinc through the scalp while shampooing their hair. In addition, zinc oxide is used extensively to treat minor inflammatory skin conditions from diaper rash to sunburn."[34]

In a double-blind crossover study, reported in *The Journal of Applied Nutrition* in 1991, Michael Colgan, Ph.D., and colleagues at the Colgan Institute of Nutritional Science in Encinitas, California, supplemented 12 male and 11 female endurance athletes with the RDA for all vitamins and minerals, and compared the same protocol plus 48 mg of iron, 60 mg of zinc, 2.4 mg of folic acid, 150 mg of vitamin B6, 500 mg of vitamin C and 100 mcg of vitamin B12. Compared to the baseline values, the RDA-supplemented group showed declines in serum ferritin, iron, zinc, vitamin C and vitamin B6 status. The high-dose supplemented group had increases in serum cobalamin, ferritin, red cell folate, zinc, B6, vitamin C, whole blood hemoglobin, MVO_2 and time to exhaustion on the cycle ergometer. The research team concluded that the absence of increases in blood levels of B12, folic acid, zinc and vitamin C during supplementation at the level of the RDA, and lack of improvement of MVO_2 and time to exhaustion during these periods, suggests that the RDAs for these nutrients are insufficient for optimal performance in endurance athletes.[35]

Elaborating on the role of zinc, Colgan said that the average zinc level of a 2,850-calorie American diet is 13.2 mg or 88 percent of the male RDA of 15 mg. But studies of actual zinc intake in adults reveal a daily level of only 8.6 mg. Therefore, he said in *Optimum Sports Nutrition: Your Competitive Edge*, zinc deficiency is probably widespread.[36]

"Because adequate zinc is essential for normal testosterone levels and sperm counts, some researchers suggest that the high incidence of impotence in American men is partially caused by chronic zinc deficiency," Colgan added. "Athletes certainly need more zinc than couch potatoes, for their high production of red blood cells to replace cells lost by hemolysis, for losses of zinc in sweat, for the increased fatty acid metabolism caused by exercise, for multiple interactions of zinc in iron metabolism, and for the added testosterone they need for muscle growth. There is also direct evidence that exercise reduces zinc status. With the low level of zinc in average diets, athletes are doubly at risk. No surprise then that zinc deficit is rampant in sports including marathon running, triathlon, track and field, wrestling, gymnastics and dance."[36]

As I reported in *Happy Feet*, Linda Strause, Ph.D., and Paul Saltman, Ph.D., of the University of California at San Diego, said that their interest in trace minerals and bone metabolism developed when they were introduced to the orthopedic problems of Bill Walton, the professional basketball player.[37]

"Several years ago (Walton) was plagued by frequent broken bones, pains in his joints and an inability to heal bone fractures," Strause and Saltman said. "We hypothesized that he might be deficient in trace elements as a result of his very limited vegetarian diet."[37]

In cooperation with Walton's physician, the San Diego researchers analyzed Walton's blood and found no detectable manganese. His serum concentrations of copper and zinc were also below normal. The researchers supplemented his diet with trace elements and calcium, and over a period of several months his bones healed and he returned to professional basketball. In cooperation with several other orthopedic physicians, the San Diego researchers analyzed serum from other patients with slow bone healing and found that several of these patients also had abnormally low zinc, copper and manganese levels.

The San Diego researchers added that it is not surprising that trace minerals can affect the growth and development of bone, since deficiencies in these nutrients profoundly alter bone metabolism in animals, either directly or indirectly. When trace elements are not provided in the diet, this can lead to inefficient functioning of a certain enzyme or enzymes that require the transition nutrient as a cofactor. For example, copper and iron are required in the cross-linking of collagen, the connective tissue between bone, and elastins, which are tissue proteins. As a result of their animal studies, the two researchers conclude that various trace minerals, especially manganese, may play a significant role in the development of osteoporosis.[37]

Saltman recalled looking at X-rays of one of Walton's ankles that was not healing and exclaiming, "This guy has osteoporosis or an osteoporosis-type disease." Saltman said that, although Walton was deficient in manganese, zinc and copper, he had lots of calcium, suggesting that the athlete "was not synthesizing bone well." He concluded that Walton had a remarkable imbalance of nutrients.[37]

A recap on the importance of zinc to the immune system was reported by A. S. Prasad, of Wayne State University School of Medicine in Detroit, in the

Journal of the American College of Nutrition in October 1992. He pointed out that a zinc deficiency leads to thymic atrophy and a reduction of lymphocytes and macrophages in the spleen. Thymulin is a zinc-dependent hormone, and T-cell antibody responses are lowered in zinc-deficient mice. In the animal studies, the researchers found that zinc deficiency results in insufficient production of lymphocytes from the bone marrow. Prasad added that patients with acrodermatitis enteropathica, the zinc-related skin condition, have reduced parameters of immune function and increased secondary infections. He added that there are similar findings in zinc deficient sickle-cell anemia patients. A zinc deficiency can, therefore, decrease serum thymulin activity and decrease interleukin-2.[38]

COMMON COLD SYMPTOMS EASED

Although previous studies concerning zinc and the common cold were inconclusive, J. C. Godfrey, M.D., and colleagues reported in *The Journal of International Medical Research* in June 1992, that zinc lozenges were beneficial. The research team used zinc gluconate-glycine lozenges in which 23.7 mg of zinc were in each 4.5/g lozenge. At their initial visit to the clinic, volunteers were given 16 lozenges. When they returned two days later, 64 lozenges were prescribed if symptoms persisted. The participants were instructed to chew, not suck, the lozenges at two-hour intervals, but not to exceed eight lozenges per day. The researchers reported that the disappearance of cold symptoms occurred after an additional 4.9 days of zinc treatment, versus 6.1 days for the controls who did not receive zinc. Cold duration was an additional 4.3 days in the zinc-treated group, compared with 9.2 days for the placebo group. Mild side effects were reported, and cough, nasal discharge and congestion were the symptoms that were helped.[39]

Researchers at the U.S. Department of Agriculture/Nutrition Research Center in Grand Forks, North Dakota, reported in *Clinical Research* that low zinc intake, coupled with alcohol consumption, might cause prolonged tissue exposure to alcohol. But adequate zinc intake helps the body to metabolize alcohol and remove it from the blood, lessening its impact on health.[40]

TO TREAT WILSON'S DISEASE

Wilson's disease is an autosomal recessive disorder associated with copper accumulation in the body. Zinc therapy is becoming well established as a treatment for this disorder, especially when it is for the presymptomatic condition or for maintenance, according to George J. Brewer, M.D., and colleagues at the University of Michigan at Ann Arbor, in the *Journal of the American College of Nutrition* in 1990. Dosages of 75 mg of zinc divided into three daily doses is more effective than taking 75 mg at once, they reported.[41]

Writing in *Hepatology* in 1990, Irmin Sternlieb, M.D., of the Albert Einstein College of Medicine, Bronx, New York, reviewed the role of zinc and vitamin B6 in the treatment of Wilson's disease. When the drug D-penicillamine is utilized, vitamin B6 at 25 mg/day should be included, since the drug has a mild antipyridoxine effect. Zinc, ranging in doses from 75 to 300 mg/day has been recommended for patients with neurologic symptoms, as well as those who are asymptomatic to maintain wellness. Sternlieb said that zinc theoretically works by synthesizing intestinal metallothionein, which enhances the ability of copper binding by epithelial cells. The copper is thus trapped in the intestinal mucosa and absorption is inhibited. He noted that side effects include headaches, abdominal cramps, gastric irritation and appetite loss, and that zinc can interfere with iron absorption.[42]

Z. T. Cossack, Ph.D., of Odense University in Denmark, reported in the *New England Journal of Medicine* in 1988, that he and other researchers have found zinc to be a beneficial long-term treatment for Wilson's disease. Results from the Danish study showed that oral zinc alone is effective in maintaining a negative or zero copper balance in children, and that the children have been doing well on zinc therapy for seven years, with no side effects or complications.[43]

Cossack added that there are a number of conditions in which zinc can be an effective alternative to penicillamine:

1. In renal failure in Wilson's disease;
2. In pregnancy, since the risk is great enough that a pregnant woman may discontinue penicillamine therapy during at least part of her pregnancy (moreover, such a woman is unprotected from copper accumulation);
3. As adjunctive therapy to prevent zinc deficiency resulting from chelation therapy;
4. As adjunctive therapy to reduce the amount of chelation therapy required in the presence of toxicity from the chelating agent; and
5. As alternative therapy in the face of intolerable toxicity from the chelating agent.[43]

Researchers often prescribe Captopril and Enalapril, two ACE inhibitors, for patients with high blood pressure. Writing in the July 1990 issue of *Metabolism*,

A. Golik, M.D., and colleagues at the Assaf Harofeh Medical Center, Zerifin, Israel, discussed 13 essential hypertensive patients being given the two drugs, compared with six untreated hypertensives and nine healthy controls. The researchers found that zinc losses in urine were significantly increased in the Captopril-treated patients, and the zinc-creatinine urinary ratio was significantly increased in both of the medication groups. Blood levels of zinc were comparable in all groups, but red blood cell levels of zinc were low in the Captopril group. The research team noted that intracellular zinc depletion is associated with weakness, impotence and loss of taste.[44]

Zinc supplementation may be useful in treating patients with acute myocardial infarction, according to Tomoyuki Katayama, M.D., and colleagues at the Nagasaki Citizens Hospital in Japan. The researchers reported in *Angiology* in June 1990 that serum zinc levels were assessed within 24 hours after 61 patients had been stricken with acute myocardial infarction. Serum zinc levels dropped in 84 percent of the patients, and these levels fell sharply as early as three hours after the onset of the problem. Zinc levels were at their lowest two or three days after the infarction and then rose to normal values within five to 10 days. The extreme low-serum zinc concentrations were associated with more severe clinical findings, the researchers said, and the prognosis seemed to be worse. They suggested that following zinc levels may be a good diagnostic and prognostic parameter in acute myocardial infarction.[45]

Since zinc is required for normal insulin structure and secretion, it may have benefit in diabetics and help to prevent future complications, according to B. Winterberg, M.D., et al. in *Trace Elements in Medicine* in 1989. The researchers, from the University of Munster, Germany, studied the zinc, fasting glucose, glycosylated hemoglobin and alkaline phosphates and insulin in 24 insulin-dependent and 45 non-insulin dependent diabetics. Significantly lower serum zinc levels were found in 55 percent of the diabetic patients compared to controls. And the mean serum level was lower in the insulin-dependent diabetics as compared to those not needing insulin. It was determined that zinc was seven percent lower in females than in males. Those without any diabetic complications had higher zinc levels than those with various complications. And zinc was inversely correlated with glycosylated hemoglobin and fasting blood glucose.

The researchers also reported that there was a positive correlation between serum zinc levels and the duration of the diabetic disease. Twenty-four insulin-dependent (Type I) diabetics were given 50 mg/day of zinc for three weeks, and there was a substantial increase in their serum zinc levels with a significant decrease in blood glucose. Significant reductions in cholesterol and an increase in alkaline phosphates were also noted.[46]

An enzyme that enables the body to use folic acid, the B vitamin, has been discovered, purified and characterized by researchers at the University of California at Davis. Added Charles H. Halsted, M.D., the lead researcher, "What we have found is that this enzyme, called folate conjugase, works best in the normal intestine and that it seems to be more active in the presence of zinc. Our laboratory findings raise many questions, such as, 'How important is zinc in folate absorption? If zinc activates the enzyme, do zinc deficient people have less of the enzyme and develop folate deficiency?'

"Folate deficiency is a significant factor in alcoholism, in certain intestinal diseases such as celiac sprue and in patients who have had intestinal surgery," Halsted said. "Its primary symptom is anemia, but because it affects the gut, diarrhea is also associated with it. Folate deficiency is prevalent in alcoholics mainly because of an inadequate diet, but also because they don't absorb folate normally. We find folate deficiency in people with diseases such as celiac sprue because these diseases interfere with intestinal absorption."

He added that, in clinical studies, the researchers found that the amount of folate conjugase in patients afflicted with celiac disease is so low that it can barely be detected. And drugs such as sulfasalazine, a drug used to treat ulcerative colitis and Crohn's disease, and phenytoin sodium, a drug to treat epilepsy, can also lead to folic acid deficiency.[47]

ZINC FOR MEN

Since the prostate gland is a rich storehouse of zinc, both anecdotal and clinical studies have suggested that zinc in the diet and supplements might prevent or lessen disorders of this gland in men.

As explained by Andrew Weil, M.D., in *Natural Health, Natural Medicine*, the prostate gland is a walnut-sized organ surrounding the urethra at the neck of the bladder in males. Its secretions are one component of semen. Prostatitis, or inflammation of the gland, is a common ailment in young men who get urinary tract infections. Unfortunately, this condition easily becomes chronic and is difficult to treat. Older men, he added, are subject to a different sort of problem, enlargement of the gland, which can interfere with urination.

"Prostatitis causes pain on ejaculation and urination, urinary frequency and sometimes urethral discharge; chronic prostatitis can be a cause of low backache," Weil said. "This condition resists treatment because the gland has a poor blood supply, making it hard for the immune system to defend it against infection and making it hard for antibiotics to reach the site. Regular doctors can do little except give antibiotics; too often the condition recurs whenever the drugs are stopped."

Weil added that you can get over prostatitis if you follow these suggestions:

1. Eliminate all prostatic irritants (coffee, decaffeinated coffee, other caffeine sources, alcohol, tobacco and red pepper).
2. Drink more water—dehydration is one of the great stresses on the prostate.
3. Avoid jarring motion to the perineal (seat) area, such as riding a horse, motorcycle or bicycle, and avoid prolonged sitting.
4. Take 60 mg/day of zinc picolinate until symptoms subside. Then cut the dose in half and continue on this therapy indefinitely.
5. Take 2,000 mg of vitamin C three times a day.
6. Adjust your frequency of ejaculation (both too much and too little encourage prostatitis).
7. Try a warm sitz bath.
8. Prostatic massage is helpful; this can be done by inserting a finger in the rectum and gently pressing on the gland. This helps to drain the gland and increases blood flow to it.
9. Use antibiotics if you have acute symptoms but do not remain on them for more than two weeks.
10. Use an herbal remedy, saw palmetto (*Serenoa repens*) for benign prostatic hypertrophy (BPH). Try the standardized extract, 160 mg, twice a day. It is nontoxic and can be used indefinitely. It protects the prostate from the irritating effects of testosterone and, by promoting shrinkage of the gland, improves urinary function.[48]

"Most men over the age of 50 develop benign prostatic hypertrophy, an enlargement of the gland that may be due to accumulation of testosterone in it," Weil added. "This condition can be asymptomatic or it can cause a number of urinary problems; increased frequency, decreased force of urination and nighttime awakening to empty the bladder. If these symptoms become severe, doctors will urge surgery to remove all or part of the gland."[48]

Zinc is the backbone of his treatment for men with prostate problems, according to Robert M. Giller, M.D., in *Natural Prescriptions*. Men with BPH have low levels of zinc in prostatic fluids, and supplements can raise these levels and reduce the enlargement. In one study, 14 out of 19 patients treated with zinc supplements had shrinkage of the prostate after two months, he said.

"Essential fatty acids are also helpful in relieving an enlarged prostate," Giller added. "Researchers postulate that essential fatty acids work by influencing prosta-glandin production; prostaglandin deficiency may be a cause of BPH. The best common sources of essential fatty acids are flaxseed oil, sunflower oil and soy oil."

As a natural prescription to prevent prostate problems, Giller recommends:

1. Eat a low-fat diet and keep your cholesterol below 220.
2. Avoid margarine, hydrogenated vegetable oils and fried foods, since they can interfere with prostaglandin metabolism.
3. Cut down on alcohol consumption, especially beer.
4. If your frequent urination is irregular, you may be allergic to a particular food.
5. Always empty your bladder completely when you feel the urge.
6. In addition to your daily supplements, take one to two tablespoons of flaxseed oil daily for several months, adding sunflower oil or soy oil to your diet; take 400 mg/day of vitamin E; take 60 mg/day of zinc; and use 160 mg of saw palmetto extract twice a day (it is available in health food stores).[49]

At a meeting of the American Medical Association in Chicago in 1974, I. M. Bush reported that 200 male volunteers with prostatitis, with no evidence of a bacterial infection, were given zinc supplements. Seventy percent of the men reported relief from their symptoms. The zinc dosages ranged from 50 to 150 mg/day.[50]

In *Improving Your Health with Zinc*, Ruth Adams and I reported that most American men are brought up on diets in which processed cereals, white bread and other foods made with white flour are staples. Since the zinc has been removed from these and never replaced, could this not explain why prostate gland problems are so prevalent in Western society and almost unknown among the so-called primitive people eating their ancestral diet? We quoted Richard J. Turchetti and Joseph M. Morella as saying that 23 of the 50 states are devoid of zinc and that "the food grown in those soils is subsequently devoid." It is possible that the zinc-deficient prostate, by swelling, is reacting the same way the thyroid gland reacts when it is deprived of iodine.[51]

ZINC AND WOMEN'S HEALTH

At the 46th annual meeting of the American Fertility Society in Washington, D.C., in 1990, C. James Chuong of the Baylor College of Medicine in Houston evaluated 10 patients with premenstrual syndrome and 10 controls for zinc levels throughout the menstrual cycle every two or three days. During the luteal (egg-releasing) phase of the cycle, there were significantly lowered zinc levels in the blood of the women with PMS compared to the controls. The researchers theorize that a zinc deficiency may lead to decreased secretion of progesterone, opiates or endorphins. PMS patients often have lower levels of endorphins during the luteal phase. The Texas researchers said that, in another study, progesterone levels dropped in the afternoon, which brought on cravings for sweet and salty foods. In still another study, six female patients with PMS had a steep drop in progesterone in the first few hours after lunch.[52]

In a study by Estelle Thauvin and colleagues in Grenoble, France, it was found that vitamin and mineral supplemented pregnant females had a decreased incidence of muscular cramps and other complications of pregnancy. They reported in *Biological Trace Element Research* in 1992 that it appears that multivitamin and mineral supplementation, particularly with zinc (15 mg/day) and copper (2 to 2.65 mg/day) is necessary during pregnancy. Concerning zinc, the supplementation allows for the normalization of biological status as well as preventing deficiencies. Copper supplementation is important to insure adequate copper retention as well as preserving the balance of trace minerals supplied during pregnancy.[53]

Preeclampsia, which often occurs during pregnancy, is characterized by high blood pressure, protein in the urine and swelling of the body. It can develop into eclampsia, a life-threatening problem involving convulsions and coma. In the placentas of 18 women in which eight developed preeclampsia, Michael H. Brophy, M.D., of the Veterans Administration Medical Center in Dallas, Texas, found that there were significantly higher copper levels and lower zinc levels in the preeclamptic women.[54]

Brophy elaborated on his theories concerning preeclampsia in the *American Journal of Obstetrics and Gynecology* in July 1990. He believes that low zinc status may increase the risk of preeclamptic seizures because the mineral is involved in the maintenance of pyridoxal phosphate (vitamin B6) concentrations by the activation of pyridoxal kinase. He explained that the latter enzyme is involved in decarboxylation (the removal of a molecule of carbon dioxide from an organic compound) and lowers brain gamma-aminobutyric acid (GABA), which is an inhibitory neurotransmitter that might lower the seizure threshold. Brophy added that plasma levels of GABA, an amino acid, have been shown to be lower in preeclamptic patients.[55]

Writing in *Trace Elements in Medicine* in 1989, E. A. Wright and colleagues at the University of Illinois at Urbana evaluated 20 women using Copper T-200 IUDs and 25 women who did not use the contraceptive. After 12 months there were lower levels of serum zinc, iron, hemoglobin and hematocrit in the IUD users. As might be expected, there was a significant increase in serum copper. The researchers believed that low zinc status was the probable cause of the menorrhagia (prolonged menstruation), which was probably responsible for the anemia in 50 percent of the women using the IUD. The research team suggested that women using the Copper T-200 IUD should be monitored closely, and if menorrhagia develops, they should be given iron supplements with zinc to help replace blood loss and the menorrhagia.[56]

A zinc deficiency seems to be involved when infants fail to thrive, according to Philip A. Walravens and colleagues at the University of Colorado Health Sciences Center in Denver. Their study, reported in *Pediatrics* in 1989, involved 25 pairs of infants and toddlers, ranging in age from eight months to 27 months. The researchers believe that a slowing of weight velocity while length velocity remains the same can be an early sign of a mild zinc deficiency. They recommend 5 mg/day of zinc as a diagnostic test and treatment when infants fail to thrive.[57]

In a later study, reported in *Lancet* in 1992, the same Colorado researchers evaluated 56 breast-fed infants between four and nine months of age, who were randomly given either 5 mg/day of zinc or a placebo for three months. The babies given zinc in a beverage gained about 3.6 pounds and grew 2.5 inches. In the placebo group, the infants grew 2.8 pounds and gained two inches in height.[58]

Birth defects, stunted growth and delayed sexual maturation are common problems found among laboratory rodents fed diets severely deficient in zinc. This prompted Mari Golub of the University of California at Davis to study rhesus monkeys, whose development and metabolism are similar to human beings, to determine if severe zinc deficiencies might impact on human health, according to the July 9, 1988 issue of *Science News*. The study, originally reported in the *American Journal of Clinical Nutrition* (June 1988), followed 10 monkeys from birth to adolescence. Half of the animals were given four parts/ppm of zinc in their daily diet, both *in utero* and postpartum, a level that was deemed "marginal zinc deprivation." The others received 100 ppm of zinc in their diet, which was said to be far more than they needed.[59]

"Compared with monkeys getting plenty of zinc, monkeys on the deficient diet had blood zinc levels 38 percent lower and immune function depressed 20 to 30 percent," *Science News* reported. "Significant learning impairments also were found. For example, it took zinc-deficient animals two to three times longer to discriminate between a circle and a cross."[59]

ZINC AFFECTS MEMORY

Diets mildly deficient in zinc caused memory and learning impairments in the offspring of laboratory rats fed the diets during pregnancy and suckling periods, reported Edward S. Halas, a research psychologist at the U.S. Department of Agriculture's research center in Boston, Massachusetts. Impaired learning of the animals continued into adulthood, and these results may have implications for humans, he said.[60]

The study, which was done at the USDA's facilities in Grand Forks, North Dakota, found that the hippocampus areas were less well-developed in the zinc-deficient rats with memory and learning impairments than they were in the rats on control diets. Other researchers have found that injuries to the hippocampus area of the brain impairs short- and long-term memory. Halas noted that, in both rats and humans, the hippocampus normally has high concentrations of zinc, which is essential for the formation of nucleic acids and protein. As to whether a zinc deficiency occurs in human fetuses and interferes with the rapidly developing hippocampus during pregnancy and postnatal periods, that is still being investigated, Halas said. But he suggested that it may be prudent for pregnant women to consume foods rich in zinc.[60]

"Only a few studies have involved the effect of zinc deficiency on brain function in humans," according to James C. Wallwork, Ph.D., of the University of Texas Medical Branch at Galveston, in the July 1988 issue of *The Nutrition Report.* "Mental lethargy has been observed in humans suffering from zinc deficiency. In addition, various psychological and behavioral abnormalities have been described in humans who were subjected to severe zinc deficiency by feeding large amounts of histidine. This chelator apparently caused a high loss of zinc in the urine. Upon refeeding zinc the psychological responses and behavior of these human subjects returned to normal."[61]

Tartrazine (FD&C Yellow Dye No. 5) is used to color over 300 foods and drugs. It can pose a problem for asthmatics, hyperactive children and others who are sensitive to food additives. In the *Journal of Nutritional Medicine* in 1990, Neil I. Ward, Ph.D., of the University of Surrey in England, studied tartrazine's effect on the zinc status of 10 hyperactive males, compared to 10 age-matched controls. He found that the additive reduced serum and saliva zinc concentrations as well as increasing zinc in the urine. This resulted in a corresponding deterioration of the child's behavior/emotional response in the hyperactive children but not in the controls.[62]

Focus on Zinc for Better Vision

Zinc may play a key role in the development of age-related macular degeneration, which causes gradual loss of vision and leads to blindness in many elderly people, according to David Whitley, M.D., and Don Samuelson, M.D., of the University of Florida at Gainesville. In a year-long study, pigs receiving a diet low in zinc were found to have changes in the eye similar to those occurring in the early stages of macular degeneration. The eyes of pigs are similar to those of humans, in that they both contain the same number of rods and cones, and they are distributed in basically the same way. There is no current treatment for macular degeneration, which affects one in three women and one in four men past 75 years of age. Whitley said:

> In humans, clear vision is due primarily to a small area in the center of the retina called the macula. But by age 52, nearly one of every 10 persons shows some sign of degeneration of the macula in one or both eyes. At the conclusion of our study, we found subtle alterations in the retinas of the pigs fed the low-zinc diet. These are the same sort of changes found in humans with age-related macular degeneration. We really can't say these changes are caused by a lack of zinc, but zinc clearly plays some role. Zinc is involved with many of the body's enzyme systems, and macular degeneration may be related to one or more of these systems.[63]

Zinc appears to play such a key role in the metabolism of the retina, because the elderly are at risk for zinc deficiency, and because there is no reason to believe that oral intake of zinc could possibly lead to a decrease in visual acuity, David A. Newsome, M.D., and colleagues at the Louisiana State University Medical Center School of Medicine in New Orleans undertook a two-year prospective, randomized, double-masked, placebo-controlled trial of zinc sulfate to individuals with drusen (retinal pigment cells) or varying degrees of visual reduction due to macular degeneration.

"Our data indicate that in our study group of persons with macular degeneration, the use of oral zinc sulfate was associated with a retardation of visual loss," Newsome said. "Because of the public health importance of this common visually disabling disorder, further investigation, including the testing of multiple dose levels, are warranted in a larger group of patients from a more varied population." (During the study, the participants were instructed to take two 100 mg tablets of zinc each day with food. Based on a 40-percent bioavailability, this dose represented 5.3 times the 15 mg/day that is the Recommended Dietary Allowance.)[64]

Many researchers believe that abnormal chemicals are involved in damaging the retina, reported Gina Kolata in the March 10, 1988 issue of *The New York Times*, discussing the LSU study. Normally, she said, enzymes in the retina neutralize the abnormal chemicals. But the enzymes need zinc to function properly.[65]

"In women," Kolata continued, "these retinal cells have the highest concentration of zinc of any tissues in the body. In men, the retinal cells are second only to the prostate in their zinc concentrations. Moreover, according to Dr. Newsome, Federal surveys have revealed that most older people do not have enough zinc in their diets. Good sources of zinc are red meats, nuts and oysters."

Kolata quoted Dr. John Weiter of the Eye Research Institute in Boston as saying that researchers had theorized that vitamins C and E and selenium, as well as zinc, could also help absorb the abnormal chemicals in the eye. He added that some doctors had already advised patients to take these vitamins or minerals as dietary supplements even though, until now, there had been no studies showing they were effective.[65]

After several researchers questioned Newsome about the seemingly large doses of zinc (200 mg/day), he and Clement L. Trempe, M.D., responded in the November 1992 issue of *Archives of Ophthalmology* that describing 200 mg of zinc per day as "toxic" is an exaggeration. They have not been any toxic effects of this amount of zinc, and reported that some clinicians have given this dosage for many years without "toxicity." Zinc sulfate is an emetic and, to get a toxic dose, one would have to retain large amounts of zinc, which would be very difficult with this supplement, Newsome said.[66]

Evidence strongly suggests that age-related macular degeneration is influenced by zinc deficiency and the progression of the disease can be slowed significantly with daily supplementation of 100 mg of zinc sulfate, reported the May/June 1992 issue of *Geriatric Consultant*. These studies were carried on at the Utah State University. The researchers added that, in addition to macular degeneration, a zinc deficiency is associated with diabetes, malignant melanoma and frequently thickening of the esophagus.[67]

In addition to supplements, Michael E. Farber, M.D., and Andrew S. Farber, M.D., reported in the August 1990 issue of *Postgraduate Medicine* that patients with macular degeneration might benefit from laser treatment, low-vision devices such as magnifiers or telescopic attachments to glasses and vocational rehabilitation. They added that nutritional therapies include zinc, natural vitamin E (d-alpha tocopherol) and vitamin C. Zinc is used as therapy, while the vitamins are suggested preventive agents because of their antioxidant capabilities.[68]

Researchers at the National Institute of Nutrition in India reported in *Nutrition Reports International* in 1988 that deficiencies of chromium, copper and zinc produce ocular changes. They found that levels of copper and zinc were lower in patients with cataracts. Zinc levels were correlated with age, with the older patients exhibiting more severe deficiencies than the younger patients.[69]

Some of the best food sources of zinc are fish, shellfish, liver, meat, eggs, whole grains, nuts, peanuts, lentils, soybeans, peas, corn, brewer's yeast, whole-grain rice, oatmeal and milk.

TABLE 22.1

RECOMMENDED DIETARY ALLOWANCES FOR ZINC

AGE AND CATEGORY	MILLIGRAMS OF ZINC PER DAY
Infants to one year	5 mg
Children, one to 10	10 mg
Males, 11 and over	15 mg
Females, 11 and over	12 mg
Pregnant women	15 mg
Breast-feeding women, first to 6 months	19 mg
Breast-feeding women, second 6 months	16 mg

From *Recommended Dietary Allowances*, 10th Edition. Washington, D.C.: National Academy Press, 1989.

REFERENCES

1. Ensminger, Audrey H., et al. *Foods and Nutrition Encyclopedia*. Clovis, Calif.: Pegus Press, 1983, pp. 2366ff.
2. Kies, Constance, Ph.D. "Copper, Manganese and Zinc: Micronutrients of 'Macrocon-cern,'" *Food and Nutrition News*, March/April 1989, pp. 12ff.
3. Watson, Ronald Ross, Ph.D. "B-Complex Vitamins and Trace Elements: A Role in Immunomodulation and Cancer Prevention?" *Food and Nutrition News*, May/June 1989, pp. 15ff.

4. Pennington, J., and Young, B. "Total Diet Study Nutritional Elements, 1982–1989," *Journal of the American Dietetic Association* 91:179–183, 1991.

5. Odeh, M. "The Role of Zinc in Acquired Immunodeficiency Syndrome," *Journal of Internal Medicine* 231:463–469, 1992.

6. Murray, Frank. "AIDS: Holistic Therapies Are Showing More Promise Than Ever," *Better Nutrition*, January 1990, pp. 10ff.

7. Coodley, Gregg, M.D. "Nutritional Deficiency and AIDS," *Annals of Internal Medicine* 113(10):807, November 15, 1990.

8. Gordon, A. M. De. "Effects of Adjuvant Therapy with Zinc in Human Immunodeficiency Virus Infection," *Journal of the American College of Nutrition* 11(5):601/Abstract 17, October 1992.

9. Singer, Pierre, M.D., et al. "Nutritional Aspects of the Acquired Immunodeficiency Syndrome," *American Journal of Gastroenterology* 87(3):265–273, March 1992.

10. Debartolo, Hansel M., Jr., M.D. "Zinc and Diet for Tinnitus," *Clinical Pearls*, 1990, p. 341.

11. Dreno, B., et al. "Low Doses of Zinc Gluconate for Inflammatory Acne," *ACTA Derm. Venerol Stockh.* 69:541–543, 1989.

12. Schachner, Lawrence, M.D., et al. "A Clinical Trial Comparing the Safety and Efficacy of Topical Erythromycin-Zinc Formulation with a Topical Clindamycin Formulation," *Journal of the American Academy of Dermatology* 22(3):489–495, March 1990.

13. Boukaiba, N., et al. "A Physiological Amount of Zinc Supplementation: Effects on Nutritional, Lipid and Thymic Status in an Elderly Population," *American Journal of Clinical Nutrition* 57:566–572, 1993.

14. Kunz, Jeffrey R. M., M.D., editor-in-chief. *The American Medical Association Family Medical Guide.* New York: Random House, 1982, p. 473.

15. Sjogren, A., et al. "Evaluation of Zinc Status in Subjects with Crohn's Disease," *Journal of the American College of Nutrition* 7:57–60, 1988.

16. Fernandez-Banares, F., M.D., et al. "Serum Zinc, Copper and Selenium Levels in Inflammatory Bowel Disease: Effect of Total Enteral Nutrition on Trace Element Status," *The American Journal of Gastroenterology* 82(12):1584–1589, December 1990.

17. Crofton, Richard W., et al. "Zinc Metabolism in Celiac Disease," *The American Journal of Clinical Nutrition* 52:379–382, 1990.

18. Statter, M., et al. "Zinc and Copper Status in Childhood Celiac Disease—Inflammatory Response or Malabsorption," *Trace Elements in Medicine* 70(1):8–10, 1990.

19. Kunz, Jeffrey, R. M., M.D., editor-in-chief. *The American Medical Association Family Medical Guide.* New York: Random House, 1982, p. 710.

20. Bakan, Rita, Ph.D., et al. "Dietary Zinc Intake of Vegetarian and Non-Vegetarian Patients with Anorexia Nervosa," *International Journal of Eating Disorders.* New York: John Wiley & Sons, Inc. 13(2):229–233, 1993.

21. Bryce-Smith, D., and Simpson, R. I. D. "Case of Anorexia Nervosa Responding to Zinc Sulphate," *Lancet* 2:350, 1984.

22. Humphries, Laurie, M.D., et al. "Zinc Deficiency and Eating Disorders," *Journal of Clinical Psychiatry* 50(12):456–459, December 1989.
23. Ward, Neil I., Ph.D. "Assessment of Zinc Status in Oral Supplementation in Anorexia Nervosa," *Journal of Nutritional Medicine* 1:171–177, 1990.
24. Van Voorhees, Abby S., and Riba, Michelle, M.D. "Acquired Zinc Deficiency in Association With Anorexia Nervosa: Case Report and Review of the Literature," *Pediatric Dermatology* 9(3):268–271, 1992.
25. Safai-Kutti, S. "Oral Zinc Supplementation in Anorexia Nervosa," *ACTA Psychiatr. Scand.* 361(82):14–17/Suppl., 1990.
26. Hunt, C., et al. "Effects of Dietary Zinc Depletion on Seminal Volume and Zinc Loss, Serum Testosterone Concentrations and Sperm Morphology in Young Men," *American Journal of Clinical Nutrition* 56:148–157, 1992.
27. Favier, Alain-Emile. "The Role of Zinc in Reproduction: Hormonal Mechanisms," *Biological Trace Element Research* 32:363–382, 1992.
28. Kuhnert, B., et al. "Association Between Placental Cadmium and Zinc and Age and Parity in Pregnant Women Who Smoke," *Obstetrics and Gynecology* 71:67–70, 1988.
29. Riley, Patrick A., and Willson, Robert L. "Leukemia and Lymphoma Among Young People Near Sellafield," *British Medical Journal* 300:676, March 10, 1990.
30. Faure, Henri, D.Pharm.Sci., et al. "Zinc in Surgery," *The Journal of Nutritional Medicine* 3:129–136, 1992.
31. "Zinc Deficiency Tied to Neurofibrillary Tangles in Alzheimer's," *Family Practice News* 20(20):7, October 15–31, 1990.
32. Jeandel, C., et al. "Lipid Peroxidation and Free Radical Scavengers in Alzheimer's Disease," *Gerontology* 35:275–282, 1989.
33. "Experiments Link Alzheimer's Condition to Zinc," *The New York Times*, September 6, 1994, p. C3.
34. Levere, Richard D., M.D. "Zinc and Alzheimer's," *The New York Times*, September 13, 1994, p. A22.
35. Colgan, Michael, et al. "Micronutrient Status of Endurance Athletes Affects Hematology and Performance," *The Journal of Applied Nutrition* 43(1):16–30, 1991.
36. Colgan, Michael. *Optimum Sports Nutrition: Your Competitive Edge.* Ronkonkoma, N.Y.: Advanced Research Press, 1993, pp. 199–200.
37. Murray, Frank. *Happy Feet.* New Canaan, Conn.: Keats Publishing Inc., 1990, pp. 88–89.
38. Prasad, A. S. "Zinc and Lymphocyte Immune Functions," *Journal of the American College of Nutrition* 11(5):597/Abstract 3, October 1992.
39. Godfrey, J. C., et al. "Zinc Gluconate and the Common Cold: A Controlled Clinical Study," *The Journal of International Medical Research* 20(3):234–246, June 1992.
40. Milne, D., et al. "Effects of Short-Term Dietary Zinc Intake on Ethanol Metabolism in Adult Men," *Clinical Research* 39:A652, 1991.
41. Brewer, George J., M.D., et al. "Use of Zinc-Metabolic Interactions in the Treatment of Wilson's Disease," *Journal of the American College of Nutrition* 9(5):47–97, 1990.

42. Sternlieb, Irmin. "Perspectives on Wilson's Disease," *Hepatology* 20(5):1234–1239, 1990.

43. Cossack, Z. T., Ph.D. "The Efficacy of Oral Zinc Therapy as an Alternative to Penicillamine for Wilson's Disease," *The New England Journal of Medicine* 318(5):322–323, February 4, 1988.

44. Golik, A., et al. "Zinc Metabolism in Patients Treated with Captopril Versus Enalapril," *Metabolism* 39(7):665–667, July 1990.

45. Katayama, Tomoyuki, M.D., et al. "Serum Zinc Concentration in Acute Myocardial Infarction," *Angiology*, June 1990, pp. 479–485.

46. Winterberg, B., et al. "Zinc in the Treatment of Diabetic Patients," *Trace Elements in Medicine* 6(4):173–177, 1989.

47. Weaver, Ralph D. "Scientists Describe Enzyme Involved in Folate Absorption: Zinc May Have Role in Its Activity," *Bristol-Myers Company News*, December 4, 1985.

48. Weil, Andrew, M.D. *Natural Health, Natural Medicine.* Boston: Houghton Mifflin Co., 1990, pp. 317–318.

49. Giller, Robert M., M.D., and Matthews, Kathy. *Natural Prescriptions.* New York: Carol Southern Books, 1994, pp. 284ff.

50. Bush, I. M. "Zinc and the Prostate." Paper read at annual scientific convention, American Medical Association, Chicago, 1974.

51. Adams, Ruth, and Murray, Frank. *Improving Your Health with Zinc.* New York: Larchmont Books, 1978, pp. 45ff.

52. Fackelmann, K. A. "PMS: Hints of a Link to Lunch Time and Zinc," *Science News* 138:263, October 27, 1990.

53. Thauvin, Estelle, et al. "Effects of a Multivitamin Mineral Supplement on Zinc and Copper Status During Pregnancy," *Biological Trace Element Research* 32:405–413, 1992.

54. Brophy, Michael H., et al. "Elevated Copper and Lowered Zinc in the Placentae of Preeclamptics," *Clin. Chimica ACTA* 145:107–112, 1985.

55. Brophy, Michael H., M.D. "Zinc, Preeclampsia and Gamma-Aminobutyric Acid," *American Journal of Obstetrics and Gynecology* 163:1, July 1990. (Part I):242–243.

56. Wright, E. A., et al. "Zinc Depletion and Menorrhagia in Nigerians Using Copper T-200 Intrauterine Device," *Trace Elements in Medicine* 6(4):147–149, 1989.

57. Walravens, P., et al. "Zinc Supplementation in Infants with a Nutritional Pattern of Failure to Thrive: A Double-Blind, Controlled Study," *Pediatrics* 83:532–538, 1989.

58. Walravens, Philip A., et al. "Zinc Supplements in Breast Fed Infants," *Lancet* 340:683–685, September 19, 1992.

59. Raloff, J. "Zinc Has Roles in Learning, Immunity," *Science News* 134:22, July 9, 1988.

60. Halas, Edward S. "Zinc Deficiency Retards Brain Development in Rat Studies," *USDA Research News*, November 10, 1983.

61. Wallwork, James C., Ph.D. "Zinc, Brain Development and Function," *The Nutrition Report*, July 1988, p. 51.

62. Ward, Neil I., Ph.D., et al. "The Influence of the Chemical Additive Tartrazine on the Zinc Status of Hyperactive Children—A Double-Blind, Placebo-Controlled Study," *Journal of Nutritional Medicine* 1:51–57, 1990.

63. Dyson, Patrick. "Zinc Deficiency May Play Important Role in Sight-Robbing Disease," *University of Florida News*, June 17, 1988.

64. Newsome, David A., M.D., et al. "Oral Zinc in Macular Degeneration," *Archives of Ophthalmology* 106:192–198, February 1988.

65. Kolata, Gina. "Zinc Shows Promise in Slowing Disease That Causes Blindness," *The New York Times*, March 10, 1988, p. B7.

66. Trempe, Clement L., M.D., and Newsome, David A., M.D. "Zinc and Macular Degeneration," *Archives of Ophthalmology* 110:1517, November 1992.

67. "Zinc Sulfate for Macular Degeneration," *Geriatric Consultant*, May/June 1992, pp. 23, 28.

68. Farber, Michael E., M.D., and Farber, Andrew S., M.D. "Macular Degeneration: A Devastating But Treatable Disease," *Postgraduate Medicine* 88(2):181–183, August 1990.

69. Bhat, K. "Plasma Calcium and Trace Metals in Human Subjects with Mature Cataracts," *Nutrition Reports International* 17:157–163, 1988.

PART III

Other Minerals That Keep You Healthy

23

Boron Helps to Build Strong Bones

BEFORE 1981, boron was considered unimportant for human nutrition, according to Michael Colgan, Ph.D., in *Optimum Sports Nutrition: Your Competitive Edge.* However, Drs. Curtiss Hunt and Forrest Nielsen at the U.S. Department of Agriculture's Human Nutrition Research Center in Grand Forks, North Dakota, reported that boron is essential for normal growth of chicks. By 1990, along with other researchers, they showed that the mineral is probably an essential nutrient for humans. Boron apparently provides biochemicals called hydroxyl groups, which are essential for manufacture of the active forms of some steroid hormones, especially hormones associated with calcium, phosphorus and magnesium metabolism in bone, as well as in muscle growth. This created an interest in boron as a possible anabolic supplement for athletes, Colgan said.

LINKED TO HORMONE PRODUCTION

Although there are no studies as yet with athletes, clinical research suggests that adequate boron status is necessary for normal testosterone production, Colgan added. Postmenopausal women supplemented with 3 mg/day of sodium borate showed increased blood levels of testosterone and 17-beta-estradiol, the most active form of estrogen. In some of the women, the increase in estrogen levels was as large as is achieved with estrogen replacement therapy.

The hormonal demands on the bodies of male and female athletes indicate that their nutrition should be optimal in every nutrient that is involved in hormone production, Colgan continued. As to whether or not the average athlete's diet contains enough boron to meet those demands, the answer is "probably not."

In 1987, the Colgan Institute near San Diego, California, did an analysis of the boron content of the American diet, based on an analysis of 200 commonly eaten foods. They found that the average boron intake of a good mixed diet in America is only 1.9 mg/day, which is comparable to a recent analysis of 1.7 mg/day in the average diet in Finland. However, the California researchers added that individual diets can be much lower because high boron foods—soybeans, almonds, peanuts, prunes, raisins, dates and unprocessed honey—may be seldom eaten. For example, a recent analysis of the self-selected diets of adults showed boron intakes of only 0.42 and 0.35 mg/day.

The Institute supplements athletes with 3 to 6 mg/day of boron citrate and aspartate. Toxicity of boron is low, however, intakes above 50 mg/day may interfere with phosphorus and vitamin B2 metabolism.[1]

Colgan went on to say that, "Boron supplements of up to 10 mg/pill are currently sold to athletes as anabolics, with wild claims that they increase testosterone levels. Give me a break! Boron may be an essential part of the process, but it doesn't cause the body to produce testosterone. Testosterone levels are tightly controlled by multiple mechanisms. If you are getting sufficient boron, then adding a megadose more does nothing but interfere with your metabolism of other nutrients."[1]

When it comes to minerals, the amounts in foods depend on how many of the minerals are in the soils where the foods are grown, whether there naturally or added by fertilizers. And, as we know, soils in various parts of the United States are deficient in a variety of minerals. According to J. I. Rodale and staff in *The Complete Book of Minerals for Health*:

In a large part of America, extending from Maine across the top of the country to Washington, iodine deficiencies are widespread, particularly in Montana. There are also extensive areas where the soil is low in manganese, copper and zinc. A lack of boron in plants is found along the Atlantic coastal plain, the northwest Pacific and also in Wisconsin. Manganese deficiencies are especially acute in Florida, and are also found in the muck soils of Michigan, the Atlantic coastal plain and California. A lack of copper is prevalent in the Great Lakes region, Washington, South Carolina, Florida and California. Recent studies indicate that trace element shortages are more extensive than previously thought, and some are growing even more pronounced because modern agricultural practices withdraw soil reserves without replacing them.[2]

Interestingly, in areas deficient in trace elements, local flora and fauna have usually made adaptations. Adapted local plants may be healthy, but imported or transplanted species may not do well at all. Those plants which need less of a certain trace element will become dominant as other life forms fail to develop when that element is lacking. One researcher estimates that 50 million acres of croplands require boron fertilization right now and only one-quarter are getting it. In Australia, the authors added, well-known for its trace-element deficiencies, about 300 million acres of adequately watered land are undeveloped, primarily due to lack of trace elements. These regions, which could be readily reclaimed, would quadruple the present agricultural area of all Australia.[2]

BORON IS FOR BRAINS

New research shows that a boron deficiency results in changes in brain wave patterns which indicate a drop in alertness, according to James G. Penland, Ph.D., of the USDA's Human Nutrition Research Center in Grand Forks, North Dakota, in *USDA News Feature*, April 19, 1990. The two studies involved 13 women in one case and laboratory animals in the other.[3]

"When you reduce dietary boron, you're almost certainly going to get a drop in alpha-wave activity and an increase in theta-wave activity from what we've seen on electroencephalograms (EEG)," Penland said. "That's the same type of change you see when people become more drowsy or less alert."[3]

The human volunteers in the studies ate meals containing roughly 0.25 mg of boron daily. During half of each study, a 3 mg supplement was added so that the women would have an adequate intake of the mineral. This meant, said dietitian Loanne Mullen, meals without fruit or natural fruit juices and only small portions of vegetables. Fast-food fare would contain very little boron, even if it were accompanied by a lettuce and tomato salad, she said. The studies dovetail with earlier studies on the mineral which show that it affects motor function. For example, when some of the women were given various tests their reaction time was slowed when their boron intake was very low.[3]

"A lack of boron seems to have an effect on motor performance," Penland continued. "The women could not tap their fingers as fast, follow a target as accurately using a joy-stick or respond as quickly when asked to search a field of letters for specific items."[3]

In an earlier study, Penland gave 15 older men and women 0.23 mg of boron daily for four months. During part of the study they were supplemented with 3 mg/day of boron, which is equated to what an average person might get from a balanced diet that included fruits and vegetables. At regular intervals, Penland measured the volunteers' brain activity with an EEG. Although the volunteers were less alert when they were on a low-boron diet, the brain activity was more coherent among some regions and less coherent among other regions, which could be interpreted as good or bad, depending on the task being done.

"This is the first study to show that boron depletion alters the function of an organ system," Penland concluded.[3]

Forrest H. Nielsen, a nutritionist and director of the Grand Forks center, said that, based on his nine years of studies, boron qualifies as an essential element.[3]

Commenting on the just-named study in *Scientific Research News* in 1989, Nielsen found that the volunteers had less available copper and calcium while on the low-boron diet. This was the first time that the researchers had seen an effect of boron on copper status. He explained that copper is thought to be important in preventing heart disease and bone and joint disorders. But blood levels of copper dropped during the low-boron period as did levels of two copper containing enzymes, both of which are sensitive indicators of a person's copper status. Although Nielsen did not know how boron affects copper at the biochemical level, he suggested that "any decline in a person's copper status is probably undesirable."

TO PREVENT OSTEOPOROSIS

In an earlier study, Nielsen said that eating a boron-rich diet may help to prevent osteoporosis in postmenopausal women. He said that an adequate boron intake prevents the loss of calcium, which is important for maintaining healthy bones and preventing osteoporosis. Boron depletion raised levels of a hormone that increases the loss of calcium in the urine.[4]

Elaborating on the Nielsen study, Sheldon Saul Hendler, M.D., Ph.D., in *The Doctors' Vitamin and Mineral Encyclopedia*, said that the USDA researchers evaluated the effects of dietary boron in 12 postmenopausal women ranging in age from 48 to 82. The study lasted 24 weeks. During the first 17 weeks, the volunteers were given a low-boron diet. In the next seven weeks, the diet was supplemented with a 3 mg/day of boron in the form of sodium borate capsules. About eight days after being given the boron supplement, the women markedly reduced their excretion of both calcium and magnesium. They also had significant increases (about twofold) in the production of an active form of estrogen and testosterone. The research, Hendler added, suggests that supplementation of a low-boron diet with boron causes changes in postmenopausal women consistent with the prevention of calcium loss and bone demineralization.

"The finding that supplementary boron reduces magnesium excretion is also of potential great interest," Hendler continued. "Suboptimal magnesium appears quite common, particularly in those taking diuretics and digitalis. Low magnesium status may be an important factor in schemic heart disease and other forms of cardiovascular disease. The magnesium-sparing effect of boron could have enormous significance in these matters."[5]

In his practice, Robert M. Giller, M.D., recommends boron for patients with arthritis, osteoporosis and menopausal complaints. He recaps these recommendations in his book, *Natural Prescriptions*.

"There are several nutritional supplements that I have found successful in treating patients with arthritis," Giller said. "One is the mineral boron. It seems that people who live in places where there is a minimal amount of boron in the soil have a much higher incidence of arthritis. I tell my patients to supplement their diet with 2 mg/day of boron." (His other recommendations are detailed in his book.)[6]

Boron has also proved helpful for his menopausal patients. The mineral naturally elevates estrogen levels, and he originally recommended it to help fight osteoporosis. Many women told him that it had an immediate beneficial effect on their hot flashes.

He added that zinc and boron seem to help reduce swelling in the joints of patients with rheumatoid arthritis, as well as morning stiffness. In addition to his other recommendations, he prescribes 2 mg/day of boron.

Writing in the *Journal of Nutritional Medicine* in 1990, Richard L. Travers, M.D., and colleagues in the United Kingdom, conducted a double-blind study with arthritics in which some received 6 mg/day of boron and the others a placebo. Of the 10 patients given the mineral, five improved while only one of 10 in the placebo group showed improvement. During the eight-week study, no side effects were reported, and the researchers concluded that the boron had a significant benefit in severe osteoarthritis. The 6 mg of boron was contained in two tablets containing 25 mg of borax (sodium tetraborate decahydrate).[7]

In addition to affecting calcium and magnesium metabolism, boron deficiency signs may be related to the level of vitamin D and possibly other nutrients in the diet, according to *Recommended Dietary Allowances*, 10th Edition, 1989. Boron has long been known to be essential for the growth of most plants.[8]

The richest sources of boron are fruits and vegetables. Health food stores have boron supplements.

REFERENCES

1. Colgan, Michael, Ph.D. *Optimum Sports Nutrition: Your Competitive Edge*. Ronkonkoma, N.Y.: Advanced Research Press, 1993, pp. 205ff.
2. Rodale, J. I., and Staff. *The Complete Book of Minerals for Health*. Emmaus, Pa.: Rodale Books, Inc., 1972, pp. 612–613.
3. McBride, Judy. "Diets Deficient in Boron Can Dull the Senses," *USDA News Feature*, April 19, 1990.
4. McBride, Judy. "Boron: A New Essential Element?" *Scientific Research News*, USDA, April 1989.
5. Hendler, Sheldon Saul, M.D., Ph.D. *The Doctors' Vitamin and Mineral Encyclopedia*. New York: Simon and Schuster, 1990, pp. 114ff.
6. Giller, Robert M., M.D., and Matthews, Kathy. *Natural Prescriptions*. New York: Carol Southern Books, 1994, pp. 20, 22, 245, 247, 299.
7. Travers, Richard L., M.D., et al. "Boron and Arthritis: The Results of a Double-Blind Pilot Study," *Journal of Nutritional Medicine* 1:127–132, 1990.
8. *Recommended Dietary Allowances*, 10th Edition. Washington, D.C.: National Academy Press, 1989, p. 177.

24

Chromium Helps to Balance Blood Sugar Levels

ALTHOUGH chromium was discovered in 1797 by the French chemist Vauquel, it was not until 1959 that researchers determined that the mineral impacts on the health of animals and man. Vauquel made the discovery while studying the properties of crocoite, an ore that is rich in lead chromate. Its common name of chrome was derived from the Greek word *chroma*, which means color, since the mineral is found in many colored compounds. In the early 1900s, chromium became an important ingredient of corrosion-resistant metals.

Because of this, people living in or near industrialized areas are likely to be exposed to air, food and water contaminated by traces of chromium compounds. But, unfortunately, much of the inorganic chromium in the environment is harmful rather than helpful to the body, because certain compounds of the element injure body tissues.

"It was not until 1959 that the medical scientists W. Mertz and K. Schwarz—who came to the United States from Germany—discovered that the feeding of chromium salts corrected the abnormal metabolism of sugar in rats, which resulted from the feeding of diets based on torula yeast," the *Foods and Nutrition Encyclopedia* said. "Later work by these researchers, and by H. Schroeder of the Dartmouth Medical School, established chromium as a cofactor with insulin, necessary for normal glucose utilization and for growth and longevity in rats and mice."

Schwarz had studied the nutritional effects of various types of yeasts, and, in 1957, he had discovered that selenium was present as a vital factor in the American-type of brewer's yeast.[1] According to *Foods and Nutrition Encyclopedia*:

Shortly thereafter, it was found that the inorganic salts of chromium were utilized poorly, compared to an organically bound form of chromium present in brewer's yeast, which was utilized well by both animals and man. The chromium-containing substance from yeast was named the "glucose tolerance factor" (GTF), because it sometimes restored the metabolism of sugars to normal when diabetic-like tendencies were present. (The term GTF denotes the ability of the body tissues to take the sugar glucose from the blood. Hence, it is measured by the rate at which the blood sugar drops back to normal after a test dose of the sugar has been administered to the patient. The blood sugar of diabetics remains abnormally high during the test of glucose tolerance.) Diabetic animals and people were not always helped by either inorganic chromium or the glucose tolerance factor, because their disease may have been caused by factors other than a deficiency of chromium.[1]

One-fifth of an ounce of chromium is a bountiful lifetime supply, reported Gary W. Evans, Ph.D., professor of chemistry at Bemidji State University in Minnesota, in the January 1991 issue of *Better Nutrition for Today's Living*. That equates to slightly more than 200 micrograms daily, which is the high end of the 50 to 200 mcg/day recommended by the National Academy of Sciences.[2]

NEVER ENOUGH FROM DIET

The problem, Evans said, is that nine out of 10 Americans don't get even the minimal 50 mcg/day in typical U.S. diets. Compounding the problem of inadequate supply is the fact that both exercise and high sugar consumption markedly increase urinary loss of chromium. And the mineral is an absolutely essential cofactor for the hormone insulin. Insulin, in turn, regulates the metabolism of carbohydrates, fats and protein. When chromium, in an appropriate biologically active form, is undersupplied, insulin can't perform its job normally, he added.

When there is a chromium deficiency, carbohydrate (in the form of blood sugar) tends to build up in the bloodstream (hyperglycemia), rather than being absorbed by bodily cells, Evans said. Within the cells it is "burned" to produce carbon dioxide, water and energy. Blood sugar supplies almost all human energy. Extreme hyperglycemia is called diabetes, which now afflicts roughly 10 million Americans.

In addition to elevated blood sugar, there are other symptoms of chromium deficiency, Evans continued. And supplemented chromium improves every one of these deficiency symptoms, including lowering cholesterol and increasing longevity. These symptoms are:

1. Impaired glucose tolerance (inability of the cells to pick up and use blood sugar);

2. Elevated insulin levels;
3. Glycosuria (blood sugar spilling into the urine);
4. Impaired growth;
5. Decreased fertility and sperm count;
6. Aortic plaques;
7. Elevated cholesterol levels; and
8. Decreased longevity.[2]

Drinking a sugary soda after eating a starchy meal and then ice cream smothered with chocolate fudge can drain your body of chromium, according to Richard A. Anderson, Ph.D., of the USDA's Agricultural Research Service in Beltsville, Maryland. He added that the more insulin we secrete to process sugars from a meal, the more chromium we use and lose. And once used, the mineral is discarded like a wet paper towel. As might be expected, when there's not enough chromium available, the body simply pumps out more insulin.

VOLATILE COMBINATION OF SUGARS

Anderson indicated that chronically high insulin levels (an early warning sign for adult-onset diabetes) are probably due to low body stores of chromium. Studies at the USDA facility show that the biggest rise in insulin levels and, consequently, the greatest loss of chromium, result from eating glucose followed by fructose. They are the two most common sugars in our diets.

"We seldom eat just one sugar," Anderson said. "For example, the high-fructose corn sweeteners found in many prepared foods and soft drinks are nearly half glucose. And table sugar is composed of both sugars. It's hard enough to get the minimum suggested intake—50 micrograms (millionths of a gram) per day—through a fairly well-balanced diet. Most people don't."[3]

Anderson went on to say that few foods provide more than 10 to 15 percent of the minimum suggested chromium intake. A handful of breakfast cereals provide more than 25 percent; one cereal brand provides about 60 percent. Beer and wine are also good sources of chromium. He recommends eating a variety of fresh fruits, vegetables, dairy and whole-wheat products and meat. Some foods and beverages, such as beer, pick up chromium during processing from the stainless steel equipment. But, he added, other foods lose natural chromium in the refining process.

Anderson and his colleagues conducted a study at the Beltsville facility to assess the effects of consuming glucose, fructose and starch (many glucose units linked together) alone and in combination, on a range of blood indicators. The 11 men and nine women in the study had the greatest rise in blood insulin and the greatest loss of chromium when they drank a glucose solution followed 20 minutes later by a fructose solution. Although the sugar levels in the study were much higher than people would normally consume in a meal, Anderson said, the combination of sugars is analogous to eating a meal. He noted that glucose taken alone caused the second highest rise in insulin and loss of chromium, followed by fructose taken 20 minutes after starch. However, fructose taken alone produced the smallest rise in insulin and loss of chromium.[3]

Sheldon Reiser, Ph.D., who heads carbohydrate research at the Maryland facility, who coordinated the study, said that fructose consumed on an empty stomach doesn't raise blood insulin levels because the body metabolizes it differently than glucose. However, once blood glucose levels are elevated, fructose somehow stimulates insulin secretion. Reiser added that, for fructose to kick in, blood glucose has to be elevated.

Based on earlier studies, Anderson said that when they supplement people with chromium, they definitely see an improvement in glucose metabolism. But, he added, physicians rarely if ever use such a treatment.[3]

At another time, Anderson said that chromium helps keep blood sugar from climbing too high as well as dipping too low. He added that, "I don't know of any other nutrient that affects both high and low blood sugar. In fact, I don't know of any drug that raises low blood sugar." He noted that the standard treatment for hypoglycemia, or low blood sugar, is to eat smaller meals more frequently and avoid a lot of sugar.

Anderson and his colleagues confirmed that chromium helps to raise low glucose by studying women being treated for hypoglycemia at Georgetown University Hospital in Washington, D.C. Patients with low blood sugar often complain of feeling drowsy, sweaty, shaky, fatigued and mentally dull a few hours after eating. The symptoms are not so much a result of how far blood sugar drops, but how rapidly it drops.[4]

Speaking at a meeting of the Federation of American Societies for Experimental Biology in New Orleans in March 1989, Gary W. Evans, Ph.D., discussed a study in collaboration with Raymond I. Press, M.D., and Jack Geller, M.D., of the Mercy Hospital and Medical Center in San Diego, California. In the double-blind, cross-over study, 11 volunteers with diabetes who were not taking insulin received 200 mcg/day of chromium picolinate or a placebo for 42 days. When the subjects were ingesting chromium picolinate, their fasting blood glucose, glycosylated hemoglobin, total cholesterol and low-density lipoprotein cholesterol

(LDL, the harmful kind) went down considerably. Eight of the 11 showed a positive response to the chromium supplements. Their blood glucose range decreased by 24 percent; glycosylated hemoglobin decreased by 19 percent; total cholesterol decreased 13 percent and LDL-cholesterol went down 11 percent.

"These results demonstrate that chromium picolinate is effective in regulating blood glucose and lipids in adult onset diabetes," Evans said.[5]

Chromium supplements improved glucose tolerance and the various subjective symptoms of low blood sugar, according to Jorgen Clausen, M.D., in *Biological Trace Element Research* in 1988. During the study, at the Institute for Life Sciences and Chemistry, Roskilde University, in Denmark, 20 hypoglycemic patients received 125 mcg/day of chromium for three months. During the treatment, which consisted of yeast chromium, glucose tolerance curves were improved in 40 percent of the patients. Thirty days after the treatment period, glucose tolerance curves were improved in 72 percent of the patients. There were also improvements in symptoms of chilliness in 47 percent and a total disappearance of chilliness in 15 percent of the patients. The researchers also reported that 50 to 90 percent of the subjective symptoms improved, such as trembling, emotional instability and disorientation.[6]

In an animal study reported in *Annals of Nutrition and Metabolism* in 1991, G. Mahdi, et al., found that chromium-rich barley is effective in treating the diabetic animals. Barley contains about 5.69 mcg of chromium per gram.[7]

In a review article in the *South African Medical Journal* in 1992, N. Silvis, M.D., said that the ideal diet for diabetics is high in complex carbohydrates and fiber and low in fat. And appropriate supplements can improve glucose tolerance, immune function and wound healing in diabetic patients, while decreasing the risk of cardiovascular disease and other complications. The suggested nutrients included chromium, selenium, zinc, vitamin C, vitamin E and the vitamin B-complex.[8]

In a detailed article in *Biological Trace Element Research* in 1992, Richard A. Anderson, Ph.D., reviews the role of chromium in helping diabetic patients. Since all of those who develop maturity-onset diabetes will have initially impaired glucose tolerance, the prevention of impaired glucose tolerance could lead to the prevention of maturity-onset diabetes. Chromium supplements could, therefore, be very valuable in these patients, he said.[9]

E. G. Offenbacher, Ph.D., of Columbia University in New York, reported in *Biological Trace Element Research* in 1992, that the diets of many healthy seniors are below recommended levels. This places them at risk for developing chromium-related disorders. While the daily recommended amount of chromium is supposed to be between 50 and 200 mcg, some of the elderly patients were only getting 30 mcg/day.[10]

Researchers at the Israel Institute of Technology in Haifa, reported in the *American Journal of Clinical Nutrition* in 1992, that an impaired utilization of chromium might be an etiological factor in women who develop diabetes during pregnancy.[11]

In the October 12, 1991 issue of *USDA News*, Richard A. Anderson, Ph.D. said that, after analyzing 22 well-balanced diets, he found that most of them did not contain the recommended daily intake of 50 mcg/day of chromium. The average chromium content of the diets was 13.4 mcg per 1,000 calories.

"At that level," Anderson said, "a person would have to eat close to 4,000 calories a day to get 50 mcg of chromium. Typical daily intakes in the USDA studies were 2,273 calories for women and 2,950 for men. It's difficult to get enough chromium from foods."

Anderson added that a significant amount of the chromium present in foods is likely to be added during growing, handling and processing. Or it may sneak in through fortification with calcium or other minerals or through preparation in stainless steel containers, which are about 18 percent chromium. One cup of broccoli contained 22 mcg of chromium in one of their studies, which is at least 10 times more than other fruits and vegetables they analyzed. He suspects the mineral may have come from chemical sprays. The peeling of apples reduced chromium content by 70 percent (from 1.4 to 0.4 mcg per apple) bringing it close to the content of peeled oranges. And three ounces of turkey ham, a processed luncheon meat, contained 10 mcg of chromium, which is at least five times more chromium than the same amount of beef, chicken, turkey or ham, he added.[12]

DEFICIENCY MAY DEVELOP WITH AGE

During the 1970s and 1980s, researchers reported that many vitamin and mineral deficiencies in the U.S. were found in both young and old alike, but they also found that deficiencies were most prominent in older people, according to Judy Shabert, M.D., in *The Ultimate Nutrient: Glutamine*. As an example, she said, a survey of people in the Boston area showed that about 65 percent of older people living at home took in less than two-thirds of the Recommended Dietary Allowances for vitamin B6, vitamin B12, folic acid, vitamin D, zinc, calcium and chromium.

"One explanation," Shabert added, "is that as people age, they require fewer calories, and they often sacrifice nutritious foods in favor of more high-calorie, fatty foods and/or alcohol. Another part of the problem is that many elderly people do not have the resources or the energy to shop or cook for themselves."[13]

She added that deficiencies can lead to numerous problems that complicate aging and, in some cases, accelerate the aging process. When inadequate intake of nutrients is combined with poor absorption of nutrients from the gastrointestinal tract, potentially serious problems with accelerated aging can occur.

Many seniors are addicted to antacids, and this can contribute to a chromium deficiency. C. Seaborn and colleagues at Oklahoma State University in Stillwater, writing in *Nutrition Research* in 1990, said that many people are consuming less than the current recommended amount of chromium, while the use of calcium-containing antacids is increasing in an attempt to prevent osteoporosis. Using animals, the researchers found that chromium chloride absorption is poor and that calcium carbonate antacids further reduce chromium absorption.

During the study, the animals were fasted and then given either water, vitamin C or a calcium-based antacid followed by chromium chloride. While the absorption of chromium chloride is low, it is even further reduced when coming in contact with calcium carbonate antacids. It is believed that the antacid might form insoluble complexes with chromium in the intestinal tract or perhaps alter the intestinal pH.[14]

A PILL THAT FIGHTS FAT?

Chromium picolinate supplements may help to reduce body fat without cutting calories, according to the May 19, 1994 issue of *Medical Tribune*. The study, reported at a meeting of the Experimental Biology Conference in Anaheim, California, on April 25, was done by Deborah Hasten, a Ph.D. candidate at Louisiana State University in Baton Rouge. For maximum benefit, she recommends 500 mcg/day. She added that "chromium picolinate is extremely safe, with extensive studies showing no adverse effects."[15]

In his book, *The Chromium Program*, Jeffrey A. Fisher, M.D., said that chromium picolinate may promote weight loss because high blood levels of insulin, which occur as a consequence of tissues' resistance to insulin, promote excessive disposition of fat. Chromium reduces insulin resistance, he said, which in turn decreases the storage of adipose (fatty) tissue and increases its metabolism.

"Another way could be by decreasing hunger," Fisher added. "By helping to stabilize blood sugar levels, chromium diminishes the desire to eat. In addition, insulin stimulates the synthesis in the brain of serotonin, a member of a family of chemicals called neurotransmitters, which facilitate communication between brain cells. Increased amounts of serotonin in the brain can help promote a feeling of satiety. Increasing chromium intake should help insulin perform the job better as well."[16]

The results of early research suggested that chromium picolinate by itself—in the absence of increased exercise—could increase fat loss, according to Richard A. Passwater, Ph.D., in *The Longevity Factor: Chromium Picolinate*. By the end of 1991, he added, three other studies were completed, all supporting the premise that chromium picolinate does indeed decrease body fat and build muscle even without dieting or increased exercise. And he reported on a study by Gilbert Kaats, M.D., at a San Antonio, Texas clinic, in which those getting chromium picolinate averaged a loss of 4.2 pounds of fat and a gain of 1.4 pounds of muscle. Intakes of the mineral ranged from 200 to 400 mcg/day.[17]

Writing in *The Nutrition Report* in May 1989, Elizabeth Somer, M.A., R.D., said that a recent study by Richard Anderson and colleagues (*Journal of Applied Physiology* 64:249–252, 1988) found that strenuous exercise produces increased urinary loss of chromium in trained athletes. She explained that the function of chromium is directly linked to the function of insulin, muscle synthesis, glucose and lipid metabolism, and therefore energy substrate metabolism during exercise.[18]

"Even marginal deficiencies of chromium are associated with impairment of lipid metabolism, in particular elevated serum cholesterol and triglycerides," Somer said. "Chromium supplementation improves glucose intolerance, lowers total serum cholesterol and increases HDL-cholesterol concentrations, and lowers serum triglycerides. The short-term and long-term effects of even marginal chromium status on athletic performance and substrate utilization could be pronounced."[18]

If athletic rats are any indication, human athletes may be able to endure a little longer and compete a little better with a little more chromium in their bodies, according to Richard A. Anderson, Ph.D., in *USDA Quarterly Report of Selected Research Projects*, January 1 to March 31, 1989. Marathoners and other long-distance athletes prepare for competition by eating a high-carbohydrate diet to stockpile all the glycogen (the storage form of glucose) their muscle tissue will hold. However, Anderson said that how fast the glycogen disappears during competition may determine who finishes first—or who finishes at all. Rats that were fed adequate chromium for five weeks lost significantly less muscle glycogen during strenuous exercise than those fed a low-chromium diet, Anderson said.[19]

Exercise results in an accelerated excretion of chromium, zinc and copper, according to Wayne W. Campbell and Richard A. Anderson, of the USDA research facility in Beltsville, Maryland, in *Sports Medicine*. Those who train intensively may be at special risk due to repeated losses of the minerals, they said. In other words, when large losses are coupled with low dietary intakes of the minerals, the body may be placed in a compromising nutritional state. With suboptimal amounts of these minerals, many body processes involving carbohydrate, fat and protein metabolism are altered and may affect performance, they added.

"An athlete's diet should contain a variety of foods, including foods rich in trace minerals, such as whole grains and cereals, legumes, green leafy vegetables, meats and fish," the researchers said. "Highly processed and refined foods should be limited; trace minerals are often lost during processing. It may be difficult to consume adequate trace minerals strictly from dietary food sources; supplementation may be necessary to obtain the recommended dietary levels for chromium, zinc and copper."

They added that this may be especially true for those on low-calorie diets, such as people on weight-reducing programs and athletes who must control their weight for competition. They recommended that the multivitamin or multimineral supplement should contain from one to two times the Recommended Dietary Allowance for each nutrient.[20]

In *The Chromium Program*, Jeffrey A. Fisher, M.D., reported on the work of Gary Evans, Ph.D., who has researched chromium picolinate in relation to weight loss, the lowering of cholesterol, etc. Evans used to be with the U. S. Department of Agriculture facility in Grand Forks, North Dakota and, as previously mentioned, is currently with the Minnesota State University system in Bemidji.[21]

Working with Muriel B. Gilman, Evans conducted two separate studies at the university. In the first one, he recruited 10 freshmen who had enrolled in weight-training classes. In the double-blind study, one group received 200 mcg/day of chromium picolinate for six weeks. The other group was given an inactive placebo. Both groups followed a prescribed weight-lifting protocol for three hours a week. Measurements were taken at the beginning and end of the study and included percent of body fat, lean body mass and circumferences of the biceps and calf muscles.[21]

"In the group on the placebo the lean body mass increased only about 0.008 lbs (less than two ounces), which was not significant," Fisher said. "In the group given chromium picolinate, the lean body mass increased (about 3.5 pounds)—30 times more than those on the placebo. The calf and biceps circumferences of the group on chromium also increased significantly."[21]

In a second study, Fisher reported, Evans selected 31 football players, who received either 200 mcg/day of chromium picolinate or a placebo for six weeks, Fisher reported. In the group on chromium, the lean body mass increased significantly after only 14 days and continued to increase to 5.69 pounds at the end of the study.

"The magnitude of muscle gain in some of the participants in Dr. Evans's studies with safe and natural chromium paralleled that seen with dangerous anabolic steroids," Fisher said.

Since all volunteers were on a weight-training program, the placebo group also gained lean body mass, but it was 42-percent less than the chromium group.

"In the group on chromium," Fisher continued, "total body fat decreased by 22 percent, from 15.8 percent to 12.2 percent. Just as remarkable, the group on chromium actually lost weight, 2.63 pounds during the six weeks. Since they gained 5.69 pounds of lean muscle mass, and since muscle weighs more than fat, they lost more fat than they gained muscle. These are ideal results for anyone who wants to shape up—an increase in lean muscle, a loss of body fat and a loss of weight."[21]

Reporting on the various studies involving weight reduction, Richard Anderson, Ph.D., said in the June 1993 issue of *The Nutrition Report* that, "The effects of supplemental chromium on lean body mass, percent body fat and weight loss are controversial. However, there is an overriding theme that supplemental chromium leads to improvements in lean body mass, percent body fat and possibly weight loss. The improvements from both human and animal studies support a role for chromium in increasing lean body mass and decreasing body fat. Studies reporting weight loss in nonexercising subjects simply taking a chromium tablet need to be confirmed. These studies are consistent with the functions of chromium but need to be documented in independent laboratories."[22]

Insulin's effect upon muscle development and energy production is vital to athletic performance and development, but, without GTF-chromium, it is ineffective, according to Michael E. Rosenbaum, M.D., in *Sports Science Update*. He added that experiments have shown that GTF or insulin alone are unable to significantly affect glucose intake by body tissues, but together they can dramatically increase (sugar) uptake and utilization. As we know, GTF stands for Glucose Tolerance Factor, and it is the chromium-containing substance from yeast that was isolated by Dr. Walter Mertz and colleagues in the 1950s.

"When exercise-enhanced chromium loss is coupled with diets high in refined carbohydrates and low in biologically active GTF-chromium, the nutritional status for GTF and overall health for exercising individuals is likely to be suboptimal," Rosenbaum said.[23]

HELPS METABOLIZE FATS AND LIPIDS

Chromium appears to be essential for the metabolism of dietary fats and lipids as well as glucose, according to H. DeWayne Ashmead, Ph.D., in *Conversations on Chelation and Mineral Nutrition*. If we were to look at people who had hardening of the arteries, he said, we would see that their serum cholesterol and other lipid levels were elevated. In this condition, there is less tolerance to ingested or injected glucose, and sometimes a mild state of diabetes is fostered, he added.

And eventually, since these fats cannot be metabolized properly, plaques begin to grow on the arterial walls.[24]

"I think that it is worth noting that scientists can duplicate these biological and pathological changes under experimental conditions simply by introducing a chromium-deficient diet," Ashmead explained. "Dr. Henry A. Schroeder did something else that incriminated chromium and tends to substantiate the connection between its deficiency state and atherosclerosis. He and his associates obtained aorta tissue samples from people all across the United States who had died from atherosclerosis heart disease. They also obtained tissues from people who had died from other forms of cardiovascular diseases."

These tissues were assayed along with tissues taken from healthy individuals who had died in accidents. And the researchers found that those who had died of atherosclerosis had chromium levels significantly lower than those otherwise healthy people who had died in accidents.

"When you consider that atherosclerosis can be induced experimentally by creating a chromium deficiency, it is only logical to conclude that a definite relationship exists between chromium deficiency and atherosclerosis," Ashmead said.[24]

In a study involving rabbits, researchers at Shaare Zedek Medical Center in Jerusalem, Israel, reported in *Annals of Nutrition and Metabolism* in 1991, that the animals fed 20 mcg of chromium chloride had the greatest regression of atherosclerosis. They added that chromium supplementation lowers and regresses atherosclerotic plaque independent of any changes in blood lipids or lipoproteins.[25]

Writing in *Trace Elements in Medicine* in 1992, Indian researchers reviewed the role of chromium, sodium, potassium, calcium, magnesium, phosphorus, copper, zinc, selenium, cadmium, lead and mercury in the cardiovascular system. As might be expected, cadmium, lead and mercury are toxic to the system. Most of the other minerals have a protective role. For example, they pointed out that chromium and copper may have a cholesterol-lowering effect, and chromium can increase high-density lipoprotein cholesterol (HDL, the beneficial kind) while controlling high blood sugar.[26]

In an extensive review in *Biological Trace Element Research*, Walter Mertz, Ph.D., explained the role of chromium in human health. The significance of chromium nutrition may extend well beyond the importance of impaired glucose tolerance tests, he said. Normal glucose tolerance is maintained at the expense of increased insulin production, he added, which gradually deteriorates with advancing age. This increase in insulin levels, along with impaired glucose tolerance, are increased risk factors for both diabetes and cardiovascular disease, he said.[27]

In a double-blind study reported in the *American Journal of Clinical Nutrition* in 1981, 13 of 23 healthy males were given 200 mcg/day of chromium while the rest received a placebo. After 12 weeks, the chromium-supplemented men demonstrated increased serum triglycerides and total cholesterol, along with HDL-cholesterol and improved glucose tolerance.[28]

The fact that a high-sugar diet can contribute to chromium losses was once again demonstrated by Adriane S. Kozlovsky, et al., at the Beltsville Human Nutrition Research Center in Maryland and reported in *Metabolism* in 1986. The study involved 19 men and 18 women, who were studied for 12 weeks. Compared to the reference diets, consumption of the high-sugar diets increased urinary chromium losses from 10 to 300 percent for 27 of the 37 volunteers. The authors agreed that their data demonstrate that consumption of diets high in simple sugars stimulates chromium losses. And this, coupled with marginal intake of dietary chromium, might lead to marginal chromium deficiency, which is associated with impaired glucose and lipid metabolism.[29]

Chromium supplementation is suitable for lipid modulation therapy because of its low cost (about $5 per month), easy administration and the fact that it has virtually no risk, according to John R. Roeback, Ph.D., in *Annals of Internal Medicine* in 1991. He added that these features make chromium supplementation appealing for those who are interested in natural, inexpensive and nontoxic modes of health care.[30]

Chromium is just one of the nutrients that play a role in preventing degenerative diseases in the elderly, according to Kathleen Johnson, M.S., R.D., and Evan W. Kligman, M.D., in *Geriatrics* in 1992. Other important vitamins and minerals, they said, include magnesium, potassium, calcium, copper, zinc, selenium, vitamin C, vitamin E, beta-carotene, vitamin A, folic acid, vitamin B6, vitamin D, pantothenic acid and others.[31]

Richard Doisy, M.D., of the State University of New York Upstate Medical Center in Syracuse, studied the effect of GTF in 10 grams of brewer's yeast on the cholesterol levels of 16 of his medical students over a month, reported Richard A. Passwater, Ph.D., in *GTF-Chromium*. One-half of the students had blood cholesterol levels above 240 milligram-per-deciliter, which is in the upper limit of the "normal" range. After one month of brewer's yeast supplementation, the students having elevated blood cholesterol had a decrease of an average of 56 milligram-per-deciliter. The others, who had normal blood cholesterol levels, had a lesser decrease. The average for the entire group of students was a 36 milligram-per-deciliter decrease, Passwater reported.

Doisy also studied the effects of GTF on nine persons over the age of 75 and found their blood cholesterol dropped from an average of 245 mg/dl to an average of 205 mg/dl.

"Another example is the study of Dr. Ester Offenbacher of Columbia University that documents significantly improved blood cholesterol in both diabetic and nondiabetic persons receiving chromium-rich brewer's yeast," Passwater continued. "Dr. Victoria Liu found a test group with a blood cholesterol level averaging 216 mg/dl to have a decrease of 90 mg/dl with brewer's yeast supplementation. In 1968, Dr. Henry Schroeder found that two milligrams of inorganic chromium lowered blood cholesterol levels by 14 to 17 percent. Similar results were reported by Dr. H. W. Staub."[32]

Also in the news is chromium polynicotinate which, as the name suggests, is chromium combined with niacin (vitamin B3). Niacin has often been recommended for lowering cholesterol levels, but the megadoses that are sometimes suggested (500 to 4,500 mg/day) can cause skin flushing, itching, rashes, nausea, diarrhea and other complications in susceptible people. The jury is still out concerning the value of timed-release niacin in this application.

At any rate, the yeast-free chromium nicotinate, in which the mineral is bound to nicotinic acid, another form of vitamin B3, is being studied for possibly lowering cholesterol levels, curbing carbohydrate cravings and other chromium attributes.

Writing in the *Journal of Family Practice* in 1988, Martin Urberg, M.D., of Wayne State University in Detroit, found that 200 mcg of chromium and 100 mg of niacin daily decreased low-density lipoprotein cholesterol (LDL) by 23 and 30 percent in the two patients evaluated. Although the study is admittedly small, it suggests that niacin may enhance chromium's ability to lower cholesterol.[33]

In a more recent double-blind study, Robert Lefavi, Ph.D., of Georgia Southern University in Statesboro, reported that 200 mcg of chromium as niacin-bound chromium complex lowered blood cholesterol levels by an average of 14 percent and improved total cholesterol/HDL ratios by seven percent. The chromium-niacin supplement included 200 mcg of chromium bound to two mg of niacin and, at these low niacin levels, there were no side effects such as skin flushing, the researchers said.

The study, which involved 34 male athletes, was performed at Auburn University in Alabama in conjunction with Richard A. Anderson, Ph.D., and others at the U.S. Department of Agriculture. During the eight-week study, the volunteers were assigned to three groups. Each group received either 200 mcg of niacin-bound chromium, 800 mcg of the same supplement or a placebo.

After eight weeks, the average serum cholesterol in the first group (200 mcg) dropped from 147.9 mg/dl to 126.8 mg/dl or a decrease of 14.3 percent. In the second group (800 mcg, including 7.2 mg of niacin), the cholesterol dropped from 159.2 mg/dl to 131.3 mg/dl. In the placebo group, the cholesterol increased from 139.9 mg/dl to 153.4 mg/dl.[34]

In an article in *Cardiovascular Research* in 1984, Monique Simonoff of Centre National de la Recherche Scientifique, Bordeaux-Gradignan, France, said that recent measurements have demonstrated that blood chromium levels in patients with coronary artery disease are very much lower than in normal subjects. She added that a review of the literature concerning the physiological functions of chromium (or GTF) shows it to be implicated in most of the known factors of cardiovascular risk, such as insulin levels and activities. Chromium deficiency results in impaired fat and glucide metabolism and results in high circulating insulin levels, "the probable consequence of which suggest that chromium deficiency may be a primary risk factor in cardiovascular disease." She added that the literature suggests that it would be eminently reasonable to combat the incipient chromium deficiency found in Western societies by increased intake of chromium, especially of biologically active GTF, since some individuals appear to lose their ability to convert inorganic chromium to a biologically active form.[35]

In a study reported in the *Journal of Nutritional Medicine* in 1992, Richard Cook, Ph.D., and David Benton, Ph.D., of University College in Swansea, United Kingdom, discussed their evaluation of an adult female who was bothered by recurring headaches. Over a period of 13 months, they gave her at varying intervals zinc, manganese, chromium, magnesium, copper, vitamin C and vitamin B6 and found that her condition improved when she was given the supplement. They suggested that chronic headaches respond to supplementation and that the active ingredient in this instance was chromium.[36]

Breastfed infants consume less than two percent of the estimated safe and adequate recommendations for chromium, which is 10 mcg, according to Richard Anderson, Ph.D., and colleagues in the *American Journal of Clinical Nutrition* in 1993. The USDA researchers suggested that the mineral's content of breastmilk is independent of dietary chromium intake by the mother as well as serum and urinary levels, but that it falls far below current recommended levels for infants.[37]

CAN CHROMIUM BOOST LONGEVITY?

Following a four-year study with rats, Gary W. Evans, Ph.D., said that the animals that received chromium picolinate throughout their life, and allowed to eat as much or as often as they wanted, had a median life span of 45 months. This contrasted with 33 months for the rats receiving less effective forms of chromium. He told a meeting of the American Aging Association and the American College of Clinical Gerontology, October 19, 1992, in San Francisco, that this represents a 12-month or 36 percent increase in life span. While the implications for human longevity remain to be seen, Evans said that this would be equivalent to extending human life from the current age of 75 years to about age 102.[38]

Since high blood sugar levels are believed to impact on the aging process, Evans measured the rats' blood sugar and glycated hemoglobin (an average blood level measurement) and found glycated hemoglobin in the older rats to be about 60 percent lower in those receiving chromium picolinate than in the other animals. Several researchers have also theorized that caloric restriction may also be beneficial in reducing blood sugar levels. Blood sugar is known to interact with tissue or blood proteins in the so-called glycation reaction, and these reactions may alter protein and nucleic acid function, resulting in changes that are associated with the normal aging process.

"Chromium picolinate enhances insulin function and may, therefore, produce the same glucose-lowering benefits as underfeeding, but without restricting calorie intake," Evans said.[38]

Dried liver and brewer's yeast are two of the richest sources of chromium in the diet. Others are blackstrap molasses, eggs, cheese, liver, wheat bran, beef, whole wheat, apple peel, wheat germ, potatoes and oysters.

Since diabetes and heart disease are major health problems in the United States, most of us probably need to evaluate our chromium intake.

As Julian M. Whitaker, M.D. reported in *Reversing Diabetes*, "As early as 1854, it was reported that brewer's yeast improved the diabetic condition. Later, researchers found that the active ingredient in brewer's yeast is a complex of chromium and several amino acids that has become known as the Glucose Tolerance Factor (GTF)."

Be Patient . . .

He added that when Dr. Walter Mertz gave chromium supplements to six diabetics, three of them demonstrated improved control ("Effects and Metabolism of Glucose Tolerance Factor," *Nutrition Review* 33:1929, 1975). GTF chromium does not act like insulin but rather seems to enhance insulin sensitivity. Whitaker added that Dr. Mertz has noted that chromium concentration in tissues of Americans declines with age and that this may be a reason for the significant increase in diabetes as we get older. Mertz also reported that chromium supplementation can sometimes take two to three months before any beneficial changes are noted.[39]

REFERENCES

1. Ensminger, Audrey H., et al. *Foods and Nutrition Encyclopedia.* Clovis, Calif.: Pegus Press, 1983, p. 416.

2. Evans, Gary W., Ph.D. "Chromium: A Basic Ingredient for Good Health," *Better Nutrition for Today's Living*, January 1991, pp. 26, 28.
3. McBride, Judy. "Too Many Sweets Can Set Off Chromium Alert," *Scientific Research News*, USDA, July 10, 1989.
4. Becker, Hank. "To Balance Blood Sugar, Chromium Swings Both Ways," *Scientific Research News*, USDA, November 1986.
5. Press, Raymond I., M.D., Geller, Jack, M.D., and Evans, Gary W., Ph.D. "The Effect of Chromium Picolinate on Serum Glucose, Glycosylated Hemoglobin and Cholesterol of Adult Onset Diabetics." Paper read at a meeting of the Federation of American Societies for Experimental Biology, New Orleans, Louisiana, March 21, 1989.
6. Clausen, Jorgen, M.D. "Chromium Induced Clinical Improvement in Symptomatic Hypoglycemia," *Biological Trace Element Research* 17:229–236, 1988.
7. Mahdi, G., et al. "Chromium-Rich Barley Effective Treatment for Diabetes," *Annals of Nutrition and Metabolism* 35:65–70, 1991.
8. Silvis, N. "Nutritional Recommendations for Individuals with Diabetes Mellitus," *South African Medical Journal* 81:162–166, February 1, 1992.
9. Anderson, Richard A. "Chromium, Glucose Tolerance and Diabetes," *Biological Trace Element Research* 32:19–24, 1992.
10. Offenbacher, E. G. "Chromium and the Elderly," *Biological Trace Element Research* 32:123–131, 1992.
11. Aharoni, A., et al. "Hair Chromium Content of Women with Gestational Diabetes Compared with Nondiabetic Pregnant Women," *American Journal of Clinical Nutrition* 55:104–107, 1992.
12. McBride, Judy. "Chromium Is Hard to Come By, Well-Balanced Diet or Not," *USDA News*, October 21, 1991.
13. Shabert, Judy, M.D., and Ehrlich, Nancy. *The Ultimate Nutrient: Glutamine.* Garden City Park, N.Y.: Avery Publishing Group, 1994, pp. lff.
14. Seaborn, C., et al. "Effects of Antacid or Ascorbic Acid on Tissue Accumulation and Urinary Excretion of Chromium," *Nutrition Research* 10:1401–1407, 1990.
15. "Chromium Supplements May Help Reduce Body Fat," *Medical Tribune*, May 19, 1994, p. 19.
16. Fisher, Jeffrey A., M.D. *The Chromium Program.* New York: Harper and Row, 1990, pp. 33–34.
17. Passwater, Richard A., Ph.D. *The Longevity Factor: Chromium Picolinate.* New Canaan, Conn.: Keats Publishing, Inc., 1993, pp. 65–69.
18. Somer, Elizabeth, M.A., R.D. "Athletes at Risk for Chromium Deficiency," *The Nutrition Report*, May 1989, pp. 34, 38.
19. *Quarterly Report of Selected Research Projects*, USDA, January 1 to March 31, 1989, p. 10.
20. Campbell, Wayne W., and Anderson, Richard A. "Effects of Aerobic Exercise and Training on the Trace Minerals Chromium, Zinc and Copper," *Sports Medicine* 4:9–18, 1987.

21. Fisher, Jeffrey A., M.D. *The Chromium Program.* New York: Harper and Row 1990, pp. 13ff.

22. Anderson, Richard A., Ph.D. "Chromium and Its Role in Lean Body Mass and Weight Reduction," *The Nutrition Report*, June 1993, pp. 39, 46.

23. Rosenbaum, Michael E., M.D. "GTF-Chromium and Athletic Performance," *Sports Science Update*, March 1988.

24. Ashmead, H. DeWayne, Ph.D. *Conversations on Chelation and Mineral Nutrition.* New Canaan, Conn.: Keats Publishing, Inc., 1989, pp. 85ff.

25. Abraham, A., et al. "Chromium and Cholesterol-Induced Atherosclerosis in Rabbits," *Annals of Nutrition and Metabolism* 35:203–207, 1991.

26. Singh, R. B., et al. "Macro and Trace Mineral Metabolism in Coronary Heart Disease," *Trace Elements in Medicine* 9(3):144–156, 1992.

27. Mertz, Walter, Ph.D. "Chromium History and Nutritional Importance," *Biological Trace Element Research* 32:3–7, 1992.

28. Railes, R., et al. "Effect of Chromium Chloride Supplementation on Glucose Tolerance and Serum Lipids Including High Density Lipoprotein of Adult Men," *American Journal of Clinical Nutrition* 34:2670–2678, 1981.

29. Kozlovsky, Adriane S., et al. "Effects of Diets High in Simple Sugars on Urinary Chromium Losses," *Metabolism* 35(6):515–518, June 1986.

30. Roeback, John R., Ph.D. "Effect of Chromium Supplementation on Serum High-Density Lipoprotein Cholesterol Levels in Men Taking Beta-Blockers: A Randomized, Controlled Trial," *Annals of Internal Medicine* 115(12):917–924, December 15, 1991.

31. Johnson, Kathleen, M.S., R.D., and Kligman, Evan W., M.D. "Preventive Nutrition: Disease-Specific Dietary Interventions for Older Adults," *Geriatrics* 47:39–49, October 1992.

32. Passwater, Richard A., Ph.D. *GTF-Chromium (Glucose Tolerance Factor).* New Canaan, Conn.: Keats Publishing, Inc., 1982, pp. 7ff.

33. Urberg, Martin, M.D., et al. "Hypocholesterolemic Effects of Nicotinic Acid and Chromium Supplementation," *The Journal of Family Practice* 27(6):603–606, 1988.

34. Lefavi, Robert, Ph.D., et al. "Lipid-Lowering Effect of a Dietary Nicotinic Acid-Chromium (III) Complex in Male Athletes," *FASEB Journal* 5(6):A1645, 1991.

35. Simonoff, Monique. "Chromium Deficiency and Cardiovascular Risk," *Cardiovascular Research* 18:591–596, 1984.

36. Cook, Richard, Ph.D., and Benton, David, Ph.D. "Chromium Supplementation Involves Chronic Headaches: A Case Study," *Journal of Nutritional Medicine* 3:61–64, 1992.

37. Anderson, R., et al. "Breast Milk Chromium and Its Association with Chromium Intake, Chromium Excretion and Serum Chromium," *American Journal of Clinical Nutrition* 57:519–523, 1993.

38. Evans, Gary W., Ph.D. Address before a joint meeting of the American Aging Association and the American College of Clinical Gerontology, October 19, 1992, San Francisco.

39. Whitaker, Julian M., M.D. *Reversing Diabetes.* New York: Warner Books, 1987, pp. 89–90.

25

Cobalt: The Mineral Within a Vitamin

COBALT has the distinction of being one of the few minerals inside a vitamin. It is an essential constituent of vitamin B12 (cyanocobalamin). Since B12 is derived from bacterial synthesis, inorganic cobalt can be considered essential for animal species that depend totally on their bacterial flora for their vitamin B12, according to *Recommended Dietary Allowances*, 10th Edition. This is the case for ruminant animal species in whom cobalt deficiency is well known; it might also have some relevance for strict vegetarians whose intake of the preformed vitamin is severely limited. However, there is no evidence that the intake of cobalt is ever limiting in the human diet, and there is no RDA for the mineral.[1]

Cobalt is derived from the German word *kobold* meaning goblin or mischievous spirit. The term originated in the 16th century, when arsenic-containing cobalt ores were dug up in the silver mines of the Harz Mountains. Thinking that the ores contained copper, miners heated them and were injured by the toxic arsenic trioxide vapors that were released. These evils were attributed to the goblin or kobold.

George Brandt, the Swedish chemist, first isolated the mineral in 1742, although cobalt had been used for centuries for the blue color in decorative glass and pottery.

"The discovery, in 1948, that vitamin B12 contains four percent cobalt proved this element to be essential for man," the *Foods and Nutrition Encyclopedia* said. "It is noteworthy that cobalt's essential role in ruminant animal nutrition was known much earlier. In 1935, Australian scientists discovered that lack of cobalt, resulting from its deficiency in the soil and thus in the herbage grazed, produced a wasting disease. Much earlier, and long before the cause was known, stockmen in different areas of the world learned that this peculiar malady could be prevented and/or cured by transferring animals from 'sick' to 'healthy' areas."[2]

Cobalt is readily absorbed in the small intestine, but the retained cobalt serves no physiological function since human tissues cannot synthesize the vitamin. Most of the absorbed cobalt is excreted in the urine and little of it is retained. However, small amounts are concentrated in the liver and kidneys. Vitamin B12 is synthesized by E. coli, a species of bacteria found in the colon. However, the microorganisms of the colon do not make sufficient B12 to meet human needs. Actually, little of the vitamin can be absorbed past the small intestine.[2]

"A cobalt deficiency as such has never been produced in humans," the encyclopedia added. "The signs and symptoms that are sometimes attributed to cobalt deficiency are actually due to lack of vitamin B12, characterized by pernicious anemia, poor growth and occasionally neurological disorders."[2]

In *The Nutrition Desk Reference*, Robert H. Garrison, Jr., M.A., R.Ph., and Elizabeth Somer, M.A., R.D., said that cobalt has several functions in the body, including:

1. Acting as a substitute for manganese in the activation of several enzymes (such as glycylglycine dipeptidase);
2. Replacing zinc in some enzymes (such as carboxypeptidase A and B; and bovine, human and monkey carbonic anhydrase);
3. Activating phosphortransferases and other enzymes (even though these enzymes are activated in the presence of other metals or in the absence of any metal);
4. Participating in the biotin-dependent oxalacetate transcarboxylase.[3]

The average intake of cobalt is five to eight mcg/day, the authors said. Normal cobalt concentrations in the blood range from 80 to 300 mcg/ml. Foods containing about 0.2 ppm cobalt include figs, cabbage, spinach, beet greens, buckwheat, lettuce and watercress.[3]

Henry Schroeder, M.D. said that the milling of wheat into refined flour removes 40 percent of the chromium; 86 percent of the manganese; 76 percent of the iron; 89 percent of the cobalt; 68 percent of the copper; 78 percent of the zinc; and 48 percent of the molybdenum.[4]

Dr. D. Behne, of Berlin's Hahn-Meitner Institute, told a conference in Montreux, Switzerland, that cobalt and selenium might be essential to the proper functioning of insulin, since they vary in plasma concentration with both glucose and insulin administration.[4]

A DEADLY BREW

In 1966, a strange disease, which culminated in heart failure, struck heavy beer drinkers in Quebec City, Canada; Leuven, Belgium; Omaha, Nebraska; and Minneapolis, Minnesota, according to Carl C. Pfeiffer, M.D., Ph.D., in *Zinc and Other Micro-Nutrients*. Some researchers attributed the disease of the heart muscle to an excess of cobalt. Others thought other dietary factors were involved and that cobalt was not solely responsible. C. A. Alexander, M.D., noted that many of the victims had inadequate diets that were especially low in protein.[5.]

"These tragic victims were consuming between six and 30 bottles of beer per day, and the *Annals of Internal Medicine* (February 1969) reported that 1.2 ppm of cobalt were found in the Canadian beer," Pfeiffer said. "The film left on the glassware by synthetic detergents kills the foamy 'head' of beer. Therefore, cobalt was added to beer to preserve the foamy head and keep the product aesthetically pleasing."[5]

Pfeiffer added that, as "beer drinkers' cardiomyopathy" illustrates, too much cobalt may be toxic. Administering too much cobalt has caused polycythemia (too many red blood cells) in rats, mice, guinea pigs, ducks, chickens, pigs, dogs and humans. In *Clinical Toxicology* September 1969, G. S. Wiburg and colleagues found that a high-quality protein diet gave considerable protection against the toxicity of cobalt.[5]

Memory function was impaired in 12 adult, former hard metal workers who were exposed to tungsten carbide and cobalt in the form of dust powder, mist and an organic solvent, according to Catherine Jordon, et al. in *Toxicology Letters* in 1990.[6]

In *Let's Eat Right to Keep Fit*, Adelle Davis said that cobalt forms part of vitamin B12 and that as little as three micrograms of B12 daily can prevent pernicious anemia. This small amount could have kept thousands of people from suffering fatigue which tortured every cell in their bodies and prevented a crippling paralysis and finally a bedridden living death during the years before Drs. George R. Minot and William P. Murphy found that raw liver could control the disease.

"Thousands of cattle, sheep and other animals, grazed on land deficient in cobalt, especially in Florida and Australia, sickened and died from a crippling anemia. Deaths like these could be prevented if a few pounds of cobalt were added to each acre of land. Such anemia, however, was never confined to Florida or Australia."[7]

Studies conducted at the University of Florida Agricultural Experiment Station showed that 81 percent of the children living in the area suffered from anemia, just as did the animals, Davis added. Fifty percent showed definite anemia, whereas 31 percent were borderline cases. When the land is deficient, she continued, the plants grown on that land are deficient; the animals which eat the plants are deficient; the people who eat the animals and the plants are deficient. It cannot be otherwise.[7]

CASES OF DEPRESSION

Thirty-five patients (21 males and 14 females) suffering from depression were compared to 35 controls. R. L. Narang and colleagues at the Dayanand Medical College in India reported that plasma cobalt levels were lower in the depressed patients. And cobalt levels in recovered patients were considerably higher when compared to levels in depressed patients, suggesting that cobalt levels increased after they recovered from depression. Plasma manganese levels were unchanged during depression and following recovery. The researchers noted that cobalt is in the center of the vitamin B12 molecule, and that pernicious anemia and subacute combined degeneration of the spinal cord are well known symptoms of vitamin B12 deficiency. The predominant symptoms of the depressed patients were headache, malaise and neurasthenia. And the researchers noted that psychological changes—depression, irritability and neurasthenia—are often precursors of anemia. It was unclear whether cobalt deficiency produces depression or is a result of the depression, however.[8]

REFERENCES

1. *Recommended Dietary Allowances*, 10th Edition. Washington, D.C.: National Academy Press, 1989, pp. 267–268.
2. Ensminger, Audrey H., et al. *Foods and Nutrition Encyclopedia.* Clovis, Calif.: Pegus Press, 1983, p. 434.
3. Garrison, Robert H., Jr., M.A., R.Ph., and Somer, Elizabeth, M.A., R.D. *The Nutrition Desk Reference.* New Canaan Conn.: Keats Publishing, Inc., 1990, p. 62.
4. Rodale, J. I., and Staff. *The Complete Book of Minerals for Health.* Emmaus, Pa.: Rodale Books, Inc., 1972, pp. 410, 499.
5. Pfeiffer, Carl C., M.D., Ph.D. *Zinc and Other Micro-Nutrients.* New Canaan, Conn.: Keats Publishing, Inc., 1978, pp. 137–138.
6. Jordon, Catherine, et al. "Memory Deficits in Workers Suffering from Hard Metal Disease," *Toxicology Letters* 54:241–243, 1990.
7. Davis, Adelle. *Let's Eat Right to Keep Fit.* New York: New American Library, 1970, p. 197.
8. Narang, R. L., et al. "Plasma Cobalt and Manganese in Depression," *Trace Elements in Medicine* 9(1):43–44, 1992.

26

Copper: Worth More Than a Few Cents

WHEN you think of copper, you are apt to focus on the shiny copper tubing in your home, perhaps the copper kettle on the stove, or even the jar full of pennies you don't know what to do with. As useful as these copper instruments are, the mineral plays a significant role in human nutrition as well. It may offer protection against cardiovascular disease and some forms of cancer, and as an antioxidant it can help to boost the immune system and provide some comfort against arthritis. It may also help to stave off diabetes. Of course, copper is somewhat schizophrenic, in that too little copper in the diet may result in heart complications, while too much of the mineral has a deleterious effect. And copper and zinc have an age-old feud going on, in which one or the other tries to annihilate its competitor.

Copper was discovered and used some time during the Stone Age, probably around 8000 B.C. The chief source of the mineral for those living near the Mediterranean Sea was the Island of Cyprus, and the metal was known as Cyprian metal. Therefore, both the word for copper and the chemical symbol (Cu) are derived from *cuprum*, which is the Roman name for Cyprian metal.

In a series of studies at the University of Wisconsin in 1925, Hart and associates discovered that a small amount of copper is necessary, along with iron, for hemoglobin formation. In 1931, Josephs reported that copper was more effective than iron alone in overcoming the anemia of milk-fed infants. Now the mineral is considered an essential nutrient for all vertebrates and some lower animal species.[1]

About 30 percent of the ingested copper is absorbed, mostly in the stomach and upper part of the small intestine. Following absorption, the mineral enters the bloodstream, where 80 percent or more becomes bound to ceruloplasmin, a protein (globulin-copper) complex. The remaining amount is bound to albumin and transported to various tissues, reported *Foods and Nutrition Encyclopedia.*

The role of copper in hemoglobin formation is generally recognized as that of facilitating the absorption of iron from the intestinal tract and releasing it from storage in the liver and the reticuloendothelial system, the reference book continued. Although not necessarily a part of hemoglobin, copper is necessary for the formation of hemoglobin. As a constituent of several enzyme systems, copper is required for normal energy metabolism. And it is needed for the development and maintenance of skeletal structures (bones, tendons and connective tissue). Copper is also essential for the development of the aorta and vascular system, and it is necessary for the formation and functioning of the brain cells and the spinal cord. Copper is also required for normal pigmentation of the hair.

"Dietary copper deficiency is not known to occur in adults under normal circumstances," the encyclopedia reported. "But it has been diagnosed in Peru in malnourished children and in the United States in premature infants fed exclusively on modified cow's milk and in infants breast-fed for an extended period. Fortunately, the liver of newborn babies contains five to 10 times as much copper as the liver of adults—a reserve that is drawn upon during the first year of life."[1]

WHY WE NEED IT

A copper deficiency is related to a variety of abnormalities, such as anemia, skeletal defects, demyelination and degeneration of the nervous system, defects in the pigmentation and structure of hair, reproductive failure and pronounced cardiovascular lesions.

"Copper is also involved in the production of collagen, the protein responsible for functional integrity of bone, cartilage, skin and tendon; elastin, the protein that is mainly responsible for the elastic properties of the blood vessels, lungs and skin; the neurotransmitter noradrenalin, a key molecule in the working of the nervous system; and melanin formation (pigment found in the skin and hair)," according to Sheldon Saul Hendler, M.D., Ph.D., in *The Doctors' Vitamin and Mineral Encyclopedia.*

He added that copper helps protect against the ravages of oxidant damage through the enzyme copper-zinc superoxide dismutase, as well as ceruloplasmin. By oxidizing iron, he explained, ceruloplasmin inhibits free-radical formation from reduced iron. And it is one of the most important blood antioxidants, since it prevents peroxidation (rancidity) of polyunsaturated fatty acids and maintains the integrity of cell membranes.

Hendler said that a copper deficiency in young men (produced by taking 160 mg/day of zinc, a copper antagonist, for a protracted period) contributed to a significant lowering of the level of high-density lipoprotein cholesterol (HDL), the beneficial kind. And it has been reported that there was an increase in cholesterol levels in rats when they were fed diets high in zinc and low in copper, suggesting that an imbalance in the zinc-to-copper ratio increases the risk of coronary heart disease by lowering the amount of protective HDL. In a study involving 24 male volunteers fed a copper-deficient diet, it was found that they had significant increases in low-density lipoprotein cholesterol (LDL), the harmful kind, as well as total cholesterol and significant decreases in HDL after 11 weeks.

"The use of copper bracelets in the folk-remedy treatment of arthritis has persisted despite the skepticism of most doctors," Hendler continued. "It turns out there might be something to it, after all. Researchers have discovered: a) that the clinical condition of those suffering from arthritis (mainly osteoarthritis, or degenerative joint disease) who habitually wore the copper bracelets became significantly worse after discontinuing their use; b) the worsening effects were not seen in those subjects who had worn placebo bracelets; and c) there was evidence that copper from the bracelets, when dissolved in sweat, could be absorbed through the skin."[2]

Forrest H. Nielsen, Ph.D., director of the Human Nutrition Research Center, USDA, in Grand Forks, North Dakota, and Leslie M. Klevay, M.D., a physician and research leader at the facility, said that a copper deficiency is one that may have major implications for public health, reported Judy McBride in *Scientific Research News*, October 1992. Klevay pointed out that his review of the scientific literature has identified more than 60 similarities between animals deficient in copper and people with heart disease.[3]

Recent Center studies on copper deficiency have found that:[3]

- It more than doubled the time it takes mice to dissolve blood clots, which can accumulate in and constrict arteries. Heart disease patients also take longer to dissolve clots when assessed by the same test that was done on the animals.
- It decreased release of a substance that prompts rats' arterial muscles to relax. This is apparently how the mineral deficiency raises blood pressure in adult rats, stated Jack T. Saari, Ph.D., a physiologist at the North Dakota facility.
- It appears that copper increases the potential for oxidative damage to tissues when combined with high intakes of fructose—which constitutes half of

table sugar and nearly half of high-fructose corn sweeteners. Six men developed lower levels of protective antioxidant enzymes from eating diets low in copper and higher in fructose than currently consumed.

"We're getting all kinds of evidence that copper deficiency has pathological consequences," Nielsen said. "I think low copper intakes typical in the United States and other industrialized countries can lead to problems, particularly in older people."[3]

Jack T. Saari, Ph.D., of the North Dakota research center, has shown that a copper deficiency in test animals causes symptoms that resemble human diabetes and aging, according to the *USDA's Quarterly Report of Selected Research Projects*, July 1 to September 30, 1994. These findings support the hypothesis that copper deficiency increases the spontaneous attachment of glucose molecules to proteins, known as protein glycation.[4]

Saari went on to say that, if left unchecked, the dangling glucose molecules attach to a second site on the protein, producing "cross links." Protein glycation is known to increase as we age and to cause tissue damage in diabetics.[4]

Earlier work at the facility suggests that the average American is getting 50 to 60 percent of the recommended dietary levels of copper, reported *Medical Tribune*, October 18, 1990. This may place people at risk to free-radical damage and cause problems with cardiovascular disease and immune function. Copper-rich foods include nuts, seeds, oysters, liver, cocoa, blackstrap molasses and organ meats.[5]

Leslie M. Klevay, M.D., reported in *Nutrition Reviews*, May 1992, that elevated levels of homocysteine are associated with coronary, cerebral and peripheral hardening of the arteries. Homocysteine is a natural amino acid metabolite of the essential amino acid methionine, but, if it is not converted into a harmless substance, it can be dangerous as cholesterol in leading to hardening of the arteries.[6]

Klevay said that, in animal models, homocysteine produced a decrease in both cardiac copper and cardiac activity of copper-zinc superoxide dismutase, which resulted in increased oxidative damage to the heart. He added that 10 surveys showed that 35 percent of the daily diets probably contain less than 1 mg, an amount that proved insufficient for some men and women in depletion experiments. Some two-thirds of the daily diets contain less than 1.5 mg of copper, which is the lower limit of the recommended safe and adequate intake for adults. If homocysteine metabolism is abnormal, then daily intakes of copper of greater than 1 mg can be insufficient, Klevay said.[6]

Abnormal amounts of zinc can bring a copper deficiency, as illustrated by Edwin J. Gyorffy, M.D., and Hung Chan, M.D., in the August 1992 issue of *The American Journal of Gastroenterology*. A 57-year-old man was admitted to the hospital with microcytic anemia. He had been given the equivalent of 810 mg/day of elemental zinc for over 18 months "on the advice of a nutritionist." (The RDA for this age group is 15 mg/day.) Eight weeks after discontinuing the excess zinc, his copper deficiency was corrected. Four weeks after the zinc supplement was discontinued, his hemoglobin and white blood cell count went up appreciably.[7]

Women at risk for developing osteoporosis should get sufficient amounts of copper, zinc and manganese, in addition to calcium, according to P. Saltman in the October 1992 issue of the *Journal of the American College of Nutrition*. These minerals are cofactors for enzymes involved in the organic matrix metabolism. The researchers induced osteoporosis in animals by copper and manganese restricted diets, which resulted in lower calcium and trace mineral content of the bone. In a two-year, double-blind study involving 200 postmenopausal women, the researchers found that there was no significant bone loss in the group getting calcium and the three trace minerals when compared to the placebo group. In addition, they found, there was a strong indication of increased bone mineral density in the calcium citrate-malate plus trace element group. The treatment group was given each day 1,000 mg of calcium; 15 mg of zinc; 2.5 mg of copper; and 5 mg of manganese.[8]

FOLK REMEDY FOR ARTHRITIS?

"There's long been a connection between copper and reduction of arthritic pain," according to Robert M. Giller, M.D., in *Natural Prescriptions*. "Perhaps you've seen or heard of people wearing copper bracelets for this purpose. Copper is an effective anti-inflammatory agent that may be more potent than aspirin. It is known to reduce morning stiffness and help joint mobility, sometimes reducing the need for other drugs. Studies have suggested that rheumatoid arthritis patients are marginally deficient in copper, and supplementation may help relieve symptoms."

In addition to your usual supplements, Giller provides this anti-rheumatoid arthritis formula:

- 1,000 mg three times a day of fish oil and increase your intake of fish;
- 2 mg/day of boron;
- 1,000 mg three times a day of evening primrose oil;
- 100 mcg/day of selenium;

- 2,000 mg/day of vitamin C;
- 400 IU/day of vitamin E;
- 22.5 mg/day of zinc;
- 2 mg/day of copper salicylate with meals and 50 mg of zinc two times a day with meals (discontinue after six weeks if there is no improvement);
- 500 mg powdered ginger three times a day.

If you take nonsteroidal anti-inflammatory drugs (NSAIDs) for pain relief, take 100 mg/day of vitamin B1; and 1,000 mcg/day of vitamin B12 dissolved under the tongue. These supplements may allow you to reduce your drug use, he said.[9]

Without copper, nerves would fray like worn toaster cords, reported *The Complete Book of Minerals for Health.* In other words, copper helps to forge the protective myelin sheath around each of the millions of nerve fibers in our bodies. Calm nerves and clear thinking depend on copper, and the mineral also builds proteins that give blood vessel walls the strength and flexibility to accommodate the forceful rivers coursing through our veins and arteries. In addition, the publication said, copper activates a number of enzymes important to energy metabolism. And copper apparently shares some of zinc's anti-inflammatory powers, augmenting zinc's role in healing. Taste perception may also be partially influenced by copper.[10]

IMPORTANT FOR CONNECTIVE TISSUE

The publication added that copper is the key mineral in a special enzyme (lysyl oxidase) which intertwines the tough, elastic fibers of collagen and elastin, two main connective tissue proteins in the body. A combination of collagen and elastin is essential for tissues such as tendons and blood vessels, which must be both strong and flexible. In the aorta, the large artery leading from the heart, as well as other primary coronary arteries, collagen buttresses the vessel walls; elastin provides elasticity.[10]

"A diet totally devoid of copper would cause hemorrhage severe enough to end life," the publication added. "That's not likely, though. The practical question is, can major blood vessels—particularly the heart's aorta—survive short periods of low copper without serious harm? Or do the patches heal over?"[10]

The authors quoted Edward D. Harris, Ph.D., a Texas A&M University biochemistry professor, who speculates that copper deficiency during the early stages of growth could leave a person more susceptible to damaged blood vessels later on in life.[10]

Addressing the 30th Annual Texas Nutrition Conference in 1975, Harris said: "It is reasonable to suspect that lysyl oxidase must function continuously in the early development of the aorta. A [short lull] in activity during development could give rise to an adult protein structure with intrinsic weaknesses throughout, much the same as a bricklayer who, in constructing a wall, omits certain bricks, leaving gaps in the wall."[10]

There are many reasons why people have poor sleep habits, but the inadequate consumption of certain essential trace minerals, especially copper, for an extended period may be a contributing factor, according to James G. Penland, Ph.D., of the USDA research facility in North Dakota. In the study, reported by Judy McBride in *Scientific Research News*, April 1 to June 30, 1988, Penland asked women in a series of five carefully controlled studies of trace element nutrition to answer eight questions each morning concerning how long and how well they slept the night before. Their responses were then correlated with dietary intake and blood plasma levels of the mineral being studied. Penland added that the results do not mean that a supplement can act as a sleeping pill.[11]

Of the seven minerals studied, copper, zinc and aluminum most strongly altered sleep patterns, Penland said. Reducing daily intake of copper or iron increased sleep time but decreased its quality. And high doses of aluminum—a nonessential element found in antacids—reduced sleep quality. He noted that regular users of antacids can easily get 1,000 mg/day of aluminum, the amount used in the study.[11]

Penland said that, according to 1985 food consumption figures from the USDA's Human Nutrition Information Service, the average copper intake for women 19 to 50 was half the amount considered adequate. Iron intake was a little over half the Recommended Dietary Allowance. Men in the same age group got 80 percent of the suggested copper intake (other studies show lower intakes) and 50 percent more iron than the RDA.[11]

Penland went on to say that a low copper intake prompted the largest number of sleep problems. When 11 women in the copper study got only 0.8 mg/day of copper (less than the 2 to 3 mg/day considered adequate), they slept for a longer period of time, but had more trouble getting to sleep and awoke feeling less rested than when they got 2.8 mg/day.[11]

"Sleep simply represents one state of consciousness and behavioral activity," Penland said. "If a lack of copper is influencing human sleep behavior, it is probably affecting waking behavior as well."[11]

The 13 women in the iron study also slept longer when their meals contained only 5 mg of iron (less than one-third the RDA) than when they contained at least 15 mg. The RDA for women prior to menopause is 18 mg/day but is difficult to get in the diet. Unlike the women on the low-copper diet, Penland added, those on the low-iron diet awoke more often during the night.[11]

In other research at the USDA facility, reported in the *Quarterly Report of Selected Research Projects*, October 1-December 31, 1987, researchers found that even a mild copper deficiency can elevate blood pressure, especially when the individual is stressed, according to Henry C. Lukaski, Ph.D. During a hand-grip test at the center, eight healthy young women, who were getting only 0.6 to 0.7 mg/day of copper for three months had above normal increases in both systolic (pumping) and diastolic (resting) pressures. There were substantial increases in the diastolic pressure.[12]

"Isometric exercises normally result in smaller blood pressure increases than those measured in the study," Lukaski said. "The women had no change in blood pressure while at rest or moving about, and the low copper intake did not affect heart rate."[12]

In the same publication, David B. Milne, Ph.D., said that many people may be suffering from a mild copper deficiency (less than 1 mg/day) because they do not eat enough copper-rich foods. Over the long run, that could be bad news for their hearts. He added that recent studies with eight men and eight women indicated that the earliest signs of copper deficiency occur after three or four months on a copper intake of 0.8 mg/day or less. Some people in the U.S. and other industrialized countries are getting only 0.8 mg/day through their diets, but he said that this can be remedied by eating liver, oysters, chickpeas, nuts, seeds, etc. He said that another study showed that two copper-containing proteins are sensitive indicators of the onset of deficiency. The enzymatic activity of ceruloplasmin (found in the blood) and cytochrome-c-oxidase (found in all body cells) dropped even though standard indicators of body copper remained unchanged, he said.[13]

COPPER/ZINC BALANCING ACT

People taking zinc tablets to increase their intake of that mineral may risk decreasing their supply of copper, also needed for good health, said Helen Anderson, Ph.D., professor of home economics at the University of Missouri-Columbia, in *UMC News*, September 14, 1983. She added that zinc tablets may reduce the body's ability to absorb copper from food, as well as cause the loss of stored copper. And copper shortage is associated with anemia in adults and children and childhood bone abnormalities.[14]

In the study, involving nine male college students, Anderson found that only slightly exceeding the RDA of zinc (15 mg) markedly reduced copper retention. She noted that zinc tablets typically contain 10 to 50 mg of zinc, and that our normal diets supply about 12 mg/day, raising zinc intake well above the recommended level.[14]

"One theory is that zinc increases the ability of certain proteins in intestinal cells to chemically bond to copper," Anderson added. "The cells, excreted from the body regularly, take the copper away with them. In some studies there is evidence that we don't get the optimal amount of copper from our diets. So, based on our small study, I'd have to caution healthy adults against taking in much more than the recommended 15 mg/day of zinc."[14]

In a study reported in the *American Journal of Clinical Nutrition* in 1991, Judith R. Turnlund, Ph.D., et al., placed women 21 to 30, who were not on oral contraceptives, on diets containing varying amounts of vitamin B6. The idea was to determine whether or not the diets affected zinc, copper and iron status. Zinc absorption and retention were greater during pyridoxine depletion, but blood zinc declined, suggesting that absorbed zinc was not available for utilization. The researchers found that copper absorption was lower during B6 depletion but that serum copper levels were not affected. Iron was not impaired significantly by B6-deficient diets, but iron status may have declined. The researchers concluded that young women on low B6 diets may have altered zinc metabolism, inhibited copper absorption and possibly an affect on iron status.[15]

In the *Journal of the American Dietetic Association* in 1991, Jean Pennington, Ph.D., R.D., of the Food and Drug Administration in Washington, D.C., discussed The Total Diet Study, an annual program conducted by the FDA, which assesses the levels of pesticide residues, industrial chemicals, radionuclides, toxic elements and nutritional elements in foods in the daily diets of eight age groups. The daily intakes of nutrients were compared to the Recommended Dietary Allowances.[16]

She found that most Americans are consuming too much sodium and not enough copper. Teenage girls are consuming inadequate amounts of calcium, magnesium, iron and manganese. In fact, most Americans are consuming inadequate amounts of essential vitamins and minerals, she said.[16]

Forty-six patients with acute proximal femoral fractures were evaluated after being admitted to the Glenfield General Hospital in Leicester, United Kingdom. D. Conlan, et al., reported in *Age and Ageing* in 1990 that 16 patients with fractures (35 percent) had serum copper levels below the normal mean level for that essay, while only four percent were recorded in the control group. The researchers noted that copper-dependent enzymes in the bone matrix are necessary for cross-linking of collagen and therefore maintain bone strength. They noted that patients with femoral neck fractures are often malnourished and may not be getting adequate amounts of copper. Dietary copper supplementation in the elderly who are at risk for malnourishment may help reduce the incidence of femoral-neck (upper leg) fracture and improve morbidity and mortality, they reported.[17]

Edward D. Harris, Ph.D., and Susan S. Percival reported in the *American Journal of Clinical Nutrition* in 1991, that a copper deficiency may produce scurvy-like symptoms. That is because vitamin C is known to antagonize the intestinal absorption of copper. The Texas A&M researchers added that vitamin C appears to directly or indirectly react with ceruloplasmin, labilize bound copper atoms and facilitate their cross-membrane transport. And, they added, vitamin C appears to inhibit the intracellular binding of copper to copper-zinc superoxide dismutase. In fact, vitamin C deficiency may impair copper metabolism and transport and regulation of copper uptake might be compromised. They suggest that scorbutic animals and humans may be suffering from copper deficiency as well as a vitamin C deficiency.[18]

In a study at the University of Medicine and Dentistry in New Jersey, 58 patients with confirmed secondary immunodeficiency syndrome were tested for plasma copper and zinc levels, according to Robert H. Garrison, Jr., M.A., R.Ph., and Elizabeth Somer, M.A., R.D., in *The Nutrition Desk Reference*. The patients had depressed cell-mediated immunity and were found to have a low serum zinc and elevated serum copper level. Garrison and Somer wrote:

> The authors conclude that zinc and copper homeostatis are significantly altered in many immunodeficiency disorders and may be important factors in host defense. Cellular immunity is known to be impaired by zinc deficiency, but it is not clear from this study whether the immunodeficiency observed in these patients is caused by the zinc/copper imbalance or whether the imbalance results from the immunodeficiency. When given zinc supplements, the patients with primary and secondary immunodeficiency conditions apparently improved. This supports the hypothesis that the alteration of zinc and copper metabolism through dietary imbalance contributes to the cause of immunodeficiency.[19]

Estelle Thauvin et al. reported in *Biological Trace Element Research* in 1992 that reasonable dosages for pregnant women are 15 mg/day of zinc and 2 to 2.65 mg/day of copper during their pregnancy. The French researchers reported that vitamin and mineral supplemented pregnant females had a decreased incidence of muscular cramps. They added that zinc supplementation allows for the normalization of biological status and prevents deficiencies, while copper supplementation is necessary to insure inadequate copper retention and to preserve the balance of trace elements supplied during pregnancy.[20]

Researchers at Ohio State University reported in the *Journal of the American*

College of Nutrition in 1992 that copper supplementation improved the antioxidant status of a group of rheumatoid arthritis patients. For the volunteers getting 2 mg/day of copper for four weeks, their red blood cell copper-zinc superoxide dismutase activity increased from subnormal levels to within the normal range for 18 of the 23 patients given gold or methotrexate. Supplementation did not affect ceruloplasmin activity or protein concentrations in either of the groups involved, although rheumatoid arthritic volunteers showed slightly lower copper activity to protein ratios, when compared to the controls before and after supplementation. The Ohio researchers concluded that RA patients may be deficient in copper and might benefit from moderate-dose supplementation.[21]

Another group of researchers at Ohio State University reported in the *Journal of Nutrition* in 1991 that a strain of lean rats susceptible to cardiac failure was placed on a copper-deficient diet. The male rats developed more severe symptoms of cardiac hypertrophy than the female animals, suggesting that the copper-deficient male rat might serve as a model for studying the effects of low-copper intakes and cardiac risk in human beings.[22]

METABOLIC ACTION

Although copper is present in the human body in very small amounts, it is involved in a large number of important metabolic functions, including respiration and the synthesis of blood hemoglobin, according to Ronald Ross Watson, Ph.D., of the University of Arizona College of Medicine at Tucson, in *Food and Nutrition News*, May/June 1989. He added that copper's role in the prevention of cancer may be partially due to its action as an antioxidant, thus protecting cells from damage by oxygen radicals which cause cancer.[23]

In *ACTA Hematologica* in 1992, Nobuhisa Hirase, et al., of Kyushu University in Japan, reported that total parenteral (through a tube) nutrition often increases the possibility of a copper deficiency. They pointed out that the mineral is necessary for maintaining normal hematopoiesis or the formation of the various types of blood cells.[24]

Forty-one patients with acute myocardial infarction, who were compared to healthy controls, had slight decreases in mean levels of blood magnesium, significantly lower zinc levels and significantly higher copper levels than the controls, according to It-Koon Tan, Ph.D., in the *Journal of Clinical Laboratory Analysis* in 1992. The research team found that the mean copper-zinc serum ratios for patients with acute myocardial infarction were 1.91, almost double the 1.02 for the controls. They added that ceruloplasmin, the copper-containing enzyme, may serve as an antioxidant, and it tends to be elevated with tissue damage. It is possible, they said, that ceruloplasmin may have two antioxidant roles; that is, the prevention of decompartmentalized iron acting as a free-radical catalyst, and a directly inactivating role against free radicals by way of the copper-containing enzyme superoxide dismutase.[25]

Dr. John Sorenson of the University of Cincinnati College of Medicine has discovered during his research on anti-inflammatory drugs for arthritis that copper chelates and complexes are potent anti-ulcer agents in laboratory animals, according to Richard A. Passwater, Ph.D., and Elmer M. Cranton, M.D., in *Trace Elements, Hair Analysis and Nutrition.* In addition to localized copper deficiency in the stomach lining, it has been found that ulcer patients average 23 percent less copper in their bodies.[26]

DO SCHIZOPHRENICS NEED COPPER?

Carl C. Pfeiffer, M.D., Ph.D., at the New Jersey Psychiatric Institute (now the Brain-Bio Center) in Stillman, New Jersey detailed a case history in the December 14, 1973 issue of *Medical World News.*[27]

Pfeiffer, who passed away several years ago, said that the patient arrived at the clinic in 1971 suffering from "an unrelenting inferno of mental and bodily suffering." The female patient had complained for years about insomnia, loss of reality, attempted suicide, seizures or convulsions, vomiting and difficulty with menstruation. She had been given nerve and psychiatric tests, all of which were normal. She had been hospitalized and tranquilized.

Pfeiffer treated her with massive doses of vitamin B6 and supplements of zinc and manganese. The woman had had trouble with knee joints when she began to menstruate, suggesting to Pfeiffer that she might need the two minerals. And he suggested group therapy and a tranquilizer. The patient improved with the supplements but relapsed when they were discontinued. Returning to the nutrients, she had been free from convulsions for two years without other medication, and she was planning to become a doctor.

As Ruth Adams and I discussed in our book *Minerals: Kill or Cure?*:

Testing urine for the presence of a "mauve factor" has become a standard test for schizophrenia among physicians and psychiatrists who use megavitamin therapy in their treatment of this severe mental illness, which disables many thousands of Americans every year. Pfeiffer said that 30 to 40 percent of all schizophrenics excrete in their urine a substance which turns a deep pink or mauve when tested on a laboratory machine. The substance has been identified as something which the disordered, unbalanced body chemistry of the mentally ill person is excreting.

This condition was reported in medical journals as long ago as 1963 by Dr. Abram Hoffer of Saskatoon, Canada, and Dr. Humphrey Osmond of New Jersey.[27]

The mauve factor (or "malvaria") seems to indicate that copper levels are normal in these people, whereas, in other schizophrenics who do not have it, copper is lacking, we continued. Other symptoms: white spots on fingernails, loss of the ability to dream or to remember dreams after waking, a distinctive sweetish odor on the breath and abdominal pain in the left upper side of the abdomen, constipation, inability to tan in sunlight, itching in sunlight, malformation of knee cartilages, joint pains. These patients may also have anemia, tremor and muscle spasms. They may also be impotent or have menstrual difficulties, low blood sugar and an anemia which does not respond to iron but is improved when they are given vitamin B6.[27]

EXCESS OF MINERAL RELATED TO WILSON'S

Wilson's disease, which affects some 7,000 Americans, is a hereditary disorder of metabolism in which there is a progressive accumulation of copper in the liver and other organs, according to *The Physicians' Manual for Patients*. When copper is released from the liver into the red blood cells, it produces anemia, and, as it keeps accumulating in the liver, it produces cirrhosis. If left untreated, it can be fatal. Therapy includes a diet that restricts the intake of copper and penicillamine, a drug that removes the mineral from the tissues and blood so that it can be excreted through the kidneys.[28]

Named after Dr. Samuel A. K. Wilson, an American-born neurologist working in England, the disorder was initially described by him in 1912, reported Lawrence K. Altman, M.D., in *The New York Times*, January 31, 1984. He was one of the first to distinguish it from multiple sclerosis, with which it had often been confused.

"Wilson's disease is a hereditary disorder that is passed on in an autosomal recessive pattern," Altman said. "In order for a case to occur, both parents must be carriers of the Wilson's disease gene. One in every 90 people, or 2.5 million Americans, is such a carrier. However, they do not develop any manifestations of the disease."[29]

Because it is so rare, Wilson's disease is often overlooked by physicians, Altman added. The accumulation of copper apparently results from a deficiency of ceruloplasmin, a protein that carries copper in the blood. The name is derived from the Latin and Greek meaning "blue blood," since the protein, when purified, is intensely blue. He added that doctors know that copper must be incorporated into ceruloplasmin or several other cooper-binding proteins to exert its normal physiologic role. When copper is not attached to protein, it is left to combine with, or impair, the function of other molecules.

"Without enough ceruloplasmin," Altman continued, "copper slowly collects in the liver and eventually destroys the organ by causing cirrhosis. Meanwhile, the copper-rich liver releases variable amounts of the metal, sometimes rapidly, causing a serious anemia. However, the release is usually gradual. Copper is deposited in the brain, kidneys, eyes and other organs and the damage takes years to develop. The damage to the brain affects motor function and not intelligence."

Altman added that mothers of children with Wilson's disease have pointed out that something was wrong with their children's eyes, only to have the doctor scoff at or ignore the observation. A 19-year-old man with Wilson's disease passed his physical for the United States Marines in spite of hand tremors and slurred speech that developed when he was 11 years old. He was later discharged because he could not salute without shaking uncontrollably. A doctor was diagnosed as having chronic viral hepatitis when he was in medical school; he actually had Wilson's disease. The hepatitis continued for several years and was only discovered when he developed pinkeye and consulted an ophthalmologist. It was then that he learned that he had Kayser-Fleischer rings as well as Wilson's disease.[29]

Penicillamine, the drug of choice for Wilson's disease, causes severe side effects in about 30 percent of the people who take it, according to the March 1984 issue of *Prevention*. But Michigan doctors have found that zinc therapy worked well in ridding the body of excess copper.[30]

"In a number of studies, zinc has been shown to be effective in the treatment of Wilson's disease," reported Z. T. Cossack, Ph.D., of Odense University in Denmark, in the February 4, 1988 issue of *The New England Journal of Medicine*. "Our studies in adults showed that oral zinc can be used as maintenance therapy after initial treatment with penicillamine. Other investigators reported promising results of using zinc as a long-term treatment for the disease. Our results showed that oral zinc alone is effective in maintaining a negative or zero copper balance in children; those we described are now in their seventh year on oral zinc and are doing well, with no side effects or complications."[31]

Writing in the *Journal of the American College of Nutrition* in 1990, George J. Brewer, M.D., and colleagues at the University of Michigan, reported that zinc acetate is an effective therapy for maintenance or treatment of the presymptomatic Wilson's disease patient and is essentially nontoxic.[32]

Lorenzo Rossaro, M.D., and colleagues of Padova, Italy, reported essentially the same thing in *The American Journal of Gastroenterology* in 1990. They stated that long-term treatment of Wilson's disease with zinc therapy can be a safe and effective alternative to copper chelating agents but that copper/zinc status should be monitored to assess compliance.[33]

An extensive review of Wilson's disease is reported by Joseph C. Yarze, M.D., and colleagues at Jefferson Medical College in Philadelphia, in the *American Journal of Medicine* in June 1992. They added that eliminating copper in the diet is difficult, since the mineral is so ubiquitous. They indicated that a negative copper balance cannot be achieved by diet alone. Patients with early Wilson's disease should avoid such high-copper-containing foods as shellfish, organ meat (especially liver), nuts, chocolate and mushrooms. They added that domestic water softeners dramatically increase the copper content of the water, so that distilled water may be recommended for drinking and cooking.[34]

REFERENCES

1. Ensminger, Audrey H., et al. *Foods and Nutrition Encyclopedia.* Clovis, Calif.: Pegus Press, 1983, pp. 476ff.
2. Hendler, Sheldon Saul, M.D., Ph.D. *The Doctors' Vitamin and Mineral Encyclopedia.* New York: Simon and Schuster, 1990, pp. 127ff.
3. McBride, Judy. "Trace Elements—Major Players on the Health Scene," *Scientific Research News*, USDA, October 1992.
4. Saari, Jack T., Ph.D. "Copper Deficiency in Test Animals," *Quarterly Report of Selected Research Projects*, July 1 to September 30, 1994.
5. "Copper Needs Surveyed," *Medical Tribune*, October 18, 1990, p. 14.
6. Klevay, Leslie M., M.D. "The Homocysteine Theory of Arteriosclerosis," *Nutrition Reviews* 155:50, May 1992.
7. Gyorffy, Edwin J., M.D., and Chan, Hung, M.D. "Copper Deficiency and Microcytic Anemia Resulting from Prolonged Ingestion of Over-the-Counter Zinc," *The American Journal of Gastroenterology* 87(8):1054–1055, August 1992.
8. Saltman, P. "The Role of Minerals and Osteoporosis," *Journal of the American College of Nutrition* 11(5):599/Abstract 7, October 1992.
9. Giller, Robert M., M.D., and Matthews, Kathy. *Natural Prescriptions.* New York: Carol Southern Books, 1994, pp. 299ff.
10. Faelten, Sharon, et al. *The Complete Book of Minerals for Health.* Emmaus, Pa.: Rodale Press, 1981, pp. 93ff.
11. McBride, Judy. "Sleep Problems Could Be Elementary," *Scientific Research News*, USDA, April 1 to June 30, 1988.
12. Quarterly Report of Selected Research Projects, USDA, October 1 to December 31, 1987.
13. Ibid.
14. Myers, Larry. "Zinc May Sink Our Body's Supply of Copper," *UMC News*, University of Missouri-Columbia, September 14, 1983.
15. Turnlund, Judith R., et al. "A Stable-Isotope Study of Zinc, Copper and Iron Absorption and Retention by Young Women Fed Vitamin B6-Deficient Diets," *American Journal of Clinical Nutrition* 54:1059–1064, 1991.

16. Pennington, Jean, Ph.D., et al. "Total Diet Study Nutritional Elements: 1982–1989," *Journal of the American Dietetic Association* 91:179–183, 1991.
17. Conlan, D., et al. "Serum Copper Levels in Elderly Patients with Femoral Neck Fractures," *Age and Ageing* 19:212–214, 1990.
18. Harris, Edward D., Ph.D., and Percival, Susan S. "A Role for Ascorbic Acid in Copper Transport," *The American Journal of Clinical Nutrition* 54:1193–1197S, 1991.
19. Garrison, Robert H., Jr., M.A., R.Ph., and Somer, Elizabeth, M.A., R.D. *The Nutrition Desk Reference.* New Canaan, Conn.: Keats Publishing, Inc., 1990, p. 112.
20. Thauvin, Estelle, et al. "Effects of a Multivitamin-Mineral Supplement on Zinc and Copper Status During Pregnancy," *Biological Trace Element Research* 32:405–413, 1992.
21. DiSilvestro, R., et al. "Effects of Copper Supplementation on Ceruloplasmin and Copper-Zinc Superoxide Dismutase in Free-Living Rheumatoid Arthritis Patients," *Journal of the American College of Nutrition* 11:177–180, 1992.
22. Medeiros, D., et al. "Copper Deficiency in a Genetically Hypertensive Cardiomyopathic Rat: Electrocardiogram, Functional and Ultrastructural Aspects," *Journal of Nutrition* 121:1026–1031, 1991.
23. Watson, Ronald Ross, Ph.D. "B-Complex Vitamins and Trace Elements: A Role in Immunomodulation and Cancer Prevention?" *Food and Nutrition News*, May/June 1989.
24. Hirase, Nobuhisa, et al. "Anemia and Neutropenia in a Case of Copper Deficiency: Role of Copper in Normal Hematopoiesis," *ACTA Hematologica* 87:195–197, 1992.
25. Tan, It-Koon, M.D., et al. "Serum Magnesium, Copper and Zinc Concentrations in Acute Myocardial Infarction," *Journal of Clinical Laboratory Analysis* 6:324–328, 1992.
26. Passwater, Richard A., Ph.D., and Cranton, Elmer M., M.D. *Trace Elements, Hair Analysis and Nutrition.* New Canaan, Conn.: Keats Publishing, Inc., 1983, pp. 147ff.
27. Adams, Ruth, and Murray, Frank. *Minerals: Kill or Cure?* New York: Larchmont Books, 1974, pp. 150ff.
28. Subak-Sharpe, Genell J., editor. *The Physicians' Manual for Patients.* New York: Times Books, 1984, pp. 185–186.
29. Altman, Lawrence K., M.D. "The Tragedy of a Confusing, Rare Disease," *The New York Times*, January 31, 1984, p. C4.
30. "Zinc May Replace Penicallamine in Wilson's Disease," *Prevention*, March 1984, p. 7.
31. Cossack, Z. T., Ph.D. "The Efficacy of Oral Zinc Therapy as an Alternative to Penicillamine for Wilson's Disease," *The New England Journal of Medicine* 318(5):322–323, February 4, 1988.
32. Brewer, George J., M.D., et al. "Use of Zinc-Metabolic Interactions in the Treatment of Wilson's Disease," *Journal of the American College of Nutrition* 9(5):47–49, 1990.
33. Rossaro, Lorenzo, M.D., et al. "Zinc Therapy in Wilson's Disease: Observations in Five Patients," *The American Journal of Gastroenterology* 85(6):665–668, 1990.
34. Yarze, Joseph C., M.D., et al. "Wilson's Disease: Current Status," *The American Journal of Medicine* 92:643–654, June 1992.

27

The Fluoride Fraud

THE RIP-OFF OF THE 20TH CENTURY

SINCE fluorine is found in small but widely varying concentrations in soils, water supplies, plants and animals, one might conclude that fluorine/fluoride has some health benefits. But those of us who have read the literature find that water fluoridation to allegedly prevent dental caries and fluoride supplements to build stronger bones are a sham that should be investigated by the U. S. Supreme Court. It should be unconstitutional for the bureaucrats to doctor our water supplies with sodium fluoride, a rat poison, in an attempt to reduce tooth decay. But fluoride has no effect whatsoever on the teeth of adults, which were formed a long time ago. In any event, we get ample amounts of fluoride from water, canned foods and beverages made with fluoridated water, air pollution, etc. Even the National Research Council has stated that, because of the conflicting information about fluoride, this does not "justify a classification of fluorine as an essential element, according to accepted standards." But it waffles by calling it "a beneficial element." Incidentally, the NRC said that "fluoride is the term for the ionized form of the element fluorine, as it occurs in drinking water. The two terms are used interchangeably."[1]

In 1984, I quoted David O. Woodbury as saying:

Fluorine, Peck's Bad Boy of the chemical underworld, made the atomic bomb possible. The only way to free the tiny quantities of fissionable Uranium-235, buried in the inert mass of its parent, U-38, was to force uranium hexafluoride gas through many acres of porous barriers, gradually concentrating the precious element. In three years of continuous battle, enough U-235 was finally collected to put an end to the Second World War. Hex is what they called the vicious stuff. Today, without a thought, 70 million Americans swallow a daily dose of sodium fluoride with their drinking water. Linked in sodium, fluorine is not as violent as

Hex, but violent enough in high concentrations to be the standard rat and roach killer and a first-rate pesticide.[2]

It has been known since the turn of the century that something in the environment causes mottling (brown spots) of teeth. In 1902, Dr. J. M. Eager, a U.S. Marine surgeon stationed in Naples, Italy, reported on the mottled teeth there. About the same time, Dr. Frederick Summer McKay found similar staining among his dental patients in Colorado Springs, Colorado, where water is naturally fluoridated. Mottling was noticed early on in Amarillo, Texas, where the water contains fluoride left there by nature. But it was not until 1930 that the causative agent was identified as fluoride. It was discovered by Dr. H. V. Churchill, who was sent to Bauxite, Arkansas, to find out why employees at the Alcoa plant had stained teeth.[2]

John Lear, then the editor of *Saturday Review*, remarked: "Fluoride then was known only as a poison. It had not been considered as a possible constituent of drinking water. The immediate reaction was one of alarm, for fluoride had a powerful effect on body tissues and nerves as well as on bones. In Colorado Springs, the municipal water supply came under taboo as a source of drinking water for the town's babies."[2]

TOXIC WASTE DISSOLVED IN WATER

In 1939, a biochemist at the Mellon Institute in Pittsburgh, C. J. Cox, was assigned by the Aluminum Company of America to find a use for the sodium fluoride wastes produced by aluminum pot lines. Another 50 industries were also interested in getting rid of the chemical, especially since some of them had been subjected to damage suits because of the effects the poisons had had on livestock and crops. (The chemical, piled up in mounds near the plants, would be blown by the wind onto nearby farms, contaminating the grass and fodder and causing animals to die or be deformed.)

"Cox decided that it was feasible to dissolve the poison in drinking water, and, although he had no medical background and had not studied the effects of fluoride on human beings, he suggested that fluoride might be needed for healthy teeth," David Woodbury said. "A number of scientists jumped on the bandwagon, proclaiming fluoride to be 'the greatest health measure of modern times.' Soon thereafter Alcoa began advertising that they had fluorides for water treatment."[2]

Woodbury added that the Public Health Service got into the fray and, in 1945, it announced that a study would be conducted to prove the effectiveness of fluoride in preventing tooth decay. Newburgh, New York was selected to have its water fluoridated, while nearby Kingston would be nonfluoridated, thus setting up a double-blind study. The test was to proceed for 10 years but, about five years into the study, the PHS gleefully announced that children in Newburgh were 100-percent free of cavities and the study was terminated.

"Soon after, cavities began to show up, but the score, compared to Kingston's was (reportedly) still 65 percent better," Woodbury continued. "This marvelous result for the price of one candy bar per year. Similar miracles were reported from Grand Rapids, Michigan and Brantford, Ontario, Canada, which had joined the fluoride-for-health parade."

Meanwhile, Woodbury added, Oscar Ewing, an Alcoa attorney, resigned his post and became head of the U.S. Public Health Service and started fluoridation in earnest. Surgeon General Leonard Scheele joined the shouting, hailing this happy scheme as "a mass application method for controlling noninfectious diseases," Woodbury said.

Although the results of the Newburgh-Kingston study had not been published, the fluoridation bandwagon was in high gear, being touted as the miracle of the century by many government agencies and professional groups. Still there were skeptics. One of these was Dr. James G. Kerwin of the Department of Health in Passaic, New Jersey. Before deciding to fluoridate his city, he asked the University of the State of New York for an analysis of the Newburgh-Kingston fluoridation project. The Bureau Chief at the university shocked a number of people by saying that the fluoridated town of Newburgh had almost 50 percent more "dental defects" than nonfluoridated Kingston. Needless to say, the water supply in Passaic was not fluoridated.

In September 1967, Woodbury said that the International Society for Research on Nutrition and Vital Substances met in Luxembourg and passed the now-famous Resolution 39. It reads: "All governments, state parliaments and city councils concerned with the problem of fluoridation . . . should refrain from fluoridating drinking water, which measure is actually a medication, as long as the scientific aspects of the problem are not satisfactorily clarified."[2]

No doubt it was that resolution, plus accumulating scientific evidence, that prompted many nations to forego fluoridation. These countries have never had fluoridated water or discontinued it for legal or other reasons: Austria, Belgium, Denmark, Egypt, France, Germany, Greece, Holland, India, Italy, Luxembourg, Norway, Spain and Sweden.[2]

In 1981, Dr. Phillip R. N. Sutton, an Australian dentist, said: "The German Association of Gas and Water Experts reported (in 1975) on the effects of fluoridation in Basel, Switzerland. They said that, in 1960, Prof. Gutherz predicted that, by 1967, as a result of fluoridation, of the 10 dentists practicing in 1960, only six would be required. However, by 1967, the number of dentists had increased to 17 and three years later, after 10 years of fluoridation, there were 18 dentists and five practicing dental auxiliaries. In 1975, the Swiss Health Department suggested that fluoridation should be discontinued due to its ineffectiveness."[2]

In the July 2, 1982 issue of *Science*, it is stated that current levels of fluoride in fluoridation are producing more than twice as much dental fluorosis as expected and that "the optimun concentration of fluoride in community water supplies needs to be reassessed."[2]

Dr. Douw G. Steyn, Emeritus Professor of Pharmacology at the University of Pretoria, South Africa, said that the American Dental Association has, for 40 years, recommended that water be fluoridated to combat dental caries.

> It recommends that drinking water be fluoridated to 1 ppm of water, that is, one milligram of fluorine (F-) as fluoride, in 1 liter of water =1 ppm fluorine. But this dilution was based on the assumption that on average an individual will take 1 to 2 liters of water daily with food and drinking water [a liter is 1.0567 quarts] This was a very grave mistake as, depending on several factors—atmospheric and environmental temperatures, humidity, physical exertion, diet, sex, state of health (diarrhea, diabetes, fever, kidney disease, etc.), drug treatment (diuretics)—one individual may, and frequently does, consume up to 40 times (or more) water daily than another. It is, therefore, obvious that instead of the recommended ingestion, with artificially fluoridated water, of 1 to 2 milligrams of fluorine (as fluoride) daily, many individuals may, and will, consume up to 15 milligrams, and more, daily, which will have disastrous effects on their health. The extreme seriousness of the above fact is fully realized when, according to reports from England, Japan, India, the United States and Israel, concentrations of less than 1 ppm fluorine in drinking water can cause chronic fluoride poisoning (mottling of teeth). In the view of the British Medical Research Council ... mottling of teeth, however mild, is the first symptom of incipient chronic fluoride poisoning. ... According to reports from several countries, concentrations of fluorine slightly higher than the recommended 1 ppm caused serious bone disease.[2]

I stated that fluoride has often been touted as a way of alleviating or preventing osteoporosis, suggesting that the fluoride concentrates in the bones and makes them stronger. But an editorial in the October 6, 1978 issue of the *Journal of the American Medical Association* cautioned that fluoride may produce toxic effects which may not surface for many years. In fact, no studies have shown that fluoride prevents bones from breaking.[2]

Testifying before the U.S. Senate Committee on Appropriations on March 10, 1980, Dr. Dean Burk, a distinguished research biochemist with the Federal government for 47 years, including 35 years with the National Cancer Institute, said: "I estimate that there now are some 40,000 cancer deaths a year in the United States that are linked with and induced by the fluoridated drinking water which 40 percent of the American population is forced to drink, whether it wants it or not. At the widely accepted figure of about $25,000 total cost per cancer patient death, this amounts to a national loss of the order of a billion dollars a year."[2]

Isabel Jansen, a nurse in Antigo, Wisconsin, has been keeping statistics on heart ailments in her city. She said that, "It appeared to myself as a nurse and to others that heart deaths in our city had noticeably increased in the years following the artificial fluoridation of the municipal water supply."

Antigo was fluoridated in 1949 and an increase in heart deaths began in 1951, according to the Wisconsin State Board of Health and Langlade County vital statistics. In a 20-year period (1950 to 1970), the national average of heart deaths rose 35.3 percent per 100,000 population. During the same time in Antigo, heart deaths rose 298.2 percent per 100,000, an increase of 744.8 percent above the national average. The increase in deaths from heart attacks in Antigo is similar to those from Grand Rapids, Michigan and Newburgh, New York.[2]

Using animal studies at the Chicago Medical School, Dr. Stephen R. Greenberg found that fluoride exposure causes degeneration of white blood cells. He added: "These data suggest an attempt by the [blood-forming] system to increase the number and maturation rate of leukocytes after significant fluoride exposure, perhaps to compensate for the destructive effect of this substance upon mature circulating cells."[2]

Dr. John R. Lee of Mill Valley, California, said that fluoridated water may be the reason for an increase from zero to four the number of his patients with Gilbert's liver disease. One patient, who monitored his serum bilirubin levels, found that they went down when he was drinking nonfluoridated water and rose again when he lived in a fluoridated town.[2]

On May 24, 1974, a three-year-old boy was taken to the Brownsville Dental Health Center in New York, where a dose of fluoride, in jelly form, was smeared on his teeth to prevent tooth decay. According to authorities, the dose was "three times the necessary amount." The child became ill almost immediately, sweating and vomiting, before going into a coma. He later died.[2]

In 1980, the late Dr. George L. Waldbott testified in a Massachusetts Superior Court case that he described his first case of chronic fluoride poisoning in 1955. During 50 years of medical practice, he had treated about 40,000 allergic patients.[2]

"Since then, I have been making a thorough study of this disease, particularly in its clinical aspects, on hundreds of patients," Waldbott said. "They recuperated once they discontinued using fluoridated water and substituted distilled water for drinking and cooking. In others the disease originated and subsided when the patients had moved into or moved away from a fluoridated community. Most of the patients had been under the care of other physicians at leading U.S. medical centers and had been undergoing numerous tests and treatments without obtaining a diagnosis or relief. The disease is difficult to diagnose because fluoride, contrary to former belief, can accumulate in, and affect, any organ of the body, causing a wide variety of symptoms."[2]

According to Dr. Albert Schatz emeritus professor at Temple University, who discovered streptomycin during his college days, statistics from fluoridated towns are often misleading because fluoride delays tooth eruption in children.

> In other words, teeth erupt later in fluoridated children than they do in nonfluoridated children of the same age. That delayed eruption, which is well-documented [has several interesting implications. Children who have fewer teeth in their mouths obviously have fewer teeth that can decay. For that reason, fluoridated children should have a lower decayed-missing-filled (DMF) ratio, even if fluoride does not prevent caries. Secondly, delayed eruption produces younger teeth. The younger teeth in the fluoridated children have been exposed to bacteria in the mouth for less time than the older teeth in the nonfluoridated children, which means there are less cavities. Therefore, fluoridated children should have a lower DMF, even if fluoride does not prevent caries.[2]

Fluoridation was started in Chile in 1953 and terminated in 1977, thanks largely to the efforts of Schatz, who was a professor at the University of Chile from 1962 to 1965. In various publications in Chile and South America, Schatz showed that fluoridation did not prevent caries but merely delayed the appearance of tooth decay. He also presented evidence that fluoridation is not safe, especially for malnourished people, reported the October-December 1980 issue of *National Fluoridation News.*[3]

"The final straw that broke the back of fluoridation in Chile was a detailed report that Dr. Schatz published in 1976," the newspaper said. "This report analyzed official demographic statistics published by the government of Chile. It conclusively proved that Briner and Carmona, the two top officials in the Dental Section of the National Health Service of Chile, had distorted and misrepresented death rates in order to convince Chileans that fluoridation was safe."[3]

Schatz's paper was called "Increased Death Rates in Chile Associated with Artificial Fluoridation of Drinking Water, with Implications for Other Countries."

Both the American Dental Association and the American Medical Association refused to publish Schatz's report. But it was later published in the Susan B. Anthony University Journal of Arts, Science and Humanities. He sent copies of this report to all medical and dental officials in the National Health Service in Chile, and one year later, fluoridation was discontinued in Chile.[3]

Writing in *Medical Hypotheses*, a British journal, in 1992, P. R. N. Sutton, of Melbourne, Australia, noted: "Observations of the behavior of a large number of fluoridation promoters over a period of more than 30 years has led to the conclusion that most of them are neurotics." He wondered whether this explains their continued "fervent advocacy of this discredited process."[4]

Sutton said that in a private conversation with a senior Italian dental professor some 20 years ago, the professor described fluoridation as an "Anglo-Saxon Madness." Sutton maintains that the 1946 recap of fluoridation trials in Evanston in the U.S., which helped to launch the worldwide fluoridation bandwagon, as well as studies in Grand Rapids and Newburgh, and Brantford, Canada, are "a first-class example of the errors, omissions and mis-statements which abound in the reports of all these fluoridation trials."

In fact, Sutton said, in an article in the *Journal of the American Dental Association*, in 1967, detailing the number of 12- to 14-year olds in the Evanston study, there were six different numbers given in the article. Various charts referred to 1,703, 1,702, 1,701, 1,697, 1,556 and 1,146 children in the study.

"No mention of these errors in the Evanston study has been found elsewhere in the very voluminous literature on fluoridation (much of which is unbridled propaganda) published in the 24 years since that 1967 special article in the *Journal of the American Dental Association*," Sutton continued. "In the manner which is common in reports of fluoridation trials, those erroneous tables have been accepted by fluoridation promoters at their face value, without investigation."[4]

From its inception, he added, the study of fluoridation has been conducted mainly by senior government officials. And, after the 10-year trials were over in the late 1950s, those with even a basic knowledge of scientific research, and who took the trouble to check the data, realized that they "contained many errors and other undesirable features which made the published claims unacceptable."

NONEXISTENT STUDIES

After considerable time had passed, Sutton said, the fluoride promoters felt comfortable about admitting the shortcomings of the earlier studies. One of these promoters, in England, reportedly said that they did not have to rely on the inadequate studies of the past to prove the efficacy of recommending fluoridation. Sutton added that an "expert" committee of the World Health Organization, in 1984, claimed that 120 worldwide studies have proven the efficacy of fluoridation.

"For five years these claims were widely disseminated but no one queried whether that number of studies existed—which they did not," Sutton added. "Nor whether even one study had established, by scientifically acceptable means, that fluoridation decreases the prevalence of dental caries. Both these claims were then shown to be false."[4]

In his book, *Fluoridation: the Aging Factor*, John Yiamouyiannis, Ph.D., reported that Grand Rapids, Michigan had its drinking water fluoridated on January 25, 1945. Muskegon was selected as a nonfluoridated control city. Although the study was supposed to last 10 years, after five years it was observed that tooth decay rate in nonfluoridated Muskegon had decreased about as much as that of fluoridated Grand Rapids. And so the Public Health Service dropped Muskegon from the study and only reported that tooth decay had decreased in Grand Rapids after fluoridation.

"Several years after this study was completed," Yiamouyiannis said, "Dr. R. L. Glass of the Forsyth Dental Center in Boston compared the tooth decay rates of children who had spent their entire life in the fluoridated cities of Grand Rapids, Michigan and Newburgh, New York, with the tooth decay rate of children from the United States, most of whom had never lived in a fluoridated area. The results . . . clearly show that fluoride does not reduce tooth decay."[5]

James W. Benfield, D.D.S. is a Fellow of the American Academy of Restorative Dentistry, a member of the American Prosthodontic Society, the American Association for Advancement of Science, the New York Academy of Science, Federation of American Scientists; chairman of the Research Committee of the New York Academy of Dentistry; and on the faculty of the Columbia School of Dental and Oral Surgery. He wrote in the July-September 1972 issue of *National Fluoridation News* that he became interested in water fluoridation after discussing it with Daniel Ziskin, D.D.S., who at the time was Chief of the Diagnosis Department at Columbia's School of Dental and Oral Surgery and widely recognized as one of the leading authorities in the United States in the field of dental research. Ziskin had been asked by the New York State Department of Health for his opinion on the proposed experiment to evaluate the efficacy of adding sodium fluoride to the public water supply of Newburgh, New York, as a means of reducing dental caries, and he read his reply to Benfield:

Dr. Ziskin's reply stated that it was inconceivable to him that the New York State Department of Health would consider subjecting 40,000 people in Newburgh to the addition of one of the most toxic substances known to mankind, even in minute quantities, without ever having done an animal experiment to prove its safety. He also pointed out that the protocol for the proposed Newburgh experiment made no provision for X-rays to be taken of the children's teeth and that no one can properly diagnose the number of cavities in a patient's mouth without X-rays. There also was no provision for the study of the possible effects on adults or for the effects on hard and soft structures of the body other than the teeth. Furthermore, there was no provision for a double-blind study such as is standard procedure in the scientific world. He concluded by stating that he was unalterably opposed to the experiment until such time as major preliminary studies had been done. He predicted that if this experiment at Newburgh were carried out as proposed, it would forever be controversial. Dr. Ziskin died in 1948, so, unfortunately, did not live to see his prediction come true.[6]

Benfield said that the fluoridating of public water supplies was given great impetus by an article in the February 1943 issue of *Reader's Digest* titled "The Town Without a Toothache." Hereford, the town in Deaf Smith County, Texas, which was the subject of the article, had a water supply which contained 1.5 to 2.5 ppm of fluorine from natural sources. The water also contained unusually high amounts of calcium and other minerals. However, all of the credit for the low incidence of dental decay was attributed to fluorine.[6]

"Dr. Heard, the local dentist, accepted this theory for a time but when the vegetables, milk, grains and meat raised locally were also analyzed and found to contain exceptionally high levels of many other minerals, Dr. Heard, in 1951, wrote a pamphlet in which he castigated the proponents as primarily interested in promoting the sale of fluoride, and for giving all the credit to it and disregarding other minerals known to be constituents of tooth structure which were found in the diets of the residents of the town," Benfield continued.

WHAT IT REALLY DOES TO TEETH

In 1931, Drs. M. C. and H. V. Smith, at the University of Arizona Agricultural Experimental Station, discovered that fluoride in drinking water was responsible for "mottled" teeth. They proved that as little as 0.9 ppm produces white flecks in tooth enamel, which turn yellow and brown later in life. For more than a decade after this discovery, municipal authorities sought to abandon water supplies which contained 1 ppm or more of fluoride.

In 1940, the Drs. Smith stated in the *American Journal of Public Health* that:

"Although mottled teeth are somewhat more resistant to the onset of decay, they are structurally weak; when decay does set in, the result is often disastrous." And in a study at St. David, Arizona, where the fluoride content in water ranges from 1.6 to 4 ppm, the Smiths found relatively few individuals beyond age 21 in whom caries had not developed; there was a high incidence of extracted teeth in all age groups. Steps taken to repair the cavities were unsuccessful in many cases. When attempts were made to anchor a filling, the tooth might break away. Their research was the subject of editorials in journals of both the *American Medical Association* and the *American Dental Association*.[6]

"The American Medical Association's editorial stated in 1943 that ill effects had been seen such as mottling of teeth and crippling arthritic skeletal problems in various parts of the world, even at levels as low as 1 ppm of fluoride," Benfield said. "In 1944, the *Journal of the American Dental Association* carried an editorial which, in essence, said much the same thing as the American Medical Association had said in 1943, yet it was at this very same time that the experiments at Newburgh and other cities were being planned."[6]

In spite of the evidence that had already been presented in the scientific literature and the warnings of Ziskin and others, the experiments in Newburgh and Grand Rapids were begun in 1945. Dr. David B. Ast, director of the Newburgh experiment, said that studies would also be done to determine the effects of fluoride on adults and persons with diabetes and kidney disease "but these have never been carried out." Benfield explained:

> It was interesting to observe that Oscar Ewing, former counsel to the Aluminum Company of America, became Director of Social Security of the U.S. Public Health Service, and that he gave fluoridation of public water supplies the green light after only four years of the experiment at Newburgh, despite the fact that the original plan called for observing the effects for 10 years. The American Dental Association endorsed the fluoridation scheme in November 1950, even before there had been time to observe the effects of the program on the first permanent (six-year) molars of children born during the experiment at Newburgh. For many years until that endorsement, the American dental profession had been urging patients to restrict their use of sugar and emphasizing the importance of tooth brushing. That emphasis quickly changed to a reliance upon fluorides as the solution to dental problems.[6]

Once the fluoridation program was sanctioned by the U.S. Public Health Service, other endorsements rapidly followed. One of these was that of the American Water Works Association, despite the fact that the majority of water engineers, then, as now, opposed the program. Another early advocate was the Sugar Research Foundation which, in its publication "The Sugar Molecule," in October 1949, acknowledged that the purpose of its caries research program was intended "to find out how tooth decay may be controlled effectively without restriction of sugar intake." The American Medical Association endorsed fluoridation "in principle," but admitted that it has conducted no experiments of any aspects of its toxicity. It also has stated that it does not guarantee its safety. Dr. Reuben Feltman of Passaic General Hospital in New Jersey administered fluoride tablets to children and to pregnant women. He reported in the *Journal of Dental Medicine* (Vol. 16, October 1961), "Prenatal and Postnatal Ingestion of Fluorides—Fourteen Years of Investigation—Final Report," that about one percent of his patients could not tolerate the drug. At 1 mg of fluoride per day (the same level as is recommended in the fluoridation program) he observed symptoms ranging from headache to gastrointestinal disturbance, skin disorders, eczema, itching and dryness of the throat creating a desire to drink increased amounts of water, in about one out of each 100 patients.

These same symptoms were described by Dr. Kaj Roholm, a Danish biochemist and physician, who died in 1948 but who is still considered the great authority on fluorine chemistry because of his classic work, "Fluorine Intoxication," published in 1937. Roholm explained that in the early stages of fluoride poisoning, the symptoms are vague and inconsistent, making diagnosis difficult.[6]

"Evidence in the world literature has shown that fluoride introduced artificially into soft water supplies, such as those of New York City, is much more toxic than the fluoride present in harder waters," Benfield said. "Most naturally fluoridated waters are high in mineral content. It has been shown that in one area of India where the fluoride level was about 3 ppm and the water soft, there was greater toxicity with respect to dental and skeletal fluorosis than in another area where the concentration was 5 to 6 ppm of fluoride but the water was hard."[6]

The New York City water supply contains chlorine, hydrofluorosilicic acid, caustic soda (to neutralize the hydrofluorosilicic acid), copper sulphate and possibly other chemicals, Benfield added. All of these are protoplasmic poisons. In addition, hundreds of tests done over a period of several years in New York City confirm the fact that the fluoride level cannot be maintained at a uniform, so-called optimum level, of 1 ppm. The tests showed that the concentration is consistently higher nearer the reservoirs than elsewhere. This has been the experience in many other cities, he said.[6]

At least 12 Nobel Prize winners throughout the world have questioned the wisdom of fluoridation of public water supplies, Benfield added. The majority of these men won their awards for their research in chemistry. But at times fluoridation has been instituted in communities without the knowledge of its citizens. In 1959, Benfield reported, Dr. Fred Wertheimer, Michigan State Dental Health Director, stated that seven communities had initiated fluoridation during the past year. But he said that the names of these communities were "top secret" as far as the department was concerned.[6]

"In cities that have adopted fluoridation, corrosion of hot water tanks, boiler pipes, water mains and meters has become a serious problem," Benfield said. "The Miami Water Heater Co. replaced 5,000 hot water tanks after six years of fluoridation. A Toronto, Canada manufacturer of hot water tanks, in business for over 40 years, announced its intention in 1962 to discontinue sales to Brantford, Ontario (fluoridated since 1945) because 90 percent of their claims of corrosion damage came from that area. Previously, corrosion damage had been negligible from even the hardest water."[6]

Benfield added that within four years after the introduction of fluorides into the New York City water supply, a standpipe and the drain fitting in an X-ray tank in his office were completely eaten through. A 1¼-inch-diameter metal waste pipe on one of the operating room units was also eaten through. All of these parts are continuously exposed to running water for eight or nine hours a day. The Picker X-Ray Supply Co. advised him they would not replace the metal standpipe and the X-ray tank with anything but plastic pipe, "which is not adversely affected by the water."[6] Benfield continued:

Fluoridation has often been compared with chlorination of water as a health measure by proponents, but they conveniently overlook the fact that there is a highly important difference between them. While both are halogens, chlorine is introduced into water as a gas and is supposed to be eliminated before it reaches the user's tap. If it is not, it can easily be eliminated by heating the water. Not so with fluorides. These are introduced as compounds which concentrate when water is boiled. The concentration doubles when water is boiled for 15 minutes. This is not an uncommon occurrence, especially in restaurants. In the preparation of soups, gravies, sauces and other foods, much greater concentration occurs.[6]

"The Fluoride Content of Some Foods and Beverages," by J. R. Marier and Dyson Rose, of the National Research Council of Canada, appeared in the November-December 1966 issue of *Food Science*. They found that the fluoride content of vegetables processed in fluoridated water rose by a factor of 3 to 5, so that instead of having the usual fluoride concentration of 0.2 to 0.3 ppm, the concentrations ranged from 0.7 to over 1 ppm. Thus, they pointed out, the total average daily dietary intake per person was markedly increased. The same was found to be true of bottled soft drinks prepared with fluoridated water. They also found that gelatin processed in fluoridated water developed concentrations of 29 to 34 ppm, as contrasted with gelatin prepared with nonfluoridated water which was found to contain only 6 to 8 ppm.[6]

High levels of fluoride for extended periods may have negative effects on bone status, according to K. R. Phipps and B. A. Burt in the *Journal of Dental Research* in June 1990. The study involved 151 women, ages 39 to 87. Sixty-nine of the women were residents of an "optimal fluoride community," while 82 lived in a high-fluoride community (3.5 ppm of fluoride in the water). Those living in the high-fluoride community had a bone mass less than that of the controls (where the water contained 0.7 ppm of fluoride).[7]

In the August 27, 1992 issue of the *New England Journal of Medicine*, B. Lawrence Riggs, M.D., of the Mayo Clinic in Rochester, Minnesota, and Melton L. Joseph, III, M.D., reviewed the prevention and treatment of osteoporosis. Concerning women treated with fluoride, they reported that one-third had gastric irritation and another one-third complained of lower extremity pain syndrome. They added that bone with excess fluoride has an abnormal structure and its fragility may be increased. In one of the studies they evaluated, there was a three-fold increase in the rate of nonvertebral fractures among those treated with fluoride, although they admitted that the 75 mg of sodium fluoride in this instance might have been too high.[8]

Low levels of fluoridation (1 ppm) may increase the risk of hip fracture in elderly men and women, according to Christa Danielson, M.D., et al. in the August 12, 1992 issue of the *Journal of the American Medical Association*. The study evaluated 6,000 people in three Utah communities over a seven-year period.[9]

In an earlier study by B. Lawrence Riggs, M.D., and colleagues at the Mayo Clinic, it was found that, although sodium fluoride increased bone mass, the new bone was too weak to prevent the fractures that occur in the vertebrae and cause the back to curve, according to the March 22, 1990 issue of *The New York Times*.[10]

"This is the most comprehensive and most carefully controlled study of fluoride treatment carried out to my knowledge," said William A. Peck, M.D., president of the National Osteoporosis Foundation and vice chancellor and dean at Washington University School of Medicine in St. Louis. "The results are disappointing, but they do not preclude the possibility that some other fluoride preparation or a lower dose that is more slowly absorbed could be effective. But there are no data that prove this to be the case. At present time we can't recommend sodium fluoride at any dose or any preparation for treatment of osteoporosis."[10]

In an editorial in the October 1991 issue of *Better Nutrition for Today's Living*, I referred to the research by MaryFran R. Sowers and her colleagues at the University of Michigan at Ann Arbor. They analyzed the bone density of 800 women in Iowa, ranging in age from 20 to 80, and concluded that women over 55 who drink fluoridated water are more prone to bone fractures.[11]

In a personal letter to me in 1984, Albert W. Burgstahler, Ph.D., Professor of Chemistry at the University of Kansas at Lawrence, said: "As further research findings emerge it is becoming increasingly clear that fluoridation was a very bad gamble. It is not proving very effective in reducing tooth decay, if at all, and its hazards to health are becoming more and more disturbing. Even such an orthodox organ as *Health and Longevity Report* has recently carried an article expressing these concerns. Similar views have appeared recently in *Research & Development* and in *American Laboratory*. The British weekly *New Scientist* has also published critical material in recent years."[12]

GROWING OLDER WITH FLUORIDE?

In the February 1984 issue of *Research & Development*, Frederic B. Jueneman, FAIC, said that, "For more than 30 years we have been treated to joyous paeans on the benefits of fluorides to our health, well-being and good looks. Hundreds of communities have voted in resolutions to fluoridate their potable waters and take advantage of the perfectly marvelous opportunity to enrich their lives and especially that of their children. Indeed. Since this subject was last discussed [R&D, March 1980, p. 17], this wonderful house of cards is on the verge of collapse. More and more medical evidence has been surfacing which excoriates the use of fluorides in any form, and fluoride is now linked with the process of aging."[13]

Jueneman referred to the book by John Yiamouyiannis, Ph.D. (*Fluoride: The Aging Factor*), and said that as a chemist he appreciated Yiamouyiannis' reference to the efforts of John Emsley and coworkers in 1981 at King's College in London, where it was found that fluoride formed the second strongest hydrogen bond known with amides, and thus was able to disrupt and destroy the enzyme activity of a whole class of proteins.[13]

"Even the most conservative estimates have confirmed that this causes genetic damage, which accelerates the aging process and promotes the onset of cancer," Jueneman continued. "The pathologic interference of fluoride cannot therefore be underestimated. Fluoride disrupts collagen synthesis that involves the formation of cartilage, and a mineralization results which develops into various arthritic and rheumatoid conditions. Similarly, the collagen necessary for fibrous liga-ments, as well as the fibroblasts in arterial cell walls, are calcified by the action of fluoride, adding to the so-called aging process."[13]

He went on to say that the ability of fluoride to form a strong hydrogen bond with amino acid links in a protein chain is being abetted by a new water treament process as well. It seems, he added, that the tried and true method of disinfecting our drinking water by chlorination results in the formation of trihalomethanes, which are thought to be bad for our continued good health.[13]

"An alternative use of hydrogen peroxide, which ultimately decomposes into water and oxygen, is considered too expensive," he said. "So, the cheap addition of ammonia to the water along with the chlorine leads to the formation of chloramine, which permits the controlled release of chlorine without forming nasty trihalomethanes. This nice new procedure has resulted in a near 100-percent fish kill when the water is changed in the fish tank, and warnings have been posted for those who are on kidney dialysis."[13]

Jueneman added that, curiously, the chloramine treatment seems to have its greatest effect in communities with fluoridated water, which "leads one to think that a synergistic relation exists between fluoride and the amine which sends the carp to the big fishbowl in the sky. The effect on humans is a study that is worthy of another million-dollar government grant."[13]

The May 1984 issue of *Health and Longevity Report* reported that, "Aside from the issue of whether fluoridation of drinking water achieves its purpose, there is the ethical question as to whether using community water supply is the proper means of administering a chemical. Some people consider fluoridation a violation of their right to decide health matters for themselves. Water fluoridation, unlike chlorination, which is done to purify, is unique as a means of involuntary mass medication for a noncontagious condition."[14]

When fluorosis of teeth becomes severe, the publication said, it causes tooth surfaces to become pitted and rough. There is evidence, in the National Institute of Dental Research study (then recently issued) and in others, that drinking water with a high fluoride content actually increases caries incidence. One explanation is that it is easier for bacteria to stick to the rough surfaces caused by fluorosis and that it's harder to clean out the bacteria.[14]

The publication discussed the work of Dr. B. Uslu of Hacettep University in Turkey, who found that leg fractures in rats fed fluoridated drinking water healed very slowly when compared with fractures in animals without fluoride in their water. In some cases the fractures still hadn't healed after 35 days. Uslu said that the slow bone healing was attributed to inhibition of collagen synthesis, a necessary process in the mending of bones. And in a study by Dr. Toshio Imai in Tokyo, Japan, it was found that fluoride inhibits cell growth, DNA synthesis and protein synthesis in cultured cells. Imai added that when cells are exposed to fluoride they multiply much slower than normal. DNA synthesis continues as before for the first 24 hours, then slows greatly, he said.[14]

"Dr. Imai hypothesizes that the cells completed the DNA synthesis already begun at the time of fluoride introduction," the publication said. "But they didn't start any new synthesis because somehow the fluoride inhibited protein production."[14]

In at least 11 animal studies, fluoride has been shown to influence enzyme activity, according to Michael E. Elsohn, D.D.S., in the November 17, 1988 issue of *Medical Tribune*. In some tests, he said, enzyme activity was depressed; in others, it was stimulated. In addition, one study indicates a transient decrease in human serum activity associated with the advent of water fluoridation. But there have been few other studies to gauge effects of typical levels of fluoride intake on enzyme activity in people, he said.[15]

In an earlier issue of *Medical Tribune*, Elsohn said that some people may react adversely to fluoride whether it is contained in pills, water or toothpaste. He reported that the 1983 *Physicians' Desk Reference* said that, " 'In hypersensitive individuals, fluorides occasionally cause skin eruptions, such as atopic dermatitis, eczema or urticaria. Gastric distress, headache and weakness have also been reported. These reactions usually disappear promptly after discontinuation of the fluoride.' This information was omitted from later editions of the reference."[16]

Hans Moolenburg is a Dutch physician who has studied hypersensitive reactions to fluoride. He believes the reactions can be explained as effects of a toxic agent rather than as allergies. In large doses, he said, everyone reacts to fluoride, but some people react to much lower levels.[16]

Elsohn continued:

The late George L. Waldbott, founder and chief of allergy clinics in four Detroit hospitals and an antifluoridation activist, reported treating at least 500 patients who reacted negatively to fluoridated water. Their symptoms included muscle weakness, chronic fatigue, excessive thirst, headaches, skin rashes, joint pains, digestive upsets, tingling in the extremities and loss of mental acuity. Waldbott used double-blind tests to determine whether fluoride was the cause of symptoms in many of his cases. In each of the patients, he said, the symptoms disappeared when the fluoride was taken away without the patient's knowledge and reappeared when it was given again, but not with the administration of other possible agents.[16]

Writing in the *Journal of Dentistry for Children* in October 1990, David G. Pendrys, D.D.S., Ph.D., and Douglas E. Morse, D.D.S., SM, said that fluoride supplements should not be used in children who drink fluoridated water. In recent years, they said, increased evidence of enamel fluorosis has been seen in children in optimally fluoridated communities.[17] Since millions of American children are drinking fluoridated water, are consuming foods and beverages made with fluoridated water, and are using all kinds of fluoride dental products, one wonders why this report by members of the School of Dental Medicine, Harvard University, in Boston, hasn't been widely publicized. Meanwhile, some members of the American Dental Association and other fluoride promoters continue to fuel the fluoride bandwagon.

Researchers at the Tufts School of Dental Medicine analyzed 24 brands of "natural" spring water and found fluoride concentrations ranging from less than 0.1 ppm to 1.25 ppm, with most in the range of 0.55 to 0.7 ppm, reported Joseph R. Hixson in the January 25, 1990 issue of *Medical Tribune.* Granted, the legal limit of 4 ppm for community water supplies is about seven-fold greater, he said, "even the modest bottled-water level may carry dental-health implications." Suppliers of "pure" water do not have to put the fluoride concentration on the label, but they must have the data on the concentration on file for inquiries, he added.[18]

"The family that adds fluoride for anti-caries protection to 'pure' bottled water may unwittingly be adding to its fluoride risk, according to Anthi Tsamtsouris, D.D.S., associate professor of pediatric dentistry at Tufts," Hixson continued. "The American Dental Association and the American Pediatric Association recommend, for children up to age three, an optimal fluoride level in water of 0.25 ppm. The recommended level for adults is 1.0 ppm."[18] Although Hixson did not mention it, those who drink a lot of water or those who live in a warm climate are probably getting much more fluoride than they need.

CONFLICT AND CONTROVERSY CONTINUE

The February 22, 1990 issue of *Medical Tribune* discussed a study of fluoride carcinogenicity in rodents, which was conducted in the laboratories of Procter and Gamble. The study was begun in the early 1980s but had not been published almost 10 years later. Asked why, a spokesperson responded, "Just bureaucracy, I guess," reported Joel Griffiths.[19]

"The P&G study seems to be the only other rodent bioassay of fluoride carcinogenicity comparable to the widely publicized—and apparently positive—study by the National Toxicology Program," Griffiths said. "Meanwhile, official release of pathology results from the NTP study confirm the possibility of a casual link between fluoride and bone cancer (and perhaps oral cancer as well)."[19]

Added Griffiths in another section of the medical newspaper, "The unexpected positive results from the National Toxicology Program's rodent study of fluoride carcinogenicity will make it difficult for the Environmental Protection Agency not to classify fluoride a carcinogen, thereby terminating 40 years of public-water fluoridation in the United States."[19] Has the EPA taken such action? Of course not!

On February 7, 1994, Secretary of Labor Robert B. Reich ordered the Environmental Protection Agency to reinstate whistleblower Dr. Bill Marcus in his former (or comparable) position at EPA, reported the April 1994 issue of *The Fluoride Report*.[20]

"Almost two years after being fired, Dr. Marcus has finally emerged victorious over the unsavory individuals who tried to punish him for challenging the false-hoods propagated by his own agency and the Public Health Service about the safety of fluoride. He will receive back pay, legal expenses and $50,000 in damages," the publication said.[20]

In reinstating Marcus, Secretary Reich said that an EPA investigator was ordered by a superior to shred evidence gathered during the investigation, and that EPA withheld evidence that would have supported Marcus in court.[20]

"Not mentioned by Rich, but recorded in the hearing before Judge Clark, is clear evidence that EPA tampered with witnesses, threatening EPA employees with dismissal if they testified on Marcus' behalf," the publication continued. "EPA management also forged some of his time cards, and then accused him of misusing his official time. . . . At a press conference, Marcus noted that all the officials who participated in his firing are still employed by EPA and 'making decisions about drinking water that affect public health.' "[20]

In its April 1994 issue, *The Fluoride Report* said that, if fluoridation were a demonstrably sound idea, "you would think that promoters would be fearless in presenting their case, and in allowing a full and open discussion on the issues. In reality, however, when the issue of fluoridation arises, public health authorities work overtime at avoiding discussion and the democratic process, while trampling on individual rights."[20]

To illustrate the underhandedness with which some fluoride promoters work, the publication discussed the approach of a health officer in Florida, who was trying to convince officials in one city to fluoridate their water supply. The most important tactic, the official said, is "Keep a low profile: the least amount of publicity the better." Next, "pick off the community officials one by one . . . have someone they know and respect convince them of the benefits of fluoridation and of their responsibility as community officials to provide the most cost-effective public health measures available to their constituency." Then, "Do not push the issue unless you're sure the majority will vote 'yes.'" And, above all, "Avoid a referendum. The statistics are that three out of four fluoridation referenda fail."[20]

Affects Fertility

In the September 1994 issue of *The Fluoride Report*, editor Robert J. Carton, Ph.D., quoted Stan C. Freni, a scientist at the Food and Drug Administration, as saying that, when the FDA examined birth rates in countries with at least 3 ppm of fluoride in the drinking water, they found a very close correlation between decreasing total fertility rates in women between the ages of 10 and 49, and increasing fluoride levels. Freni, whose article originally appeared in the *Journal of Toxicology and Environmental Health* (42:109–121, 1994), added that a review of all the animal studies done to date shows that fluoride affects fertility in most animal species.[21]

Toxins in Town Tanks

Fluoridation mishaps are fairly common but are not highly publicized in their communities. They are sometimes referred to as a "chemical spill" without mentioning fluoridation.

On November 11, 1979, a city public works employee in Annapolis, Maryland, opened a valve on a large tank of hydrofluosilic acid to refill a control chemical feeder that introduces the acid, at specified amounts, into the water system, reported the November-December 1979 issue of *National Fluoridation News*. The employee forgot to turn off the valve and the mistake was not discovered until 8:30 the next morning. City officials believed that 1,000 gallons of the acid had entered the water supply.[22]

On November 13, eight kidney patients became ill while receiving dialysis treatment at the Bio-Medical Applications Clinic in Annapolis. The treatments were halted after patients showed signs of distress, chest pain, vomiting, nausea and itching. After being sent home, one patient became severely ill but recovered; another was found dead by his wife at home.[22]

"Even though state and county health officials had learned of the spill nine days after it occurred, no public announcement was made and the Annapolis City Council was not told of the situation for six more days," the publication reported.[22]

Charles M. Yost, a deputy to the county health officer, explained that, "We didn't want to jeopardize the fluoridation program because it has been so good for the children. You have to wait until you're really sure there is a problem before you go out and panic people."[22]

In the meantime, state officials ordered two bottling plants to destroy all soft drinks produced on November 11 and 12 because of high levels of fluoride in tap water used at the plants. Two pet stores in Annapolis reported massive fish kills in aquariums due to "unusual" acid levels in the water.[22]

More recently, Paul M. Arnow, et al., of the University of Chicago Hospital, discussed in the *Annals of Internal Medicine* an outbreak of acute illness and death in a long-term hemodialysis unit. During five consecutive hemodialysis shifts, 12 of 15 patients receiving dialysis treatment in one room became acutely ill, experiencing severe pruritus (itching), multiple nonspecific and/or fatal ventricular fibrillation (stoppage of the heart). Three patients died. The researchers said that death was associated with longer hemodialysis time and increased age when compared with other patients who became ill. Serum concentrations of fluoride in the sick patients were considerably increased, and the source of fluoride was the temporary deionization system used to purify water for hemodialysis only in the affected room. The research team concluded that, since deionization systems are used widely in hemodialysis and can cause fatal fluoride intoxication, careful design of the facility and monitoring are essential.[23]

In the January 13, 1994 issue of *The New England Journal of Medicine*, Bradford D. Gessner, M.D., et al., reported that faulty fluoridation equipment in a water system in Alaska caused one death and almost 300 cases of acute fluoride poisoning. Victims ranged in age from six months to 73 years. Fluoride concentrations in two water systems ranged from 2 to 150 mg/liter. Public Health Service recommendations are 0.7 to 1.2 mg/liter.[24]

"The water-system operator had no formal training and lacked a basic understanding of the operation of the fluoridation unit," Gessner said. "Fluoride-test results had not been submitted to or monitored by state regulators. When elevated fluoride concentrations were discovered before the outbreak, the recommendation to disconnect the fluoride pump was not implemented."[24]

Fluorosis is a major public health problem in India, where about 25 million people suffer from the crippling effects of excess fluoride, said Bhupesh Mangla in the May 18, 1991 issue of *Lancet*. Thirteen states in the country have been declared endemic for the disease. In fact, fluoride levels in natural sources of drinking water in these areas are so high that the National Technology Mission on Safe Drinking Water set up a submission on control of fluorosis. The aim is to minimize, or if possible eliminate, fluoride intake from sources other than water.[25]

"Apart from pressing for a ban on the sale and advertisements of fluoridated toothpastes in areas endemic for fluorosis, the submission also advocated that all packaging for fluoridated toothpastes should indicate exact fluoride content and a warning against their use by children below seven years," Mangla said.[25]

Osteoporosis and Bone Health

Some gynecologists are skeptical about the effectiveness of new osteoporosis treatments, and are continuing to prescribe estrogen, exercise and calcium for their postmenopausal patients, according to Celia Slom in the May 30, 1991 issue of *Medical Tribune*. She was reporting on the annual meeting of the American College of Obstetricians and Gynecologists, held at that time in New Orleans. Researchers at the University of Texas Southwestern Medical Center in Dallas had previously reported that supplements of slow-release sodium fluoride and calcium spurred bone growth in the hip and spine. Other researchers had reported on the use of natural progesterone and oral etidronate therapy to reduce fractures.[26]

But some of the doctors attending the meeting were doubtful about these new therapies, Slom said. She quoted Mike Lindel, M.D., of Fairchild Air Force Base, Spokane, Washington, as saying: "I don't use the newer treatments because of conflicting reports, especially on fluoride. I prescribe estrogen and exercise to arrest continued deterioration of bone."[26]

John R. Lee said in the March 4, 1989 issue of *Science News*:

> The long-held delusion that fluoride will be a safe, effective and marketable treatment for osteoporosis concerns me. There have been many attempts to achieve this golden result but all have failed. Fluoride is simply too toxic and its benefits are too little. Its toxicity at these high doses is not limited to gastric irritation but also shows up as pain and stiffness of joints and ligamentous structures. The slightly denser bone that eventually develops in the spine after several years of fluoride medication is disordered and lacks tensile strength. As a previous article indicated [Jan. 21, 1989, p. 36], the researchers reported that the treatment failed to decrease the incidence of hip fractures, which are the major debilitating effect of osteoporosis.[27]

SIDS Connection in Australia?

There is a correlation between the highest fluoridated cities and the incidence of sudden infant death syndrome in Australia, according to Glen S. R. Walker in the February 12, 1992 issue of *The New Zealand Medical Journal*. He added that it is interesting to note that the latest National Health and Medical Research Council of the Australia Fluoridation Report in 1991 admits that babies are consuming too much fluoride because of the availability of so many sources, especially babies on formula foods made from fluoridated water.[28]

Walker went on to say that the Victorian Health Minister recently announced that one of the leading fluoridated toothpaste manufacturers is producing a new junior toothpaste with a 50-percent reduction in fluoride content. He added that this may raise the question that, if water fluoridation is so safe, then why is the amount being reduced. And he said, the old myth that fluorides have a wide safety margin is now being put to rest with new research.[28]

An objective review of water fluoridation appears in the August 1, 1988 issue of *Chemical and Engineering News*. However, the article by Bette Hileman and the Letters to the Editor that followed in later issues would require a small book to recap. Hileman reported:

Dennis Leverett, chairman of the department of community dentistry at the Eastman Dental Center in Rochester, New York, claims that the prevalence of dental fluorosis today in communities with fluoridated water is twice the level that H. Trendley Dean, a dental surgeon in the Public Health Service, reported in 1942 from his studies of communities with the same level of natural fluoride in their water supply. Leverett fears that if additional studies substantiate his findings, fluoride levels in supplements, toothpaste (most of which contain 1,000 ppm fluoride), and water may need to be reassessed. He reasons that the increase in fluorosis may result from the increased use of fluoridated toothpastes, supplements and perhaps from higher levels of fluoride in the food chain. Today, nearly all bottled drinks and canned foods in the U.S. are processed with fluoridated water. Should further studies confirm Leverett's conclusion, it would validate a warning that has been sounded by scientific critics of fluoridation for at least 25 years.[29]

Ever since the Public Health Service endorsed fluoridation in 1950, detractors have charged that PHS and the medical and dental establishment, such as the American Medical Association and the American Dental Association, have suppressed adverse scientific information about its effects, Hileman added.

"Some of those who generally support fluoridation make similar charges," Hileman said. "For example, Zev Remba, the Washington Bureau editor of *AGD Impact*, the monthly publication of the Academy of General Dentistry, wrote last year that supporters of fluoridation have had an 'unwillingness to release any information that would cast fluorides in a negative light,' and that organized dentistry has 'lost its objectivity—the ability to consider varying viewpoints together with scientific data to reach a sensible conclusion.' "

She quoted Robert J. Carton, an environmental scientist at EPA, as saying that "the scientific assessment of fluoride's health risks written by the agency in 1985, 'omits 90 percent of the literature on mutagenicity, most of which suggests fluoride is a mutagen.' "

Hileman recalled a number of distinguished researchers whose criticisms of fluoridation were not published. Other researchers were warned by their employers not to publish anything against fluoridation.

"In 1980," she continued, "Brian Dementi, then toxicologist at the Virginia Department of Health, wrote a comprehensive report on 'Fluoride and Drinking Water' that suggested possible health risks from fluoridation. This 36-page study has been purged from the department's library, even though it is the only one the department has prepared on the subject. According to current employees, no copy exists anywhere in the department. Spokesmen say the report was thrown away because it was old but also say the department will be preparing another report on the subject soon."[29]

Hileman went on to say that ADA and PHS have actively discouraged research into the health risks of fluoridation by attacking the work or the character of the investigators.

"As part of their political campaign," she continued, "they have over the years collected information on perceived antifluoridation scientists, leaders and organizations. Newspaper articles about them are stored in files, as are letters about them from various proponents of fluoridation. Little or no effort has been made to verify the accuracy of this information. It is used not only in efforts to counteract arguments of the antifluoridationists, but also to discredit the work and objectivity of U.S. scientists whose research suggests possible health risks from fluoridation."[29]

In November 1962 and 1965, ADA included in its journal long directories of information about antifluoridation scientists, organizations, leaders and others known to oppose fluoridation. Listed in alphabetical order were reputable scientists, convicted felons, food faddists, scientific organizations and the Ku Klux Klan. Information was given about each, including quotes from newspaper articles, some of which contained false data, she said. The information was published for use by proponents of fluoridation in local fluoridation referenda.[29]

"It is easy to understand why research on risks of fluoridation has never been more vigorously pursued," Hileman said. Most of the individuals and agencies involved have been promoting fluoridation policy for nearly 40 years. Research that suggests possible harm threatens them with a loss of face, she added.[29]

"For example," she continued, "PHS has historically been the principal source of funds and fluoride research; but ever since June 1950, PHS has been officially committed to and responsible for promoting fluoridation. Thus, the agency has a fundamental conflict of interest."[29]

John A. Colquhoun, former principal dental officer in the Department of Health in Auckland, New Zealand, was told after writing a report that showed no benefit from fluoridation in New Zealand that the department refused him permission to publish it, Hileman said.[29]

"Colquhoun, now teaching the history of education at the University of Auckland, offers another explanation for what appears to be the suppression of research," Hileman said. "He notes that the editorial policy of scientific journals has 'generally been to not publish material which overtly opposes the fluoridation paradigm.' Scientific journals employ a referee system of peer reveiw. But when the overwhelming majority of experts in an area from which the referees are selected are committed to the shared paradigm of fluoridation, the system, he contends, lends itself to preservation and continuation of the traditional belief that fluoridation is safe and effective. This results in 'single-minded promotion, but poor-quality research, and an apparent inability to flexibly reassess in the presence of unexpected new data,' he said."[29]

The heated pros and cons of water fluoridation will continue as long as the bureaucrats refuse to even acknowledge that there is a wealth of information available suggesting possible harm from dumping a rat poison into the public water system.

REFERENCES

1. *Recommended Dietary Allowances*, 10th Edition. Washington, D.C.: National Academy Press, 1989, pp. 235ff.
2. Murray, Frank. "Is Fluoridation Safe?" *Better Nutrition*, June 1984, pp. 22ff.
3. "Fluoridation Ends in Chile," *National Fluoridation News*, October-December 1980, p. 1.
4. Sutton, P. R. N. "Are Most Fluoridation Promoters Neurotics?" *Medical Hypotheses* 39:199–200, 1992.
5. Yiamouyiannis, John, Ph.D. *Fluoride: The Aging Factor*. Delaware, Ohio: Health Action Press, 1983, pp. 109–110.
6. Benfield, James W., D.D.S. "Observations on Fluoridation of Public Water Supplies Over a Period of 28 Years," *National Fluoridation News*, July-September 1972, pp. 3–4.
7. Riggs, B. Lawrence, M.D. "Effect of Fluoride Treatment on the Fracture Rate in Postmenopausal Women with Osteoporosis," *New England Journal of Medicine* 322(12):802–809, March 22, 1990.

8. Riggs, B. Lawrence, M.D., and Melton, L. Joseph, III, M.D. "The Prevention and Treatment of Osteoporosis," *New England Journal of Medicine* 327(9):620–627, August 27, 1992.

9. Danielson, Christa, M.D., et al. "Hip Fractures and Fluoridation in Utah's Elderly Population," *Journal of the American Medical Association* 268(6):746–748, August 12, 1992.

10. "Doubt Raised on Bone Disease Treatment," *The New York Times*, March 22, 1990, p. B15.

11. Murray, Frank. "Fluoridation Is Still a Mistake," *Better Nutrition for Today's Living*, October 1991, p. 6.

12. Burgstahler, Albert W., Ph.D. Personal letter, June 13, 1984.

13. Jueneman, Frederick, FAIC. "Fluoride: A Factor in Aging," *Research & Development*, February 1984, p. 17.

14. "More Open-Minded Approach to Fluoridation Would Benefit All," *Health and Longevity Report*, May 1984, p. 2.

15. Elsohn, Michael E., D.D.S. "The Fluoride Intangible: Its High Enzyme-Blocking Activity," *Medical Tribune*, November 17, 1988, p. 22.

16. Elsohn, Michael, D.D.S. "Froth Over Water Fluoridation," *Medical Tribune*, November 10, 1988, p. 7.

17. Pendrys, David G., D.D.S., Ph.D., and Morse, Douglas E., D.D.S., SM. "Use of Fluoride Supplementation by Children Living in Fluoridated Communities," *Journal of Dentistry for Children*, September-October, 1990, pp. 343–347.

18. Hixson, Joseph R. "Bottled Fluoride," *Medical Tribune*, January 25, 1990, p. 2.

19. Griffiths, Norman. "New Rap Against Fluoride: P&G Study," *Medical Tribune*, February 22, 1990, pp. 1, 12.

20. "Victory for the Truth," *The Fluoride Report*, April 1994, p. 1, 8.

21. "FDA Finds Significant Correlation Between Fluoride and Decreased Fertility in Women," *The Fluoride Report*, September 1994, p. 8.

22. "Fluoride Spill Kept Secret," *National Fluoridation News*, November-December 1979, p. 1.

23. Arnow, Paul M., et al. "An Outbreak of Fatal Fluoride Intoxication in a Long-Term Hemodialysis Unit," *Annals of Internal Medicine* 121:339–344, 1994.

24. Gessner, Bradford, D., M.D., et al. "Acute Fluoride Poisoning from a Public Water System," *New England Journal of Medicine* 330(2):95–99, January 13, 1994.

25. Mangla, Bhupesh. "India: Defluoridation Battle," *Lancet* 337:1213, May 18, 1991.

26. Slom, Celia. "Osteoporosis Therapy Surveyed," *Medical Tribune*, May 30, 1991, p. 2.

27. Lee, John R. "Fluoride Is Not the Answer," *Science News*, March 4, 1989, p. 139.

28. Walker, Glen S. R., "Fluoridation and Cot Death," *The New Zealand Medical Journal*, February 12, 1992, p. 44.

29. Hileman, Bette. "Fluoridation of Water: Questions About Health Risks and Benefits Remain After More Than 40 Years," *Chemical and Engineering News*, August 1, 1988, pp. 26ff.

28

Germanium: A Mineral Waiting in the Wings

ALTHOUGH frowned on by the Food and Drug Administration, germanium is an antioxidant that shows considerable promise in boosting the immune system, in fighting AIDS and possibly preventing or treating cancer. The mineral was isolated in 1886 by German chemist Clemens Winkler, who took the name from Germania, the Latin name for his country.

As I reported in the August 1988 issue of *Today's Living*, germanium was known for a long time only as a semi-conductor. Not much attention was given to its biochemical possibilities until the 1940s, when Kazuhiko Asai, Ph.D., a Japanese researcher, began to explore germanium's therapeutic properties. Since then, at the Asai Germanium Clinic, he and other researchers have used the mineral successfully to treat some forms of cancer, glaucoma, arthritis, high blood pressure, depression and other disorders.

Using data from animal experiments, Asai concluded that germanium (found in varying amounts in ginseng, garlic, pearl barley, chlorella, aloe, comfrey, sushi and suma) increases the oxygen supply to the body. Through his research, Asai has isolated an organic germanium compound (bis-carboxyethyl germanium sesquioxide). This compound leads to the cure of various diseases and produces health-sustaining effects by serving as a substitute for oxygen in combining with hydrogen ions and other waste substances in the body.[1]

"Oxygen readily combines with hydrogen, so it becomes apparent that hydrogen will strongly bind with the oxygen atoms of the compound, consequently bringing about a dehydrogenating reaction which is the mechanism by which germanium eliminates harmful substances causing disease in the body," Asai reported in *Miracle Cure: Organic Germanium*. "Consider for a moment the basic fact of the life process whereby food is burned by the body to give energy, while carbon dioxide and hydrogen are created. Carbon dioxide is discharged from the lungs when we exhale, and hydrogen combines with oxygen to form water which is discharged in the urine and sweat. Hydrogen may be referred to as a positive ion, which is as useless to the body as dust clogging the workings of a machine."[2]

To insure that the body functions normally, Asai continued, hydrogen must be removed, but for complete removal a large quantity of oxygen is needed. The germanium compound, with its strong dehydrogenating effect, takes the place of oxygen in combining with hydrogen to eliminate the latter from the body. In fact, he added, all traces of germanium are discharged from the body through the digestive tract within 20 to 30 hours.[2]

BOOSTS BRAIN CIRCULATION

"I am inclined to believe that various types of mental disorders are caused by an oxygen deficiency due to a disorder in the blood circulation in the brain," Asai said. "This view is based on the fact that relief can be obtained to an almost dramatic extent just by supplying sufficient oxygen through administration of the organic germanium compound. Thus, I have succeeded in relieving many from the complaints accompanying softening of the brain, manic-depressive psychosis, hysteria and even the after-effects of whiplash injury."[2]

Hepatitis and cirrhosis of the liver can also respond to germanium, according to Carlson Wade in the January/February 1988 issue of *Health News & Review*. And, he added, the mineral stimulates the immune system to resist the ravages of toxic mercury, cadmium and polychlorinated biphenyls (PCBs). In some patients, it has brought high blood pressure under control.

New reports of clinical application of germanium are encouraging, Wade continued. We see it has good effects against cancer of the lung and brain, digestive tract, female reproductive organs and lymph system. Germanium is able to build immunity to cancers of the lymph system. In addition, he reported, it is said to be able to assist in rheumatoid arthritis, collagen disease, hearing problems and osteoporosis.

"Germanium exerts a regulatory normalization of the immune system," Wade said. "It initiates production of gamma interferon, a powerful antitumor agent, and is also antiviral. By stimulating the immune cells, germanium causes production of protective immunostimulants, including vitamins C and E and coenzyme Q10. These life-saving immunostimulants are needed to build resistance to common and uncommon disorders. In particular, germanium prompts activity of natural killer cells to cooperate with interferon and act as an inner shield to defend the body against cancer."

Wade added that germanium does not inhibit cancerous growth or spread. Instead, it is a "spark plug" for the immune system to create this disease-fighting process. Anticancer drugs are toxic to normal cells, and have frightening side effects, but germanium works from within to help the body protect itself against cancer, Wade said.[3]

Germanium is being used in Japan to treat some AIDS patients, according to Kaneo Yamada, M.D., of the St. Marianna University School of Medicine in Japan. Five other substances were approved for treatment of the disease at the International AIDS Treatment Conference, held February 1987 in Tokyo. These included shiitake mushroom (lentinan), isoprinosine and interferon.[4]

Parris M. Kidd, Ph.D. reported in the January 1987 issue of *International Clinical Nutrition Review*:

> The apparent versatility of Ge-132 [germanium] in normalizing homeostasis, stimulating immunity and alleviating major diseases suggests that it acts at a fundamental level of the function. The question of the possible nutritional essentiality of elemental germanium remains unresolved. The known biological and clinical effects of Ge-132 are consistent with Dr. Asai's suggestion that it substitutes for or supplements tissue oxygenation. In cells which cannot utilize oxygen, e.g., cancer cells which actually are oxygen-sensitive, we might predict that its presence as an oxygen-catalyst would destabilize homeostasis. The relative contributions of this possible effect versus its stimulation of interferon production by the host remain to be sorted out.[5]

In acute, subacute and chronic toxicity studies it has been found that germanium, given orally, intravenously, subcutaneously and intraperitoneally to mice, rats, rabbits and beagle dogs, is highly safe, even when given up to the equivalent in humans of tens of grams per day, Kidd said. At the Asai Clinic, two to three percent of the patients reported minor skin eruptions, which were resolved within a few weeks. Megadosing can result in softening of the stool, "but no major side effects have yet been reported, even after exhaustive toxicopharmacological testing," Kidd said.[5]

Kidd added that, in animal studies, germanium has been found to be an antioxidant, protecting the body against the accumulation of amyloid, a free radical-oxidative end product. And germanium protects cysteine (a sulfur-containing amino acid) against oxidation in laboratory tests.[5]

In a personal letter to me from Walter Mertz, director of the Beltsville Human Nutrition Research Center, USDA, in Maryland, he said that there is presently no evidence that germanium has an essential function in animals or man, "but this does not mean that such a function may not be discovered later on." He added that the best summary and evaluation of the mineral was given by H. A. Schroeder and J. J. Balassa.[6,7]

USEFUL IN MANY CONDITIONS

Writing in *Prescription for Nutritional Healing*, James F. Balch, M.D., reported that Kazuhiko Asai found that an intake of 100 to 300 mg/day of germanium improved many illnesses, including rheumatoid arthritis, food allergies, elevated cholesterol, candidiasis, chronic viral infections, cancer and AIDS. Germanium is also a fast-acting painkiller, he said.[8]

"Germanium works by attaching itself to molecules of oxygen, which are carried into the body to improve cellular oxygenation," Balch said. "The body needs oxygen to keep the immune system functioning properly as oxygen helps rid the body of toxins and poisons. Dr. Asai believes all diseases are caused by an insufficient oxygen supply to the area of the body where it is needed. Researchers have shown that organic germanium is an effective way to increase tissue oxygenation because it acts as a carrier in the same way as hemoglobin."[8]

There are some clinical anecdotes suggesting that germanium may be of some benefit for patients with chronic fatigue syndrome, probably via immune-enhancing effects, according to Sheldon Saul Hendler, M.D., Ph.D., in *The Doctors' Vitamin and Mineral Encyclopedia*. And it has been reported that two new organic germanium compounds (not Ge-132), PCAGeS and PCAGeO, inhibited the growth of certain mouse cancers when the tumor-containing mice were given oral preparations of these compounds. Macrophage activity (type of immune cell that kills cancer cells) was enhanced by these compounds, Hendler said.[9]

The literature does contain a few reports of germanium toxicity, which has impressed the FDA and some other regulatory agencies. For example, Reto Krapf, M.D., reported in *Nefron* in 1992 that a 43-year-old woman with nonmetastatic breast cancer had died because of severe lactic acidosis after ingesting 25 grams of elemental germanium over a two-month period. Renal failure was said to be triggered by the megadose of germanium.[10] It is not clear who prescribed this amount of the mineral, or in which form it was, but 25,000 mg of germanium is obviously a megadose.

REFERENCES

1. Murray, Frank. "Germanium: The Interferon Activator," *Today's Living*, August 1988, pp. 10ff.
2. Asai, Kazuhiko, Ph.D. *Miracle Cure: Organic Germanium*. Tokyo: Japan Publications, Inc., 1980, pp. 37, 91.
3. Wade, Carlson. "Germanium, 'Electronic Key' to a Powerful Immune System," *Health News and Review*, January/February 1988, p. 12.
4. Yamada, Kaneo, M.D. Personal letter, February 20, 1987.
5. Kidd, Parris M., Ph.D. "Germanium-132 (Ge-132): Homeostatic Normalizer and Immunostimulant. A Review of Its Preventive and Therapeutic Efficacy," *International Clinical Nutrition Review* 7(1):11–19, January 1987.
6. Mertz, Walter. Personal letter. March 25, 1987.
7. Schroeder, H. A., and Balassa, J. J. *Journal of Chronic Disease* 20:211–224, 1967.
8. Balch, James F., M.D., and Balch, Phyllis A., C.N.C. *Prescription for Nutritional Healing*. Garden City Park, N.Y.: Avery Publishing Group, Inc., 1990, p. 19.
9. Hendler, Sheldon Saul, M.D., Ph.D. *The Doctors' Vitamin and Mineral Encyclopedia*. New York: Simon and Schuster, 1990, pp. 141ff.
10. Krapf, Reto M.D. "Abuse of Germanium Associated with Fatal Lactic Acidosis," *Nefron* 62:351–356, 1992.

29

Lithium Helps to Fight Depression

SINCE lithium is used as a drug by physicians to treat depression and some forms of mental illness, it probably should be segregated into a section all its own. However, it was used during World War II as a salt substitute and a lithium ointment is sold over-the-counter for treating herpes. So I am reluctantly including the mineral in this section of the book.

Although over 40 years have elapsed since its effects on mania were first described, lithium is still a mainstay in the treatment of mood disorders, according to Lawrence H. Price, M.D., and George R. Heninger, M.D., in the September 1, 1994 issue of *The New England Journal of Medicine*. It remains the standard against which new mood-stabilizing or thymoleptic drugs are measured, they added.

Lithium salts were advocated for the treatment of "uric acid diathesis" by Garrod in England in 1859 and by Hammond in the United States in 1871, the authors added. The two physicians held that alkaline salts were effective in treating several "gouty diseases," including mania and depression.

"In an attempt to identify toxins that might cause mania, J. F. J. Cade gave guinea pigs lithium urate as a soluble salt of uric acid," the authors continued. "However, the animals became sedated rather than excited—perhaps, ironically, due to the toxic effects of lithium. Attributing a calming effect to the drug, Cade tested lithium in 10 patients with mania and reported dramatic benefits in 1949."[1,2]

In that same year, the FDA banned lithium in response to the deaths of several patients from lithium intoxication. The patients, who had heart disease and high blood pressure, had been prescribed lithium chloride as a salt substitute. As a result of this unfortunate coincidence, the authors said, as well as lack of sponsorship by the pharmaceutical industry, research on the psychotropic effects of lithium progressed slowly, and it was not approved by the FDA for the treatment of mania until 1970.[1]

Price and Heninger, from the Yale University School of Medicine in New Haven, said that lithium has largely lived up to its initial promise as the first drug to be discovered in the modern era of psychopharmacology. But in some respects, this legacy has hampered the development of other thymoleptic drugs. It is extraordinarily difficult to conduct controlled studies in patients with bipolar disorder, and the availability of lithium as an effective treatment has reduced the urgency of finding other drugs, they said.

Alternative treatments now center on carbamazepine, valproate and calcium-channel antagonists. The thymoleptic properties of carbamazepine were recognized 10 years ago, but it has not replaced lithium as a first-line treatment. This may be due in part to the declining efficacy of prolonged carbamazepine therapy, but it illustrates the difficulty of developing treatments that are clearly superior to lithium, they said, despite its limited efficacy and its side effects.

"Recent findings from a randomized, controlled multi-center study involving 179 patients suggest that valproate may be as effective as lithium in the treatment of acute mania, with both drugs better than placebo," the authors concluded. "Although it seems likely that lithium will continue to have a central role in the treatment of mood disorders over the next decade, the development of more effective and safer alternatives should be a high priority."[1]

Responding to their article, Robert Stern, M.D., Ph.D., also from Yale, stated in the January 12, 1995 issue of *The New England Journal of Medicine* that lithium produces severe side effects. In essence, lithium poisoning results from therapeutic doses of lithium carbonate that are excessive because of concurrent medical conditions or drugs that alter the metabolism of lithium or because of inadequate supervision and from intentional overdoses for attempted suicide.[3]

"In the United States in 1993, according to surveillance data for 70 percent of the population, treatment with lithium led to three deaths, 184 toxic incidents that were life-threatening or resulted in important residual disability, 710 toxic incidents that necessitated medical treatment and 1,177 minor incidents in which symptoms and signs resolved rapidly. Serum lithium measurements are not a reliable indication of lithium poisoning, particularly in patients undergoing long-term treatment, in whom severe neurotoxic effects may coexist with normal serum lithium concentrations."[3]

Stern discussed the death of a man after a five-day religious fast during which he continued to take his usual dose of lithium carbonate (1,500 mg/day), suggesting the importance of educating patients. And he said that a large malpractice award went to a woman who sustained brain damage when signs and symptoms of neurotoxic effects were mistaken for psychosis and her lithium therapy was continued without a serum lithium determination. This emphasizes the need for educating physicians, he said, and that lithium carbonate needs to be prescribed with the help of an experienced psychiatrist.[3]

Although lithium therapy for overexcited patients was discovered by Cade of Australia in 1949, its medical acceptance has been slow, explained Carl C. Pfeiffer, Ph.D., M.D., et al. in *The Schizophrenias: Ours to Conquer*. To this date, lithium therapy is legal only for the treatment of the manic stage of manic-depressive disorders, although numerous publications have indicated that lithium therapy is also useful in chronic depression, premenstrual depression, excess thyroid secretion as in hyperthyroidism, treatment of alcoholics and anorexia nervosa, he said.[4]

"At the Princeton Brain-Bio Center, we have used lithium in schizophrenia and other patients for 25 years," Pfeiffer added. "Although lithium has no effect on hallucinations, it does allow the nonhallucinatory patient to reduce his effective dose of major tranquilizers. This reduces the side effects of large doses of drugs such as Prolixin. The patient is also made better able to tolerate hallucinations while on lithium therapy. Delva and Letemendia (1982) estimate that one-third to one-half of all schizophrenic patients may benefit from the use of low-dose lithium therapy. Because their study shows no patients with signs of clinical deterioration, the implementation of low-dose lithium treatment appears to be an almost no-risk situation."[4]

Dr. B. S. Levy said: "What has caused even more interest in lithium is that it appears to be active as a prophylactic agent against recurrent psychotic depression. Studies have shown that lithium given prophylactically to patients with recurrent depression is able to substantially diminish the depressive attacks. This effect holds true whether the patient has shown only depression in the past or has had alternating phases of mania and depression. If used prophylactically, lithium requires a dosage with few side effects and causes no restriction of normal emotional expression."[4]

Pfeiffer continued: "Some professionals, motivated by inexperience—and their desire to fill hospital beds—tell patients that lithium therapy can only be started in a hospital where daily lithium levels will be run. This is untrue! We and others have found that adults ranging in age from 12 to 50 years can be started on two 300 mg tablets of lithium carbonate per day. On this dose, lithium levels can safely be determined at monthly intervals. Patients frequently do well on only one or two tablets of lithium per day."[4]

USEFUL IN TREATING ADDICTIONS?

Lithium, best known for its use in the treatment of manic-depressive syndrome, may be useful at times for controlling the mania associated with cocaine addiction, according to Sheldon Saul Hendler, M.D., Ph.D., in *The Purification Prescription*. Recently, some evidence has emerged suggesting that lithium might also help alcoholics abstain from alcohol by suppressing the urge to drink, he said.[5]

"Some cocaine or amphetamine addicts have an underlying component of manic-depressive illness," he added. "For those, a trial of lithium—maintaining a therapeutic level and monitoring for any side effects—may be helpful. It is essential that this diagnosis be made by an experienced physician."[5]

Lithium carbonate may help some alcoholics to abstain from drinking, reported *Medical World News*, September 12, 1983. In a placebo-controlled, double-blind study at Rush-Presbyterian-St. Luke's Medical Center in Chicago, Jan A. Fawcett, M.D., and colleagues found that 75 percent of 84 severely alcoholic patients who complied with lithium treatment remained abstinent after 18 months. And so did 50 percent of those given a placebo, although no noncompliant patient stopped drinking.

Fawcett reported that the mineral's efficacy suggests a genetically transmitted biochemical marker for alcoholism. But Edward M. Sellers, M.D., of the Addiction Research Foundation in Toronto, Canada, said that just because lithium helps to reduce drinking, "it doesn't follow that there is any connection to the etiology of alcoholism."[6]

In a study of 30 patients with bipolar depression, researchers in the Netherlands found that eight of them had cognitive impairment while being treated with lithium carbonate. Tremor was also a complaint from the patients receiving this drug. The geriatric patients seemed to be the most susceptible to lithium carbonate supplementation, however, their cognitive impairment was improved when they were switched to lithium citrate. But these results cannot be extrapolated to younger patients, the researchers said.[7]

In treating mania, Dr. Chouinard from McGill University (1978) considers L-tryptophan, the amino acid, to be as effective as lithium and even more effective than chlorpromazine. One mechanism by which lithium works is by promoting serotoninergic neuron transmission.[8]

At the Brain-Bio Center in New Jersey, the physicians have combined their nighttime lithium therapy with one to three grams of tryptophan. Patients subjectively tell them that this tryptophan enhances the benefit of the lithium. The staff added that a recent study using 12 g of L-tryptophan alone for mania found tryptophan extremely effective in treating this condition.[8] (Tryptophan is no longer available over-the-counter in the United States; it can only be obtained from a physician. The Food and Drug Administration removed the product from store shelves after a contamination problem in a Japanese factory caused a number of American deaths and illnesses. Now that the problem has been rectified, many people feel that the FDA has erred in keeping the product off the market.)

"A number of physicians have used up to 1,500 mg/day of lithium carbonate as a treatment for anorexia, especially if there was strong evidence of a severe mood disorder such as manic depression," according to Douglas Hunt, M.D., in *No More Fears*. "Lithium has been beneficial to anorexics even without these strong signs of mood disorder (Gross and Ebert, 1981), but researchers warn that unreliable, unstable, poorly managed patients could quickly develop a toxic condition if they continued restricted food intake, vomiting and overusage of diuretics. So the benefits should be weighed against the risks."[9]

In the December 22, 1986 issue of *Medical World News*, it was reported that an article in the November issue of *Vogue* stated that lithium may help relieve anxiety in bulimics. L. K. George Hsu, M.D., on the staff of the Western Psychiatric Institute and Clinic in Pittsburgh, said that 12 of 14 patients had 75- to 100-percent fewer bulimic episodes after being given lithium therapy. Hsu added that the potential for lithium toxicity calls for careful monitoring of the therapy.[10]

USEFUL FOR MANIA AND DEPRESSION

The introduction of lithium treatment was a major advance for bipolar disorder, both for the treatment of acute manic episodes and for the prevention of recurrences of either mania or depression, reported Richard M. Glass, M.D., in *Medical and Health Annual/1992*. He noted that lithium is a naturally occurring element that alters sodium transport in cells. Its precise mode of action in relieving bipolar symptoms, however, has not been clearly established.[11]

"Patients with bipolar disorder may require treatment with one of the antidepressants plus lithium during a depressive episode but usually should not be maintained on an antidepressant, which could lead to more frequent episodes of mania or to rapid cycling," Glass said. "For patients who do not respond well to lithium, several alternative drugs, including the anticonvulsant drug carbamazepine (Tegretol), may be effective."[11]

Lithium therapy does not decrease the availability of folic acid, the B vitamin, according to Sing Lee, et al., in the *Journal of Affective Disorders*. In fact, high folate levels may enhance the mineral's benefits, they said. The study involved 46 Chinese patients, mostly manic depressives, who were given lithium in a Hong Kong clinic, and it was designed to determine the folate status of the patients.[12]

Writing in *Agressologie* in 1973, H. A. Nieper, M.D., of the Silbersee Clinic in

Hannover, Germany, said that lithium citrate and lithium carbonate are far less effective than lithium orotate in treating patients with constitutional migraine and constant headache. He added that lithium orotate, in low doses, is also effective in treating depression, alcoholism, epilepsy. It produces no side effects.[13]

As Ruth Adams and I reported in *Minerals: Kill or Cure?*, the problem with lithium, a trace mineral found in rocks, mineral water, etc., is that too much of it in the blood disturbs the balance between body fluids and certain other minerals, including potassium and sodium. The body has a very delicate mechanism for regulating this balance and any disruption can cause serious trouble—nausea, vomiting, etc.[14]

We discussed the work of Prof. Ole Rafaelsen of Copenhagen, Denmark, who has found that lithium benefits patients with Meniere's disease, Huntington's Chorea and tardive dyskinesia. For the latter patients, Rafaelsen also prescribes tryptophan.

"No one knows why lithium benefits victims of Meniere's disease," we reported. "This is a disorder of the inner ear, involving deafness, vertigo and tinnitus or ringing in the ears. Sometimes the victim also suffers from nausea, vomiting and nystagmus, the uncontrollable rolling of the eyeballs. It is believed that Meniere's disease may be caused by a disturbance of water balance and those minerals which control this mechanism—chiefly sodium and potassium."

Of the 21 patients with Meniere's disease who benefitted from lithium, 16 of the patients were still taking the mineral when the book was written. Five have been able to stop all treatment after 10 to 18 months with total disappearance of symptoms. One of the patients, a 52-year-old woman, had gained 30 pounds, but she told Rafaelson she planned to continue the lithium therapy because of the relief it had brought her. At the time Rafaelsen had not conducted controlled trials using lithium with Meniere's disease patients.

We reported that Dr. Per Dalen of St. Jorgen's Hospital, Hisings Becka, Sweden, found that 60 percent of patients with Huntington's chorea that were treated with lithium showed improvement. This is a nervous disorder, presumably inherited, which usually appears later in life. It involves irregular, involuntary movements along with disturbed speech and brain function.

We stated: "It is said that of the 1,000 or more people in America affected with Huntington's Chorea, all descended from three men, probably brothers, who came to America in about 1630. The descendants of this trio scattered over the New England states, and many were involved in early witchcraft trials, because the odd symptoms of the disease aroused the suspicions of superstitious persons."[14]

In his book, *Fighting Depression*, Harvey M. Ross, M.D., said that lithium "is one of the most significant developments in the field of psychiatry in the last 20 years." He added that it is one of the few agents that can be monitored easily by means of periodic tests to determine if the dosage is proper. When given to a patient who is able to understand the need for caution and the use of periodic blood testing, and when administered by a competent physician, lithium is a safe, effective and relatively inexpensive treatment that has already restored full life to thousands of happy and grateful people, he said. Ross often prescribes the mineral to the patients who visit his Los Angeles office.[15]

"Other researchers have followed up with systematic studies in universities and clinics," Ross continued. "Dr. Ronald Fieve at the New York State Psychiatric Institute is a prominent investigator of lithium. Many others have conducted lithium trials and now an impressive collection of data is available which confirms the original supposition of Dr. Cade that lithium is an effective agent in the treatment of disorders of the mood."[15]

Although lithium is effective in treating childhood manic-depression and some other psychiatric illnesses affecting youngsters, it is not useful in treating Attention Deficit Disorder, according to G. Robert DeLong, M.D., of the Harvard Medical School in Boston. A more detailed study appeared in the May 1987 issue of the *Journal of the American Academy of Child and Adolescent Psychiatry*.[16]

The 10-year study involved almost 200 children with various diagnoses. The largest group, 59, with an average age of 11, was diagnosed as manic-depressive. This is characterized by periods of depression alternating with manic periods. This may include irritability, "high" or happy moods, excessive energy, behavior problems, staying up late at night and making grand plans. Thirty-nine, or 66 percent, of the 59 were successfully treated with lithium.[16]

However, of the 19 with ADD who were given lithium, the medication was not successful in treating any of them. In fact, parents indicated that behavior worsened in eight of the 19 children.[16]

DeLong also reported that of the 11 children diagnosed with emotionally unstable character disorder, nine, or 82 percent, responded favorably to lithium therapy. Their average age was 13½. Of the seven children (average age of 10) who had behavior disorders, and whose parents had been successfully treated with lithium, five, or 71 percent, improved with lithium. The mineral was also responsible for significant improvement in children with extreme aggressiveness, explosive behavior and encopresis (soiling).[16]

"These results demonstrate that the beneficial effects of lithium treatment for certain childhood behavior disorders can be sustained for more than a decade,"

DeLong said. "The question of accurate diagnosis is central in deciding which children to treat with lithium. However, certain behaviors may warrant a trial of lithium regardless of diagnosis. These include especially hateful, hostile anger, manic overexcitement, a family history of manic-depressive illness, salt-craving and encopresis."[16]

TOPICAL USES

In two studies reported in *Dermatology* in 1992, C. Cuelenaere, et al., in Belgium gave a lithium succinate ointment (tradenamed LSO) to patients with seborrheic dermatitis. They reported that a significantly high portion of patients treated with LSO showed remission or marked improvement compared to placebo. There are minor side effects, such as transient skin irritation and/or stinging sensation. The authors said that topical lithium succinate appears to be safe and effective for the treatment of seborrheic dermatitis and probably works by an anti-inflammatory mechanism.[17] (LSO-1 is an over-the-counter preparation sold in some health food stores.)

Researchers at the University of Pennsylvania reported that 10 women who received 12 months of lithium therapy for herpes, at an average daily dose of 587 mg, and who had not benefited from acyclovir, showed a 3.2 percent average monthly reduction in the number of herpes episodes and a 5.1 percent cut in the episode's duration, according to *Medical Tribune*, December 12, 1991. The researchers added that, even though acyclovir reduces herpes episodes 80 to 90 percent, lithium may benefit those women who cannot tolerate the drug.[18]

Topically applied lithium succinate ointments offer substantial symptomatic relief for herpes, reported James Braly, M.D., in *Dr. Braly's Food Allergy and Nutrition Revolution*. Applied at the first sign of an outbreak (at the burning or tingling stage) it in many cases prevents blisters from forming. In addition, he said, if blisters are already formed, an application can reduce recovery time significantly. In his book, Braly gives a nutritional protocol for dealing with Herpes Simplex, Types I and II.[19]

Researchers reported in *Lancet* in 1983 that lithium ointment significantly reduced pain duration from seven to four days. The 73 patients with recurrent genital herpes were treated within 48 hours of lesion onset with the ointment, which was applied four times a day for one week. Others received a placebo. The ointment contains lithium succinate, zinc sulfate and vitamin E.[20]

REFERENCES

1. Price, Lawrence H., M.D., and Heninger, George R., M.D. "Lithium in the Treatment of Mood Disorders," *The New England Journal of Medicine* 331(9):591–598, September 1, 1994.
2. Cade, J. F. J. "Lithium Salts in the Treatment of Psychotic Excitement," *Medical Journal of Australia* 2:349–352, 1949.
3. Stern, Robert, M.D., Ph.D. "Lithium in the Treatment of Mood Disorders," *The New England Journal of Medicine* 332(2):127-128, January 12, 1995.
4. Pfeiffer, Carl C., Ph.D., M.D., et al. *The Schizophrenias: Ours to Conquer.* Wichita, Kansas: Bio-Communications Press, 1988, pp. 341ff. (Distributed by Keats Publishing, Inc., New Canaan, Conn.)
5. Hendler, Sheldon Saul, M.D., Ph.D. *The Purification Prescription.* New York: William Morrow and Co., Inc., 1991, p. 62.
6. "Some Alcoholics Trade Liquor for Lithium—But Why?" *Medical World News,* September 12, 1983, p. 47.
7. Van Gent, E. M., and Zwart, F. M. "The Effects of Lithium Carbonate and Lithium Citrate on Cognitive Function," *ACTA Therapeutica* 17:253–262, 1991.
8. Braverman, Eric R., M.D., and Pfeiffer, Carl C., M.D., Ph.D. *The Healing Nutrients Within.* New Canaan, Conn.: Keats Publishing, Inc., 1987, p. 72.
9. Hunt, Douglas, M.D. *No More Fears.* New York: Warner Books, 1988, p. 139.
10. "Lithium for Bulimia," *Medical World News,* December 22, 1986, p. 73.
11. Glass, Richard M., M.D. "Depression in Perspective," *Medical and Health Annual.* Chicago: Encyclopaedia Britannica, Inc., 1992, p. 90.
12. Lee, Sing, et al. "Folate Concentration in Chinese Psychiatric Patients on Long Term Lithium Treatment," *Journal of Affective Disorders* 24:265–270, 1992.
13. Nieper, H. A. "The Clinical Applications of Lithium Orotate: A Two-Year Study," *Agressologie* 14(6):407–411, 1973.
14. Adams, Ruth, and Murray, Frank. *Minerals: Kill or Cure?* New York: Larchmont Books, 1974, pp. 185ff.
15. Ross, Harvey M., M.D. *Fighting Depression.* Atlanta: Larchmont Books, 1984, pp. 112ff. (Revised edition distributed by Keats Publishing, Inc., New Canaan, Conn.)
16. Duprat, Melissa. "Lithium Found Effective for Children with Manic-Depression; Ineffective in Treating Attention Deficit Disorder." Press release from the American Academy of Child and Adolescent Psychiatry, Washington, D.C., August 19, 1987.
17. Cuelenaere, C., et al. "Use of Topical Lithium Succinate in the Treatment of Seborrheic Dermatitis," *Dermatology* 184:194–197, 1992.
18. "Lithium May Relieve Herpes," *Medical Tribune,* December 12, 1991, p. 2.
19. Braly, James, M.D., and Torbet, Laura. *Dr. Braly's Food Allergy and Nutrition Revolution.* New Canaan, Conn.: Keats Publishing, Inc., 1992, pp. 384–385.
20. Skinner, G. R. B. "Lithium Ointment for Genital Herpes," *Lancet* 2:288, 1983.

30

Manganese: A Little Goes a Long Way

SOMETIMES confused with magnesium, manganese is an important trace mineral, which mineral was initially recognized as an element in 1774 by Carl W. Scheele, a Swedish chemist. His co-worker, Johann G. Ghan, isolated manganese that same year, and its name is a corrupted form of the Latin word for a form of magnetic stone, magnesia.

Manganese is rather poorly absorbed, primarily in the small intestine. In the average diet about 45 percent of the ingested manganese is absorbed, and 55 percent is excreted in the feces. But absorption can be depressed when excessive amounts of calcium, phosphorus or iron are consumed.

"Following absorption, manganese is loosely bound to a protein and transported as transmanganin," the *Foods and Nutrition Encyclopedia* said. "The bones, and to a lesser extent the liver, muscles and skin, serve as storage sites. Manganese is mainly eliminated from the body in the feces as a constituent of bile, but much of this is again reabsorbed, indicating an effective body conservation. Very little manganese is excreted in the urine. The concentration of manganese in the various body tissues is quite stable under normal conditions, a phenomenon attributed to well controlled excretion rather than regulated absorption."[1]

WHO IS AT RISK?

In the November-December 1988 issue of *Nutrition Today*, Jeanne H. Freeland-Graves, Ph.D., R.D., gives an extensive overview of the role of manganese in human health. Although gross deficiencies of the mineral have not been observed in free-living populations, cases of suboptimal status of manganese have been

319

found in selected populations, she said. These populations include children with inborn errors, such as phenylketonuria, maple syrup urine disease, galactosemia and methylmalonic acidemia; children and adults with epilepsy; and patients with exocrine pancreatic insufficiency, active rheumatoid arthritis or hydralazine syndrome. Individuals with these conditions may have special needs for this trace element, she added.[2]

The author discussed a study in which she gave seven men, ages 19 to 22, a semipurified diet containing 0.11 mg/day of manganese for 39 days. On the 35th day, five of the seven men developed a finely scaling, minimally erythematous rash. She diagnosed the rash as *miliaria crystallina*, a condition in which sweat cannot be excreted through the epidermis and results in small, clear blisters filled with fluid.[2]

Freeland-Graves added:

Biochemical reasons for the dermatitis observed in these experimentally induced deficiencies could be related to the requirement of manganese for the activity of enzymes that are necessary in maintenance of the skin integrity. The first group of enzymes, glycosyltranserases, functions in the synthesis of glycosaminoglycans, compounds which are components of the mucopolysaccharides of collagen in the skin as well as other tissue. Another manganese-containing enzyme is prolidase, which is found in dermal fibroblasts. This enzyme catalyzes the final step in the breakdown of collagen. Genetic deficiencies of prolidase have been associated with a severe dermatitis and chronic cutaneous ulcers.[2]

Another consequence of the manganese-deficient diet fed to the volunteers, she said, was a decline in total and high-density lipoprotein cholesterol (HDL) in the serum. The hypocholesterolemia that was observed may be related to the requirement of manganese at five sites in the biosynthesis of cholesterol, she continued. Since both a fleeting, finely scaling rash and hypocholesterolemia were noted in both her study and that by Doisey (1972), it seems probable that these may be clinical symptoms of a manganese deficiency in humans.

"Perhaps the most provocative findings of our study were the observed increases in serum calcium and phosphorus and enhanced activity of alkaline phosphatase," she said.

"Similar findings of elevated serum calcium and phosphorus were observed in rats that were fed manganese-deficient diets for 12 months. The bones in the manganese-deficient animals were low in manganese and exhibited an osteoporotic condition. The alterations observed in both the human and animal studies suggest that stores of manganese were being mobilized as a consequence of the manganese deficiency. Dissolution of bone to release manganese would also release calcium and phosphorus in the blood. Whether or not continued manganese depletion would eventually lead to osteoporosis is an area which demands further investigation."[2]

The current estimated safe and adequate daily dietary intake of manganese is 2.5 to 5 mg/day, she said. This range is derived from studies that found positive balance when subjects were fed 2.5 mg/day or higher and a negative balance on 0.7 mg/day. However, because of limited data, there is no Recommended Dietary Allowance for the mineral at the moment. In contrast with other trace minerals, manganese has a low level of toxicity since dietary intakes of 500 to 2,000 mcg/g are required before toxicity symptoms appear, she said. Since dietary levels as high as 18 mg/day (found in India and from eating bran muffins) have not produced any toxic effects, the upper limit of 5 mg/day seems a bit too conservative.

"The manganese content of the typical diet in the United States was estimated from analysis of 234 foods in the Food and Drug Administration's Total Diet Study," Freeland-Graves continued. "Mean manganese levels were below the lower limit of 2.5 mg/day for adolescent girls (1.76 mg/day) and adult (2.05 mg/day) and elderly (2.12 mg/day) women. Estimated intakes for men in the same age groups averages 2.74, 2.72 and 2.57 mg/day, respectively. According to numerous balance studies, these levels are not sufficient to maintain positive balance."[2]

The negative influence of both fiber and phytate on manganese bioavailability was illustrated by Schwarts, et al. They found that three bran muffins a day produced negative manganese balance in spite of dietary levels of 13.9 mg/day of manganese. In a metabolic study of adult men and women, the substitution of simple sugars for complex carbohydrates resulted in negative balances of manganese in spite of dietary levels of 4.4 and 5.9 mg/day. But it was not clear whether the negative balances were caused by lower levels of manganese in the high sugar versus the high fiber diet (6.2 to 8 mg/day) or were the result of interactions with other trace elements.

DIETARY SOURCES

Some of the food sources of manganese are nuts, seeds, whole grains, green, leafy vegetables and tea. Poor sources are meats, eggs, milk, sugar and refined foods. A diet containing a variety of nuts, seeds and whole grains may contain between 8 and 17 mg/day of manganese, whereas one based on meats, dairy products, sugary and refined foods may only contain from 2 to 2.7 mg/day. The latter diets are presumably responsible for low dietary intakes of manganese, she said.

Freeland-Graves concluded:

> In the past, there was more concern about manganese toxicity from industrial exposure than deficiency. Also, dietary intakes were much higher when unprocessed foods formed the basis of our diets. But the reports of experimentally induced deficiencies and suboptimal status of manganese in humans suggest that manganese may be more critical for human nutriture than previously realized. The mineral may be particularly important for women who are prone to osteoporosis because of its role in bone formation and stability. Furthermore, physicians routinely prescribe high dose supplements of both iron and calcium for women, minerals which are reported to have an interaction with manganese. Studies of quantities found in typical diets in the United States suggest that they are often lower than that needed to maintain positive balance. As the role of manganese in human nutrition becomes more clear, greater emphasis should be directed toward maintaining optimal dietary intakes of this mineral.[2]

In his book *Nutrigenetics*, R. O. Brennan, D.O., said that today's white bread is hardly the staff of life. The grains that compose our processed white flour and breads are more of the malignant calories Americans eat that contribute to malnutrition. These are, he said, not *naturally* empty; man has made them so. While refining grains to make flour, Brennan said that 86 percent of the manganese is removed.

Manganese made news at an American Chemical Society meeting in Anaheim, California, in 1986, when Linda Strause, Ph.D., and Paul Saltman, Ph.D., of the University of California at San Diego, discussed the importance of manganese in bone metabolism. Their discussion of the low manganese levels that affected basketball star Bill Walton are discussed in another chapter in this book.[4]

Strause and Saltman also discussed their studies with J. Yves Reginster, M.D., a rheumatologist at the University of Liege in Belgium, in which they compared blood samples from 14 Belgian women with osteoporosis and a similar number of age-matched women without the disorder. Of the 25 factors that were analyzed, the researchers found that the osteoporotic women had a quarter of the manganese levels that the controls had.[4]

"There is a great deal of both popular and professional interest in the etiology, diagnosis, prevention and treatment of osteoporosis," Strause and Saltman said.

"The extent of this disease in the United States is a major public health concern. No single cause can be identified. Certainly the influence of hormones, dietary intake of calcium, fluoride and vitamin D are significant. Our results suggest that it may be prudent to consider the possibility that trace element deficiencies, particularly of manganese, may be of significance."[4]

Based on their animal studies, Strause and colleagues reported in the *Journal of Nutrition* in 1986 that the effect of long-term dietary deficiencies in manganese and copper should be considered in human bone metabolism. They found that low-manganese and low-copper diets fed to the animals produced bone abnormalities.[5]

U.S. Pharmacist, October 1987, reported that health food stores sell tablets containing 5 mg of manganese, or 50 mg of manganese gluconate, which is equivalent. This is enough to prevent manganese deficiency (and presumably osteoporosis) if taken every day. If taking a calcium supplement, it is advisable to take calcium and manganese at different times of the day, since the two minerals compete for absorption rights.[6]

Mood swings, lack of concentration, water retention and pain are common complaints among women during their menstrual cycle. Writing in the *American Journal of Obstetrics and Gynecology*, May 1993, James C. Penland, Ph.D., and Phyllis E. Johnson, Ph.D., of the USDA Human Nutrition Research Center in Grand Forks, North Dakota, said that calcium and manganese help to relieve the monthly pain associated with menstrual complaints. In their study, involving 10 women, the researchers reported that increasing calcium intake from 600 to 1,300 mg/day, and manganese from 1 to 6 mg/day, significantly reduced premenstrual pain and mood swings. The increased calcium also improved mood and concentration and reduced water retention and menstrual pain.[7]

DEFICIENCY IMPLICATED IN MENTAL ILLNESS

Patients with schizophrenia, a major form of mental illness, may be deficient in manganese and zinc, and have high levels of copper, iron, mercury or lead, according to Carl C. Pfeiffer, Ph.D., M.D., in *Nutrition and Mental Illness*. He said that not many studies have been done on how trace elements impact on schizophrenia, even though the use of various minerals to treat the disease go back to 1929.

"At that time," Pfeiffer added, "Dr. English of Brookville, Ontario, reported on the use of manganese injections in 181 schizophrenic patients and found that about half of them improved. As with drug therapy (chlorpromazine and reserpine), Dr. English reported a gain in weight in those patients who responded to manganese therapy (intravenous manganese produced a cutaneous flush like that of niacin). Dr. English got the idea of using manganese from Dr. Reiter of Denmark, who, in 1927, found that 23 of 30 patients improved with manganese."[8]

Writing in *The Practical Encyclopedia of Natural Healing*, Mark Bricklin reported that manganese seems to impart a steadying effect on neurons, and when levels fall too low, the result may be convulsions (*Neurology*, November 1979). Researchers at Cornell University and elsewhere, who compared manganese levels in the hair and blood of healthy people with those with epilepsy, found that the latter group had "significantly lower" levels of the nutrient. Tissue levels of manganese were not consistently lower; however, "most of those with frequent seizures had manganese levels falling below the lowest control level, suggesting a relationship between manganese tissue levels and high seizure activity."[9]

PROBLEMS ASSOCIATED WITH DEFICIENCY

Manganese is essential for the metabolism of amino acids and carbohydrates, and a deficiency of this mineral can cause disc and cartilage problems, glucose intolerance, reduced brain function, middle-ear imbalances, birth defects, reduced fertility and growth retardation, according to Stephen Davies, M.D., and Alan Stewart, M.D., in *Nutritional Medicine*. They added that a deficiency in manganese, chromium, magnesium, potassium, zinc and the B vitamins cause many people to develop hypoglycemia or low blood sugar, since all of these substances are involved in carbohydrate metabolism.[10]

Carlton Fredericks, Ph.D., reported in *Arthritis: Don't Learn to Live with It* that he would like to see the diets of rheumatoid arthritis patients supplemented with manganese, cod-liver oil, vitamin C, bioflavonoids, zinc and vitamin E.

"Very few physicians and medical or lay nutritionists appear to be aware of the importance of manganese to the thymus gland, though it was recognized years ago that atrophy can be traced to deficiency in this nutrient," Fredericks said.

"In both animals and human beings, the thymus gland has been reported to recover from atrophy when manganese was administered. This observation was put to use years ago in the treatment of myasthenia gravis. It has not been applied as it should to rheumatoid arthritis. In any autoimmune disease, we are obligated to learn how to stimulate the immune system, or how to readjust the proportions of its many constituents when they aren't normal.

He went on to say that very few nutritional factors don't in some way affect that system favorably, including some—like zinc and vitamin E—which are routinely removed from the processed sugars and starches which dominate most American diets.

"I write that with emphasis gained from watching the gratifying responses in rheumatoid arthritics who were weaned away from processed carbohydrates, fed increased intake of high-quality protein, and given supplements of such nutrients as the vitamin B-complex, vitamin C, bioflavonoids, mixed tocopherols (vitamin E) and zinc and manganese, among other minerals. Iron supplements and high-iron diets, incidentally, can't be recommended indiscriminately for rheumatoid arthritics, some of whom are victims of an excessive iron load," Fredericks added.[11]

Researchers at the State University of New Jersey reported in the *Journal of Nutrition* in 1990 that manganese deficiency affects glucose metabolism by reducing the number of glucose carriers available for transport. The researchers found in their animal study that the manganese-deficient rats exhibited reduced insulin activity, impaired glucose transport, as well as lowered insulin-stimulated glucose oxidation and conversion to triglycerides in adipose cells.[12]

Manganese is frequently in short supply in heavy drinkers, according to Robert C. Atkins, M.D., a New York City physician, in *Dr. Atkins' Nutrition Breakthrough*. Other nutrients often in small amounts include vitamin C, zinc, magnesium and potassium, he said.[13]

It is in the alcoholic population that we find the true vitamin deficiency diseases such as beriberi, the symptoms of which include emotional instability, shakiness, muscle tremors and depression, Atkins added. Alcoholics may ultimately develop liver problems, eye problems, a tremor and other neurologic difficulties. He reported that Dr. Nathan Brody of Laconia, New Hampshire was successful in treating thousands of alcoholics over a 25-year period with megavitamin therapy. Brody prescribed a blood-sugar controlling diet, along with manganese, vitamin B3, vitamin C, vitamin E, vitamin B1, vitamin B6, vitamin B2, pantothenic acid and zinc.[13]

"Brody then followed the protocol of Dr. Carl Pfeiffer at the Brain-Bio Center, which is based on determining the histamine level of the blood," Atkins said. (Histamine is a breakdown product of protein metabolism.) "The low-histamine patients are treated with B3, folic acid, B12 and pantothenic acid; the high-histamine patients receive calcium, methionine (an amino acid) and the folic acid antagonist diphenylhydantoin. All patients continue on zinc and manganese."[13]

ANTIOXIDANT AND ENZYME ACTION

One of manganese's principal roles is that of an antioxidant, and it, therefore, may protect human beings from toxic oxygen forms, according to Sheldon Saul Hendler, M.D., Ph.D., in *The Complete Guide to Anti-Aging Nutrients*. With regard to the aging process, he continued, manganese's probable role as an antioxidant is interesting. In this regard, it is noteworthy that all tumors examined to date (in various studies) have diminished amounts of the manganese-containing super-oxide dismutase enzyme (*Cancer Research* 39:1141, 1979). This provides a hint, he said, but certainly not proof, that manganese deficiency may play a role in degenerative processes in humans. "Manganese has a fascinating past; I suspect it has a promising future," he added.[14]

Researchers at the University of Wisconsin at Madison reported in the *American Journal of Clinical Nutrition* in 1992, that manganese supplements increased lymphocyte concentrations of superoxide dismutase (SOD). The antioxidant enzyme protects us against chemical- and radiation-induced carcinogenesis, inflammation and free-radical damage. As might be expected, a manganese deficiency reduces SOD levels.[15]

As with other trace elements, manganese has an important role in enzyme functions, reported Ronald Ross Watson, Ph.D., of the University of Arizona College of Medicine at Tucson in *Food and Nutrition*, May/June 1989. In addition, he said, some animal studies indicate that an adequate amount of this nutrient is necessary for normal antibody production, thus suggesting a role in immune function. He added that animal studies have demonstrated that manganese can have both carcinogenic and anticarcinogenic effects. Protection of the cell against free radicals through antioxidant activity is one proposed mechanism by which manganese may protect against cancer, he said.[16]

"Concern relative to possible relationships between manganese deficiencies and epilepsy have been reviewed recently," according to Constance Kies, Ph.D., of the University of Nebraska at Lincoln, in *Food and Nutrition News*, March/April 1989. "Seizures have been found to characterize manganese deficiencies in animals. Furthermore, blood manganese concentrations have been found to be significantly lower in epileptic patients than in their normal controls. However, whether this alteration in blood levels of manganese is due to a relative manganese deficiency or whether it is simply a characteristic of the pathological condition has not yet been defined."[17]

She went on to say that manganese deficiencies have been found to be characterized by a depression in blood serum cholesterol levels, both in humans and experimental animals. For example, in male weaning rats fed diets varied in manganese concentrations, progressive increases in manganese were accompanied with increased total liver lipid and blood serum cholesterol levels.[17]

"Manganese, zinc and copper are also involved in prevention of the peroxidation (breaking up) of polyunsaturated fatty acids within various tissues of the body via combination with superoxide dismutase," Kies added. "Thus, increased intake of polyunsaturated fatty acids may increase need for these trace mineral nutrients."[17]

M. J. Campbell and colleagues reported in the *Journal of Allergy and Clinical Immunology* in January 1992, that samples of manganese from normal subjects contained about four times more manganese than did samples from patients with asthma. They concluded that low levels of manganese, a calcium channel blocker and an antioxidant, may have implications in the pathophysiology of asthma.[18]

In 1962, an 18-year-old man was brought to a South African hospital in a diabetic coma. Efforts to treat him with insulin were unsuccessful and his blood sugar remained high, Ruth Adams and I reported in *Minerals: Kill or Cure?* At one point, the young man mentioned that he had been able to control his diabetes for seven years by drinking alfalfa tea. In desperation, the doctors suggested that he make some in his room. Each time he drank the tea, his blood sugar dropped amazingly. The doctors eventually surmised that it was the manganese in the tea that was doing the good work.[19]

Writing in the *Journal of Orthomolecular Psychiatry* in 1976, R. A. Kunin reported that seven out of 15 cases of withdrawal and tardive dyskinesia were cured after they were given 5 to 20 mg of manganese chelate three times daily. Three of the 15 were much improved, four were improved, while one was not improved.[20]

References

1. Ensminger, Audrey H., et al. *Foods and Nutrition Encyclopedia*. Clovis, Calif.: Pegus Press, 1983, pp. 1370ff.
2. Freeland-Graves, Jeanne H., Ph.D., R.D. "Manganese: An Essential Nutrient for Humans," *Nutrition Today*, November/December 1988, pp. 13–19.
3. Brennan, R. O., D.O., and Mulligan, William C. *Nutrigenetics*. New York: M. Evans and Co., Inc., 1975, pp. 43–45.
4. Raloff, J. "Reasons for Boning Up on Manganese," *Science News*, September 27, 1986, p. 199.

5. Strause, L., et al. "Effects of Long-Term Dietary Manganese and Copper Deficiency on Rat Skeleton," *Journal of Nutrition* 116:135–141, 1986.
6. "Manganese for Your Bones," *U.S. Pharmacist*, October 1987, p. 36.
7. Penland, James C., Ph.D., and Johnson, Phyllis E., Ph.D. "Dietary Calcium and Manganese Effects on Menstrual Cycle Symptoms," *American Journal of Obstetrics and Gynecology* 168:1417–1423, May 1993.
8. Pfeiffer, Carl C., Ph.D., M.D. *Nutrition and Mental Illness.* Rochester, Vermont: Healing Arts Press, 1987, pp. 20–21.
9. Bricklin, Mark. *The Practical Encyclopedia of Natural Healing.* New York: Penguin Books, 1990, p. 128.
10. Davies, Stephen, M.D., and Stewart, Alan, M.D. *Nutritional Medicine.* London: Pan Books, 1987, p. 83ff.
11. Fredericks, Carlton, Ph.D. *Arthritis: Don't Learn to Live with It.* New York: Putnam Publishing Group, 1981, p. 95ff.
12. Baly, D., et al. "Effect of Manganese Deficiency on Insulin Binding, Glucose Transport and Metabolism in Rat Adipocytes," *Journal of Nutrition* 120:1075–1079, 1990.
13. Atkins, Robert C., M.D. *Dr. Atkins' Nutrition Breakthrough.* New York: William Morrow and Co., Inc., 1981, p. 102ff.
14. Hendler, Sheldon Saul, M.D., Ph.D. *The Complete Guide to Anti-Aging Nutrients.* New York: Simon and Schuster, 1985, p. 167ff.
15. Davis, C., et al. "Longitudinal Changes on Manganese-Dependent Superoxide Dismutase and Other Indexes of Manganese and Iron Status in Women," *American Journal of Clinical Nutrition* 55:747–752, 1992.
16. Watson, Ronald Ross, Ph.D. "B-Complex Vitamins and Trace Elements: A Role in Immunomodulation and Cancer Prevention?" *Food and Nutrition News*, May/June 1989, p. 15ff.
17. Kies, Constance, Ph.D. "Copper, Manganese and Zinc: Micronutrients of 'Macroconcern.'" *Food and Nutrition News*, March/April 1989, p. 12ff.
18. Campbell, M. J., et al. "Low Levels of Manganese in Bronchial Biopsies from Asthmatic Subjects," *Journal of Allergy and Clinical Immunology* 89:1, January 1992.
19. Adams, Ruth, and Murray, Frank. *Minerals: Kill or Cure?* New York: Larchmont Books, 1974, p. 171ff.
20. Kunin, R. A. "Manganese and Niacin in the Treatment of Drug-Induced Tardive Dyskinesia," *Journal of Orthomolecular Psychiatry* 5:4–27, 1976.

31

Molybdenum: A Little-Known Antioxidant

IN 1955, researchers in New Zealand found that children in the city of Napier had a lower prevalence of tooth decay than children in the nearby city of Hastings, even though the water sources were similar. Further investigation revealed that, in 1931, an earthquake elevated certain areas of the Hawkes Bay coastal region and drained a five-mile-square lagoon near Napier. Later, soil from the bottom of the former lagoon was brought out for agricultural production, and it was found that home garden vegetables grown on this soil were rich in molybdenum, according to W. H. Allaway of the U.S. Department of Agriculture in Ithaca, New York.[1]

BETTER THAN FLUORIDE

"In controlled experiments," Allaway said, "additions of molybdenum to diets has decreased the incidence of dental caries in rats. The New Zealand findings on relation of molybdenum to human dental caries have been confirmed by studies of the teeth of children living in high-molybdenum areas of the British Isles."[1]

When U.S. Navy recruits from Ohio were found to be virtually free of dental caries, it was traced to the molybdenum in the foods that they ate at home.[2]

Although recognized as a new element in 1778, molybdenum (pronounced muh-lib-duh-num) did not get a name until 1782, when a Swedish researcher, P. J. Hjelm, named it after the Greek word for "lead." This trace mineral, which is a constituent of tooth enamel, is necessary for the functioning of three enzyme systems, which are related to the metabolism of fats, carbohydrates and proteins; sulfur-containing amino acids (cysteine, glutathione, taurine, methionine and ho-

329

mocysteine); iron; and nucleic acids (DNA and RNA). The three enzyme systems are sulphite oxidase, xanthine dehydrogenase and aldehyde oxidase.[3] Enzymes are a variety of protein-like substances, formed in cells, which serve as organic catalysts for initiating or speeding up various chemical reactions.

When people have a deficiency in one of the three enzymes associated with molybdenum, they are subject to a variety of symptoms, according to S. K. Wadman and colleagues in the Netherlands, France, England and Durham, North Carolina.[4]

"A deficiency of xanthine dehydrogenase, which has been described in more than 50 patients, may lead to [urinary stones] due to the low solubility of xanthine [a precursor of uric acid]," the researchers reported in the *Journal of Inherited Metabolic Disease* in 1983. "On the other hand, sulphite oxidase deficiency is a more serious disorder, which seems to be extremely rare. So far only two cases have been published. Both patients developed seizures, mental retardation, severe neurological disturbances. . . . Their urinary sulphur excretion was severely disturbed; inorganic sulphate was low, while sulphite, taurine and other things were high."[4] (Excessive uric acid in the blood is associated with gout.)

STOMACH CANCER DECLINES

Low levels of molybdenum in the Honan Province of China are related to high levels of cancer of the esophagus, according to Sheldon Saul Hendler, M.D., Ph.D., in *The Complete Guide to Anti-Aging Nutrients*. When there are low levels of molybdenum in the soil, this increases the nitrogen content, causing the formation of nitrosamines. The same deficiency has been reported in the Transkei region of South Africa, which also reports high levels of cancer of the esophagus.[5]

"In order for nitrates in the soil to be reduced to nitrogenous substances (amines) necessary for plant nutrition, the molybdenum-activated enzyme called nitrate reductase (found in nitrogen-fixing bacteria) is required," Hendler said. Molybdenum deficiency decreases the activity of the enzyme, and, instead of being converted to amines, the nitrates get transformed to nitrosamines, known cancer-causing substances."[5]

Hendler added that the Chinese of Lin Xian (in the Honan Province) were also deficient in vitamin C, which is known to convert nitrosamines to a less toxic form. Now that the soil in that area has been enriched with molybdenum and the people are taking vitamin C supplements, the incidence of esophageal cancer may be declining for the first time in over 2,000 years.[5]

In his book, *Nutrition and Mental Illness*, the late Carl C. Pfeiffer, Ph.D., M.D., recommended 500 mcg/day of molybdenum to keep the elderly in good health. In addition to the mineral and natural foods, he recommended vitamin C, zinc, selenium (200 mcg/day), manganese (10 mg at bedtime), vitamin E (400 IU in the morning), beta-carotene (15 mg), vitamin B12 (an oral lozenge daily or weekly injection), and two magnesia tablets daily. Pfeiffer predicted that molybdenum will eventually be used to modulate excessive fetal growth in humans and animals and to help easy births.[6]

K. V. Rajagopalan, Ph.D., of the Duke University Medical Center in Durham, North Carolina, agreed. "Because of the importance of [molybdenum] for normal development of the fetus, it is also conceivable that maternal molybdenum deficiency could lead to impaired fetal development. Since molybdenum toxicity does not appear to be a problem in humans, the possibility of molybdenum supplementation during pregnancy is worth considering. A careful study on the molybdenum content of processed infant foods would seem to be in order as well," he reported in the November 1987 issue of *Nutrition Reviews*.[7]

In the same issue of the magazine, it was reported that a 24-year-old man with Crohn's disease, multiple small-bowel reactions and other complications was so chronically ill that he was being fed intravenously. Unfortunately, the patient, who was at the Upstate Medical Center in Syracuse, New York, was not getting sufficient molybdenum from the feeding and was rapidly excreting what little of the mineral was available. This is thought to be the first recorded case of a molybdenum deficiency, and he began to improve once the mineral was added to his diet.[8]

Rajagopalan went on to say that, although the association of sulfite oxidase and xanthine oxidase deficiencies in genetically conditioned disorders in humans are rare, this can be life-threatening. He mentioned two newborns with molybdenum deficiencies who were suffering from congenital defects, feeding problems and other complications. The Syracuse case establishes molybdenum as an essential trace mineral in humans, he added, and provides links to genetic diseases that interfere with the utilization of this mineral.[8]

"The case also illustrates the relative ease with which short-bowel syndrome and inadequate trace-nutrient intake can disturb the homeostasis of the trace mineral," the researcher said. "It provides a warning to all physicians prescribing total parenteral [through a tube] nutrition that the human being appears to be much more fastidious when receiving nutrients by vein than by mouth."[18]

In the United States, where a molybdenum deficiency is thought to be rare, more Americans develop esophageal cancer in areas where molybdenum content of the local water supply is low, according to Oliver Alabaster, M.D., in *What You Can Do to Prevent Cancer*.[9]

"The cancer-inhibitor effect of molybdenum has also been demonstrated in animals," he said. "And the weight of the evidence certainly suggests that good sources of this mineral—liver, kidney, legumes and certain dark green vegetables—should be part of your diet." [9]

The *Columbia Encyclopedia of Nutrition* reports that animal studies have shown that an excessive intake of zinc, cadmium and molybdenum can result in a copper deficiency and that, similarly, large copper intakes can cause a zinc or molybdenum deficiency.[10]

Since there is such a great interaction between minerals, it is not surprising that xanthine oxidase is necessary for converting iron from the ferrous to the ferric form, according to *The Nutrition Desk Reference*. This conversion is involved in how much oxygen is available to the cells. Therefore, molybdenum, like copper, is necessary in iron metabolism.

"Molybdenum is sensitive to sulfur metabolism; inorganic sulfate or endogenous sulfur from amino acids can affect the mineral's tissue concentration," the publication added. "An increased sulfur intake causes a decline in molybdenum status. Molybdenum can interfere with copper absorption, as the two minerals compete for similar absorption sites in the intestines. It is excreted in the urine and bile."[11]

The New York Times reported in 1972 that worldwide changes in the incidence of cancers of the digestive tracts are pointing to meats, alcohol and a deficiency in molybdenum in the diet as possible causes of these major killers.[12]

In the March 1968 issue of *Archives of Environmental Health*, W. H. Allaway, et al., discussed the selenium, molybdenum and vanadium content of human blood collected at blood banks around the U.S. They reported that there has generally been a direct relationship in cattle and sheep between dietary molybdenum intake and molybdenum concentration in the blood. If the data from cattle and sheep can be extrapolated to humans, they said, it would appear that very few of the blood donors in their study were subject to excessively high molybdenum intake. In fact, they added, those few donors whose blood contained more than 10 mcg/100 ml of molybdenum may be approaching a marginal condition of molybdenum interference with copper metabolism.

"There is evidence that dietary molybdenum intake by humans may be useful in the prevention of dental caries," the researchers said. "On the assumption that blood molybdenum concentrations are related to molybdenum intake in humans as they are in cattle and sheep, it would appear that a majority of the blood donors in this study may be at suboptimal levels of molybdenum intake for the prevention of dental caries."[13]

In his book, *The Doctors' Vitamin and Mineral Encyclopedia*, Sheldon Saul Hendler, M.D., Ph.D., said that molybdenum may play a useful role as an antioxidant. Uric acid has been shown to be a powerful antioxidant and a scavenger of singlet oxygen and hydroxyl radicals, he said. Toxicity of oxygen radicals is thought to be a major factor in degenerative diseases and aging.

"Uric acid is produced by the molybdenum-activated enzyme xanthine oxidase," he continued. "Most clinicians see uric acid as, at best, a useless and, at worst, a very destructive molecule in that it can cause gouty arthritis. Biologic phenomena, however, often have two sides, as is the case here. Conceivably, an optimal uric-acid level (maybe just short of the point where it begins to cause problems) is essential for optimal health and to slow down the wear and tear of aging. If this is true, then molybdenum does indeed enter the realm of useful antioxidants."[14]

The concentration of molybdenum in foods varies considerably, depending where the food is grown, according to *Recommended Dietary Allowances*. Tsongas, et al. (1980) determined that the dietary intake of molybdenum in the U.S. ranged from 120 to 240 mcg/day, depending on age and sex, with the average around 180 mcg/day. The richest sources were milk, beans, breads and cereals. But Pennington and Jones (1987) found a lower molybdenum content in the 1984 collection of the Food and Drug Administration's Total Diet Study, which ranged from 76 to 109 mcg/day for adult females and males, respectively. Human milk contains very low levels of molybdenum, and after the first month of lactation, furnishes only about 1.5 mcg/day (Casey and Neville, 1987).

"Little is known about the chemical form or nutritional bioavailability of molybdenum in foods," the publication said. "Most public water supplies would be expected to contribute between 2 and 8 mcg/day of the mineral (NRC, 1980), which would constitute 10 percent or less of the lower limit of the provisional recommended intake."[15]

There is no Recommended Dietary Allowance for the mineral, but the recommended range is between 75 and 250 mcg/day for adults and older children.[15]

REFERENCES

1. Allaway, W. H. "Agronomic Controls Over the Environmental Cycling of Trace Minerals," *Advances in Agronomy* 20:235–273, 1968.

2. Passwater, Richard A., Ph.D., and Cranton, Elmer M., M.D. *Trace Elements, Hair Analysis and Nutrition.* New Canaan, Conn.: Keats Publishing, Inc., p. 209ff, 1983.

3. Ensminger, Audrey H., et al. *Foods and Nutrition Encyclopedia.* Clovis, Calif.: Pegus Press, 1983, pp. 1572–1573.

4. Wadman, S. K., et al. "Absence of Hepatic Molybdenum Cofactor: An Inborn Error of Metabolism Leading to a Combined Deficiency of Sulphite Oxidase and Xanthine Dehydrogenase," *Journal of Inherited Metabolic Disease* 6:78–83/Suppl. 1, 1983.

5. Hendler, Sheldon Saul, M.D., Ph.D. *The Complete Guide to Anti-Aging Nutrients.* New York: Simon and Schuster, 1985, p. 172ff.

6. Pfeiffer, Carl C., Ph.D., M.D. *Nutrition and Mental Illness.* Rochester, Vermont: Healing Arts Press, 1987, p. 104ff.

7. Rajagopalan, K. V., Ph.D. "Molybdenum—An Essential Trace Element," *Nutrition Reviews* 45(11):321–328, November 1987.

8. "Molybdenum Deficiency in TPN," *Nutrition Reviews* 45(11):337–341, November 1987.

9. Alabaster, Oliver, M.D. *What You Can Do to Prevent Cancer.* New York: Simon and Schuster, 1985, pp. 175–176.

10. Winick, Myron, M.D., et al. *The Columbia Encyclopedia of Nutrition.* New York: G. P. Putnam's Sons, 1988, p. 222.

11. Garrison, Jr., Robert H., M.A., R.Ph., and Somer, Elizabeth, M.A. *The Nutrition Desk Reference.* New Canaan, Conn.: Keats Publishing, Inc., 1985, p. 71.

12. Adams, Ruth, and Murray, Frank. *Minerals: Kill or Cure?* New York: Larchmont Books, 1977, p. 176ff.

13. Allaway, W. H., Ph.D., et al. "Selenium, Molybdenum and Vanadium," *Archives of Environmental Health* 16:342–348, March 1968.

14. Hendler, Sheldon Saul, M.D., Ph.D. *The Doctors' Vitamin and Mineral Encyclopedia.* New York: Simon and Schuster, 1990, p. 168ff.

15. *Recommended Dietary Allowances,* 10th Edition. Washington, D.C.: National Academy Press, 1989, p. 243ff.

32

Potassium Keeps a Healthy Heart

COMPRISING about five percent of the mineral content of the body, potassium is the third most abundant element in the body, after calcium and phosphorus. It is found in twice the concentration of sodium.

About 98 percent of the total body potassium is located intracellularly, where its concentration is 30 or more times that of the extracellular (between cells) fluid. Although the concentration of sodium in blood plasma is much higher than potassium, the potassium concentration in muscle tissue and milk is many times higher than sodium.

The history of potassium is closely intertwined with that of sodium. Materials containing both elements, especially carbonates and nitrates, were known to some of the earliest civilizations. Both compounds were used in Mesopotamia in the 17th century B.C. and in Egypt in the 16th century B.C. However, because of their primitive methods of analysis and identification, the ancient researchers who used them could not distinguish between the two.

"This problem was finally solved in 1807 by the brilliant young English chemist Sir Humphry Davy (1778-1829), who isolated the metal which he named potassium, and gave it the chemical symbol K, from Kalium, the Latinized version of the Arabic word for 'alkali,' " according to the *Foods and Nutrition Encyclopedia*. "However, more than 100 years elapsed following discovery before McCollum, in 1938—using the rat—obtained positive proof that potassium is an essential nutrient, although this had been suggested earlier."[1]

Over 90 percent of the potassium that is ingested is absorbed, mostly in the small intestine. Digestive juices contain rather large amounts of the mineral, most of which is reabsorbed. Only a small amount exits in the feces.

The kidneys are responsible for maintaining potassium homeostasis, and rather wide variations in intake are not reflected in fluctuations in plasma concentration, the encyclopedia continued. Aldosterone, an adrenal hormone, stimulates potassium excretion, as does alcohol, coffee and excess sugar. A buildup of abnormal amounts of potassium can be blamed on kidney failure or from a severe depletion of fluids.

SIGNS OF DEFICIENCY

A potassium deficiency, which is thought to be rare, can cause rapid and irregular heartbeats, and abnormal electrocardiograms; muscle weakness, irritability and occasional paralysis; as well as nausea, vomiting, diarrhea and swollen abdomen. Hypokalemia (decreased serum potassium) of dangerous degree may be caused by a prolonged wasting disease with tissue destruction and malnutrition; by prolonged gastrointestinal loss of potassium as in diarrhea, vomiting or gastric suction; or by continuous use of diuretic drugs (water pills). In rare cases the heart muscle may stop, the encyclopedia said.

A magnesium deficiency can contribute to a potassium deficiency, while abnormal levels of potassium inhibit the absorption of magnesium. Large amounts of potassium can slow the heart to a standstill if the kidneys are unable to excrete the surplus in the urine.

"Potassium is often prescribed [for] people with high blood pressure who are required to take diuretics to reduce excess water in the body because of the belief that diuretics deplete the body of potassium," the encyclopedia added.

"However, newer knowledge indicates that diuretics do not seriously deplete natural potassium levels of the great majority of patients taking these drugs for high blood pressure. Since high blood potassium concentration can cause cardiac arrest (a heart attack) and death, potassium supplements should be taken with caution and only on the advice of a physician."[1]

The fluid between the cells (interstitial fluid) always has high amounts of sodium and chloride, reported the February 1983 issue of *FDA Consumer*. The intracellular fluid—that inside the cell—always has high potassium and phosphate concentrations. However, some medical conditions can interfere with the excretion of sodium, causing excess amounts to accumulate in the body. Those undergoing treatment for hypertension (high blood pressure), heart disorders and kidney diseases have to limit their sodium intake, as well as control potassium intake, since depletion or excesses of the mineral may develop.

"Dietary deficiencies of potassium are rare but can occur among people suffering from malnutrition or living on starvation diets," *FDA Consumer* said. "Prolonged vomiting and diarrhea, severe burns or other injury, or surgery can lead to potassium losses. And individuals taking certain diuretics and purgatives can have potassium losses that require supplementation either by eating more foods high in potassium or taking dietary supplements."[2]

Since human needs vary so much, nutrition experts cannot say precisely how much sodium and potassium an individual should consume. The most reliable norms are the safe and adequate estimates suggested by the Food and Nutrition Board of the National Academy of Sciences. In its 1980 report, the board suggested a daily consumption of 1,100 to 3,300 mg for sodium and 1,875 to 5,625 mg for potassium. These estimates were cited for healthy adults, and consumption within these ranges is considered safe for most people.[2]

As shown in Table 32.1, potassium is readily available in the American diet. It is, therefore, generally easy to reach the recommended daily intake of the mineral.

Since potassium deficiencies can contribute to muscle weakness, and since the heart is a muscle, it is not uncommon for patients with heart failure to be deficient in the mineral. Writing in *Supernutrition for Healthy Hearts*, Richard Passwater, Ph.D., reported that Apollo 16 astronauts took extra amounts of potassium before lift-off and carried potassium-rich foods aboard to prevent the irregular heart rhythms that affected the Apollo 15 crew. He said that astronauts David Scott and James Irwin suffered from heart irregularities during the Apollo 15 mission. The irregularities were traced to a heavy work schedule, along with the stress of weightlessness, which usually increases potassium excretion.[3]

"Because magnesium is involved in the retention of potassium in the cells, a deficiency of magnesium results in a deficiency of potassium, which may be even worse than magnesium deficiency in terms of resulting heart damage," Passwater added. "Stress, alcohol, nicotine, caffeine and an excess of salt all tend to reduce the body's store of potassium. This deficiency produces an electrolyte imbalance directly responsible for arrhythmia, heart failure and cell death, as well as death to the individual."[3]

Sudden Onset

Passwater said that a potassium deficiency can develop rather suddenly. As an example, he reported on a study in which healthy volunteers were fed a highly refined diet. They developed potassium deficiencies and the accompanying muscular weakness and fatigue in less than a week. One of the reasons is that refined grains have been robbed of 75 percent of their potassium, he said.[3]

A correlation between potassium deficiency and heat exhaustion was noted during a prolonged heat wave in the Central Great Plains and the Mississippi Valley in 1966, reported J. I. Rodale and Staff in *The Complete Book of Minerals*

TABLE 32.1

POTASSIUM CONTENT OF EVERYDAY FOODS

Most of the items listed below are good sources of potassium. A few such as fats, oils, processed cheese, eggs and pizza are listed to show types of foods that tend to be low in potassium. The breads and rice are listed to show the difference between whole grain and refined grain and refined grain products.

	SERVING SIZE	MILLIGRAMS OF POTASSIUM
Beverages & Fruit Juices		
Grapefruit juice, frozen	1 cup	420
Orange juice, frozen	1 cup	503
Tangerine juice, frozen	1 cup	432
Tomato juice, low sodium	1 cup	549
Prune juice	1 cup	602
Dairy Products		
American pasteurized processed cheese	1 oz.	23
Milk, whole	1 cup	351
skim	1 cup	355
Eggs, Fish, Meat & Poultry		
Egg, whole	1 large	65
Tuna, chunk style, in water	3 oz.	237
Chicken, lt. meat without skin	3 oz.	369
Ground beef, lean, cooked	3 oz.	221
Pork loin, lean, cooked	3 oz.	280
Sirloin steak, lean, cooked	3 oz.	307
Fast Foods		
Pizza, frozen, cheese	1/7 of 10" pie	65
Fruits		
Apricots, fresh	3	301
dried	10 med. halves	343
Avocado	1/2	680
Banana	1 med.	440
Cantaloupe	1/2 melon	682
Dates, with pits	10	518

	SERVING SIZE	MILLIGRAMS OF POTASSIUM
Prunes	10 med.	448
Raisins, dark, not packed	2 Tbsp.	138
Raisins, packed	½ cup	553
Watermelon, diced	1 cup	160

Grain Products

Bread, white	1 slice	29
whole wheat	1 slice	68
Oatmeal, cooked	1 cup	146
Rice, brown, cooked	½ cup	69
Rice, white, cooked	½ cup	29
Spaghetti, cooked	1 cup	103
Wheat germ	1 Tbsp.	57

Legumes & Vegetables

Broccoli, cooked	½ cup	207
Brussels sprouts, cooked	½ cup	212
Cauliflower, cooked	½ cup	129
Lentils, cooked	½ cup	249
Mushrooms, raw	½ cup	145
Peanuts, roasted, with skins, jumbo, in shell	10	127
Potato, boiled in skin	1 med.	556
Spinach, cooked	½ cup	292
Sweet potato, baked	1 large	342
Winter squash, baked	½ cup	473

Fats, Oils & Sweets

Butter	1 Tbsp.	3
Margarine	1 Tbsp.	3
Molasses, light	1 Tbsp.	183
Oil	1 Tbsp.	0

From *FDA Consumer*, February 1983; USDA Handbook No. 456.

for Health. During this period, over 150 deaths were attributed to "heat prostration" or "heat exhaustion." However, an examination of hospital records showed that many of the victims had low serum potassium levels.[4]

"In every case," the publication said, "perspiration had been excessive in the days before collapse. Many who had cardiovascular disease were taking thiazide or digitalis or both. Thiazide is known to encourage potassium losses, and coupled with excessive perspiration and a lowered potassium intake due to lack of appetite in the heat, set the stage for severe potassium deficits. Observers believe that this potassium deficit could have contributed heavily to the heat-stress disease that killed these people."[4]

Researchers have reported that heart failure cases and increased incidence of heart trouble among young people have been found in high-temperature areas. Then there were the two pilots in Vietnam who were able to maintain high performance levels over long periods in spite of the heat. The explanation was that both men ate considerable amounts of ketchup at almost every meal, and tomato ketchup contains large amounts of potassium.[4]

A one-year study of 28 men and women found that they ate too much table salt (sodium chloride) and not enough potassium, reported Lloyd McLaughlin in the December 19, 1984 issue of USDA News. This prompted James C. Smith, Jr., a chemist with the USDA's Agricultural Research Service, to suggest that an adult may risk developing high blood pressure if the sodium-potassium ratio stays askew.

Smith, who is with the Beltsville, Maryland facility, added: "Our study showed that the ratio of sodium to potassium was double what it should be for adults." The sodium-potassium ratio should be about six-tenths gram of sodium for every gram of potassium. Adults in the USDA study consumed 1.3 g/day of sodium for each gram of potassium. A teaspoon of table salt contains about 2½ grams of sodium.[5]

Athletes who don't sweat don't need extra potassium, but those who do and take salt tablets need double doses, according to Ioannis S. Scarpa, Ph.D., et al. in Sourcebook on Food and Nutrition. They quoted James Knochel, M.D., a professor at the University of Texas Southwestern Medical School, as saying that he had found 50 percent of those hospitalized with heat stroke after intense exercise were potassium depleted. He said that many of the athletes had taken salt tablets, which forced potassium out of the body.

"Add that to the potassium they were already losing through sweating and the bottom line was a severe potassium deficiency and all its symptoms—nausea, muscle weakness, cramps, irritability and, finally, total collapse," the authors said.[6]

ONE SERVING PER DAY AGAINST STROKE

A high intake of dietary potassium protects people against stroke and stroke-related deaths, with the possibility that as little as one extra serving of a potassium-rich food like fruit or vegetables per day may reduce the risk of death by stroke by up to 40 percent, reported Nathan Horwitz in the August 17, 1989 issue of *Medical Tribune*.

The study, headed by Kay-Tee Khaw, B.Chir., professor of clinical gerontology at Cambridge University in England, involved 589 men and women, aged 50 to 79, living in the upscale community of Rancho Bernardo, California.

"The protective relationship offered by dietary potassium intake is consistent for both men and women, and it is independent of dietary fiber and other cardiovascular factors," Khaw said.

The study was designed to last for 16 years, but the statistics were tabulated at the 12-year point. Nutrient data showed that 24-hour potassium intake ranged from 17 mmol (664.7 mg) to 152 mmol, with a mean of 64 mmol (2,502.5 mg).[7]

Writing in *Circulation* in 1988, Khaw and Elizabeth Barrett-Connor, M.D., said that their data support the supposition that sodium and potassium intakes and their ratio are correlated with a risk for developing high blood pressure. Their findings were independent of other dietary factors, such as fiber, calories, protein, carbohydrate, alcohol, calcium and dietary fat.[8]

Researchers at Erasmus University in Rotterdam, the Netherlands, reported that in the initial management of mild to moderate hypertension, prescribing a mineral salt that is low in sodium and high in magnesium and potassium may result in better patient compliance than restricting salt intake or giving a pure potassium chloride salt substitute, reported Dan Hurley in the September 8, 1994 issue of *Medical Tribune*. The salt in question is extracted from natural sources in Iceland and contains 41 percent sodium chloride, 41 percent potassium chloride, 17 percent magnesium salts and 1 percent of other trace minerals. The product, SagaSalt, is apparently not yet available in the United States. There are salt substitutes in the U.S. which contain potassium instead of sodium, but none are thought to contain magnesium.

In the 24-week randomized trial using 100 volunteers, blood pressure fell by 8 mmHg systolic and 3 mmHg diastolic more in patients given the mineral salt compared to those using table salt.

"The diet in the trial remained largely unchanged, and the alternative salt and foods were palatable and well accepted by the participants," the researchers said. "This provides a practical and more convenient dietary intervention than trying to get patients to restrict salt intake."

When the study began, the average blood-pressure readings were 158–91 mmHg and 158/90 mmHg in the control and mineral groups, respectively. Following 24 weeks, those using the mineral supplement had a reading of 151/87 mmHg, contrasted with 156/91 mmHg in the controls. After taking the mean of the readings at eight, 16 and 24 weeks, the researchers determined that blood pressure had dropped by an average of 8/3 mmHg more in the mineral-salt group.[9]

Writing in *Magnesium Research* in 1988, Prof. A. S. Abraham of the Shaare Zedek Medical Center in Jerusalem, Israel, reported that ischemic heart disease and congestive heart failure patients should be given potassium- and magnesium-sparing drugs. He said that patients treated with magnesium intravenously for the first 24 hours after admission to a hospital have a much lower incidence of fatal tachyarrhythmias and low in-hospital mortality. Measuring serum levels of magnesium and potassium did not have any significance in predicting life-threatening arrhythmias, he said, size of infarct or mortality, but measuring lymphocyte potassium and magnesium levels has shown that treating patients with magnesium following an acute myocardial infarction dramatically reduces the incidence of arrhythmias almost to zero and in-hospital deaths to 4.1 percent.[10]

Philip J. Podrid, M.D., of University Hospital in Boston, stated in the March 6, 1990 issue of *The American Journal of Cardiology* that, since potassium is such an important electrolyte in the physiologic mechanisms of the myocardial membrane, it plays an important role in the development of arrhythmias. Hypokalemia may reduce the effectiveness of antiarrhythmic drugs, and diuretic use is the most frequent cause of hypokalemia, he said. Epinephrine can also lower serum potassium levels, and this may be the mechanism by which beta blockers prevent sudden death in patients with a recent myocardial infarction, he added.[11]

When 37 volunteers with mild hypertension were given either a placebo, potassium (60 mmol/day) alone or in conjunction with magnesium (20 mmol/day) for 32 weeks, the potassium alone or in combination with magnesium showed a significant reduction in systolic and diastolic pressure as well as a considerable reduction in serum cholesterol, according to P. S. Patki, et al., of Byramjee Jeejeebhoy Medical College and Sassoon General Hospitals in Pune, India, in the September 15, 1990 issue of the *British Medical Journal*. Magnesium did not exhibit any additional benefits. The patients tolerated the therapy well.[12]

Another study showing that a diet low in sodium and high in potassium, calcium and magnesium prevents the development of high blood pressure was reported by Jiang He, et al., in the March 1991 issue of *Hypertension*. Although the volunteers were in various parts of China, the research team was from the

Bowman Gray School of Medicine in Winston-Salem, North Carolina.[13] Birger Jansson, Ph.D., of the University of Texas, M. D. Anderson Cancer Center in Houston, reported in *Cancer Detection and Prevention* in 1990 that, since Paleolithic times, the potassium-sodium ratio in the diet has been reduced by a factor of about 20. Primitive cultures today reveal potassium-sodium ratios 100 to 200 times as great as ours, he said. He suggests that the lack of evolutionary adaptation to our present day high-sodium diet has led to many of the diseases of civilized societies, such as cancer and cardiovascular disease.[14]

Jansson continued that the decreased potassium-sodium ratio as a risk factor for cancer has been confirmed by a variety of different methodological studies. He is convinced that the dietary potassium-sodium ratio should be at least one and probably greater than five, whereas the intracellular ratio should be at least considerably more. This would bring a significant reduction in cardiovascular disease and cancer incidence. He added that five percent of our sodium comes from food naturally; 45 percent from industrial processing; 45 percent from food preparation and the remaining five percent as a condiment added at the table. But steaming as a method of cooking and consumption of fruits and vegetables significantly increases the potassium-sodium ratio.[14]

With so many foods high in potassium, no one should be deficient in this important mineral.

REFERENCES

1. Ensminger, Audrey H., et al. *Foods and Nutrition Encyclopedia.* Clovis, Calif.: Pegus Press, 1983, pp. 1812–1813.
2. Lecos, Chris. "Potassium: Keeping a Delicate Balance." Reprint from *FDA Consumer*, February 1983.
3. Passwater, Richard, Ph.D. *Supernutrition for Healthy Hearts.* New York: The Dial Press, 1977, p. 140ff.
4. Rodale, J. I., and Staff. *The Complete Book of Minerals for Health.* Emmaus, Pa.: Rodale Books, Inc., 1972, p. 135ff.
5. McLaughlin, Lloyd. "USDA Finds Salt and Potassium Intake Askew in Adult Diets," *USDA News*, December 19, 1984.
6. Scarpa, Ioannis S., Ph.D., et al. "Potassium," *Sourcebook on Food and Nutrition.* Chicago: Marquis Academic Media, 1982, pp. 104–105.
7. Horwitz, Nathan. "Dietary Potassium Is Said to Protect Against Stroke," *Medical Tribune*, August 17, 1989, p. 6.

8. Khaw, K., and Barrett-Connor, E. "The Association Between Blood Pressure, Age and Dietary Sodium and Potassium: A Population Study," *Circulation* 77:53–61, 1988.
9. Hurley, Dan. "Low-Sodium, High-Potassium Salt Improves Compliance," *Medical Tribune*, September 8, 1994, p. 16.
10. Abraham, A. S. "Potassium-Magnesium Status in Ischemic Heart Disease," *Magnesium Research* 1(1):53–57, 1988.
11. Podrid, Philip J., M.D. "Potassium and Ventricular Arrhythmias," *The American Journal of Cardiology* 65:33E-44E, March 6, 1990.
12. Patki, P. S., et al. "Efficiency of Potassium and Magnesium in Essential Hypertension in a Double-Blind, Placebo-Controlled Crossover Study," *British Medical Journal* 301:521–523, September 15, 1990.
13. He, Jiang, et al. "Relationship of Electrolytes to Blood Pressure in Men: The Yi Peoples Study," *Hypertension* 17(3):378–385, March 1991.
14. Jansson, Birger, Ph.D. "Dietary, Total Body and Intracellular Potassium-to-Sodium Ratios and Their Influence on Cancer," *Cancer Detection and Prevention* 14(5):563–565, 1990.

33

Silicon/Silica Builds Strong Bones, Hair and Nails

ALTHOUGH there is no Recommended Dietary Allowance for silicon, there is a suggestion that a silicon deficiency may be related to hardening of the arteries and heart disease, since large amounts of bound silicon are found in the arterial wall, especially the intima or inner wall. It may impact on osteoporosis and the health of bones and cartilage; it is thought to strengthen hair, nails and skin; it enhances cell regeneration; and it may rid the body of excessive aluminum. Although silicon is the second most abundant element in nature (after oxygen), we may not be getting enough of the mineral from our diet because of the refining of foods.

As a free form, silicon is not found in nature. But it occurs as oxide silica in sand and quartz; as silicates in such minerals as granite; and in foods and algae as vegetal silica and other forms. Organ meats and whole grains are primary food sources.

Silicon should not be confused with silica (silicon dioxide), which is the most abundant silicon compound. Silica is also found in foods, and it is used as silicea as a homeopathic remedy. Vegetal silica is extracted from the herb horsetail and used as a supplement.

Silicone (pronounced the same as silicon) is a plastic based on silicon that has various applications in industry, dentistry, ophthalmology, etc. Silicone has been in the news because breast implants made from this substance have reportedly caused serious health problems in some women.

Silicon was discovered in 1823 by the Swedish chemist Jons Berzelius. Its name is derived from the Latin word *silex* or *silicis*, meaning flint or hard.[1]

Silica supplements are often water-soluble extracts of horsetail, while silica gel is derived from quartz crystals, that is, a solution of minute, nondiffusable particles suspended in water. Another silica supplement is derived from purified algae.

At a meeting of the American Chemical Society in Washington, D.C., in June 1990, J. Derek Birchall of Cheshire, England, said that studies show a link between the aluminum content of drinking water and the development of Alzheimer's disease. Although some of these studies have been criticized, other investigators have reported a relationship between the silicon content of water and its limiting of the absorption of the aluminum in food. High silicon waters appear to be low in aluminum and vice versa, he said.[2]

Birchall discussed a study that he and his colleagues published in Nature, in which Atlantic salmon were placed in acidic water containing toxic levels of aluminum. When there was little silicon (as silicia acid) in the water, there was obvious damage to fish gills and 50 percent of the fish were dead within 26 hours; all were dead within 48 hours. With high levels of silicon in the water, gills remained normal and all of the fish survived.

It seems likely that silicon reduces the bioavailability of aluminum, an element which, when it gains entry, is hostile to biology, Birchall said. The balance of the two elements may be vitally important, he added.

"Recent research suggests that silicon may have no direct biological role but that it acts to limit the biological availability of aluminum," Birchall continued. "Aluminum, the third most abundant element in the Earth's crust, was considered innocuous until the 1970s, when it was determined that the mineral can cause bone disorders (oseomalacia) and dementia (encephalopathy) observed in patients on long-term dialysis in renal failure when the dialysis water contained aluminum."[2]

Elaborating on the 1989 article in Nature, Science News for September 15, 1990, said that Birchall found that, even when present in low levels, silicon- and aluminum-based oxides and hydroxides eagerly combine in a solution to form aluminosilicates, which are also commonly found in soil minerals. He theorizes that this coupling effectively imprisons—and thus detoxifies—the aluminum.

"Birchall now suggests a possible connection between Alzheimer's disease and silicon levels in the body," Science News said. "Scientists have detected abnormally high concentrations of aluminum in the autopsied brains of Alzheimer's patients, but no one knows whether the metal is a cause or effect of the disease. To help resolve this ambiguity, Birchall proposes comparing the amounts of silicon and aluminum ingested by Alzheimer's patients."[3]

Walter Mertz, M.D., director of the U.S. Department of Agriculture's Human Nutrition Research Center in Beltsville, Maryland, is especially interested in studying the consequences of chronic marginal intakes of silicon, zinc, copper and chromium, according to *The Complete Book of Vitamins and Minerals for Health*. He maintains that silicon, zinc and copper are important in maintaining bone tissue, and he wonders whether or not patients with osteoporosis may be deficient in these elements.

"We must get away from focusing just on calcium while we ignore other nutrients involved in osteoporosis," Mertz said. "This condition may be the result of multiple deficiencies and requires a total nutritional approach."[4]

In laboratory studies, Edith M. Carlisle, Ph.D., of the School of Public Health, University of California at Los Angeles, has also determined that silicon plays an important role in connective tissue, notably in bone and cartilage, she reported in the July 1982 issue of *Nutrition Reviews*. Both abnormalities of bone and cartilage have shown up in silicon-deficient animals, she said.

"Additional support for silicon's proposed metabolic role in connective tissue is provided by the demonstration of its presence in ostenogenic [bone forming] cells," she added. "Furthermore, a hitherto unknown relationship between silicon and another element, molybdenum, recently has been demonstrated. It is evident that connective tissue metabolism cannot be completely understood without taking silicon's role into consideration."[5]

AGE AFFECTS AMOUNT

Although deficiencies of silicon have not been produced in man, it has been found that silicon content of the aorta, skin and thymus decrease significantly with age, according to *Foods and Nutrition Encyclopedia*. This is apparently related to the fact that the mucopolysaccharide (the substance that binds with water to form the thick gelatinous material which cements cells together and lubricates joints and bursas) content of body tissues also declines with aging.[6]

Klaus Schwarz, M.D., of the School of Medicine at the University of California at Los Angeles, wrote in the February 26, 1977 issue of *Lancet* that in blood vessels that contain harmful deposits, which could lead to hardening of the arteries, there is much less silicon than in healthier blood vessels.[7]

To illustrate how silicon is refined out of foods, he reported that one batch of wheat bran contained only 229 parts per million (ppm) of silicon; another, 348 ppm; another, 1,720 ppm. A batch of soybean meal contained only 1,680 ppm of silicon, while the alfalfa that was studied contained 12,740 ppm.[7]

In *Wellness Medicine*, Robert A. Anderson, M.D., reported that the walls of atherosclerotic arteries contain very little silicon, compared to the walls of normal blood vessels. Two regions of Finland have been compared for the incidence of coronary heart disease, he said. In the region demonstrating a very high incidence of coronary atherosclerosis, the drinking water was found to contain low amounts of silicon compared to another area with much lower incidence of heart disease and high amounts of silicon in the drinking water. The diets of both groups were similar.[8]

In his book, *Prescription for Nutritional Healing*, James F. Balch, M.D., said that, in addition to maintaining healthy hair, skin and nails, and for calcium absorption in the early stages of bone formation, silica/silicon is needed to maintain flexible arteries. Since silicon levels decrease with aging, larger amounts are needed by the elderly, he said.[9]

Writing in *Silica: The Amazing Gel*, Klaus Kaufmann reviewed a number of case histories in which the gel is used for a variety of complaints. Although the cases are anecdotal, they illustrate the versatility of this substance.

For example, a 36-year-old female complained of frequent sprains, back pain, brittle nails and thinning hair. She also had varicose veins and was subject to frequent respiratory infections. Her therapist recommended two tablespoons of silica daily for three months. As is typical with natural substances, which do not work overnight like drugs, there was no noticeable change during the first few weeks. However, after six weeks, the patient experienced sturdier nails and healthier hair. Back pain and varicose veins subsided and there were no further complaints about sprains. Her therapist termed her prognosis "good."

A similar amount of silica gel was recommended for a 27-year-old female with chronic digestive and abdominal complaints, varicose veins, loss of hair and abnormal strain, especially following extended physical exertion. After four weeks of therapy, the patient had less hair loss and digestive upsets. These complaints improved to the extent that her health problems were considerably alleviated, Kaufmann reported.

A 60-year-old male complaining of stomach ulcers and chronic hyperacidity declined to have a surgical procedure recommended by his physician. Instead, he was given one tablespoon of silica gel two times daily for two and a half months. A noticeable improvement was noted by the patient after the first week of therapy. His symptoms continued to abate and an X-ray later revealed a complete healing of the ulcers.

A 56-year-old female suffered from chronic, bleeding gums and gingivitis. Three times daily she rinsed her mouth with one tablespoon of silica gel diluted with three parts of water. During the two months of therapy, she also massaged her gums morning and night with one tablespoon of undiluted silica gel, as well as ingesting one tablespoon of the gel twice daily. The bleeding stopped after two weeks and at the conclusion of the therapy there was no further bleeding or inflammation and the gums remained firm.

Another patient, a 53-year-old female, suffered from drooping skin and protruding veins as a result of premature aging. Her therapy consisted of one tablespoon of silica gel daily, plus a 15-minute facial mask consisting of one tablespoon of silica gel diluted with three parts of water for 10 weeks. After two weeks, the skin appeared fresher and blood circulation increased so that, after 10 weeks, good results were achieved, Kaufmann said.[10]

Silicone and Teflon jaw implants used to treat temporomandibular joints (TMJ) may cause significant pain and aggravate bone loss, according to Laura Buterbaugh in the June 25, 1992 issue of *Medical Tribune*. A popular Teflon implant was recalled by the FDA in 1988. An estimated 50,000 to 100,000 people are thought to have TMJ implants, but, even after the implants are removed, pain and bone loss may continue, the publication reported. A spokesperson for Dow Corning Corp. said that silicone implants were not designed to stay in the jaw for more than two months.[11]

Silicon is necessary for collagen and glycosaminoglycan formation, and it is a major ion of osteogenic (formation of bone) cells, reported A. A. Moukarzel, et al., of the UCLA Medical Center, in the October 1992 issue of the *Journal of the American College of Nutrition*. Their study was designed to evaluate serum silicon levels in healthy controls and in children receiving total parenteral (through a tube) nutrition in relation to the degree of osteopenia (decreased calcification or density of bone). They found that the mean serum silicon level was lower in those on parenteral nutrition when compared to the control. They added that there was contamination of silicon from the glucose-amino acid solution as well as the fat emulsion. The children were getting between 0.6 and 1.2 mg of parenteral silicon, but in 15 of the patients, the trabecular bone density was 77.5 percent of the controls. The researchers concluded that children receiving total parenteral nutrition and who have lower silicon levels may be at risk for decreased bone mineral content.[12]

The controversy over silicone breast implants is still in the news. Some women want to have the breast reconstructions, especially following a mastectomy.

References

1. Ensminger, Audrey H., et al. *Foods and Nutrition Encyclopedia*. Clovis, Calif.: Pegus Press, 1983, p. 1994.

2. Birchall, Derek. "The Biological Role of Silicon." Paper read at a meeting of the American Chemical Society, Washington, D.C., August 29, 1990.
3. "Hints of a Biological Role for Silicon," *Science News*, September 15, 1990, p. 74.
4. "Minerals for Young Bones," *Complete Book of Vitamins and Minerals for Health*. Emmaus, Pa.: Rodale Press, 1988, p. 49.
5. Carlisle, Edith M., Ph.D. "The Nutritional Essentiality of Silicon," *Nutrition Reviews* 40(7):193–197, July 1982.
6. Ensminger, Audrey H., et al. Ibid.
7. Schwarz, Klaus. "Silicon, Fibre and Atherosclerosis," *Lancet* 1(8009):454–457, February 26, 1977.
8. Anderson, Robert A., M.D. *Wellness Medicine*. New Canaan, Conn.: Keats Publishing, Inc., 1987, p. 216.
9. Balch, James F., M.D., and Balch, Phyllis A., C.N.C. *Prescription for Nutritional Healing*. Garden City Park, N.Y.: Avery Publishing Group, Inc., 1990, p. 22.
10. Kaufmann, Klaus. *Silica: The Amazing Gel*. Burnaby, B.C., Canada: Alive Books, 1992, pp. 96ff.
11. Buterbaugh, Laura. "Jaw Implants May Cause Bone Breakdown," *Medical Tribune*, June 25, 1992, p. 5.
12. Moukarzel, A. A., et al. "Silicon Deficiency May Be Involved in Bone Disease of Parenteral Nutrition," *Journal of the American College of Nutrition* 11(5):601/Abstract 5, October 1992.
13. Perrone, Janice. "Registry Established for Breast Implant Patients," *AMA News*, February 10, 1992.

34

Sodium and Chloride: Just a Pinch Will Do

THROUGHOUT most of history, salt (sodium chloride) has been in short supply. In ancient Abyssinia, slabs of rock salt were used as currency. Caravans carried salt large distances, sometimes trading it for gold, measure for measure, reported *ABC's of the Human Body*. So precious was salt that Roman soldiers were paid partly with salt, from which we get the word *salary*. If salt were accidentally spilled during the Middle Ages, it was a sign of impending doom.

"The Dead Sea is so saturated with salt that encrusted 'pillars' form above it, a product of evaporation. Before refrigeration, salting was one of the few ways to preserve food. In biblical times, it became a symbol of the covenant between God and the Jews. When Lot's wife broke God's commandment not to look back at Sodom, she was punished by being turned into a pillar of salt."[1]

Sodium is the most abundant cation (a positively charged ion) in the extracellular fluid of the body, according to Helen S. Mitchell, Ph.D., Sc.D., et al. in *Nutrition in Health and Disease*. It combines with other electrolytes, such as potassium, in the intracellular fluid, to regulate the osmotic pressure and to maintain proper water balance within the body. Sodium is a major player in maintaining acid-base equilibrium, in transmitting nerve impulses and in relaxing muscle. Sodium is also required for glucose absorption and for the transport of other nutrients across cell membranes.

"Most sodium consumed is excreted by the kidneys, with variable amounts lost through the skin and stools. In the normal individual, sodium is almost completely absorbed from the gastrointestinal tract but substantial losses may occur with vomiting and diarrhea. Sodium homeostasis (balance) is under the control of the hormone aldosterone secreted by the adrenal gland. When the need for sodium increases, increased amounts of aldosterone are secreted which increases the resorption of sodium ions by the kidney tubules (small tubes)."[2]

Chloride is the anion (an ion that carries a negative charge) most commonly combined with sodium in the extracellular fluid and, to some extent, it is also a companion of potassium in the cells. However, chlorine can pass freely between these two fluids through the cell membranes. The chlorides are among the electrolytes that assist osmotic pressure and acid-base equilibrium in the body. As digestion takes place, some of the chloride of the blood is used to form hydrochloric acid in the gastric glands. Hydrochloric acid is secreted into the stomach where it combines with gastric enzymes and is eventually reabsorbed into the bloodstream along with other nutrients. About the only time the body becomes depleted of chloride is when gastric contents are purged during vomiting. Any excess chloride is removed by the kidneys and skin, mostly as sodium chloride.[2]

Sodium has long been considered a factor in reducing the risk of, and controlling, high blood pressure, stated Paula Kurtzweil in the September 1994 issue of *FDA Consumer*. This association was spelled out again in January 1993 in the fifth report of the Joint National Committee on Detection, Evaluation and Treatment of High Blood Pressure. The committee concurred that numerous studies have shown that reducing sodium intake can reduce blood pressure.[3]

HOW MUCH IS TOO MUCH?

Camille Brewer, a registered dietitian and nutritionist with the Food and Drug Administration's Office of Food Labeling, said that therapeutic sodium-restricted diets can range from below 1,000 to 3,000 mg/day.

"American adults, on average," Brewer said, "eat too much sodium—between 4 to 6 grams (4,000 to 6,000 mg/day). Most people would benefit from moderately reducing their sodium intakes."

Under the FDA's food labeling rules, the Daily Value for sodium is 2,400 mg. Daily Value is a new designation established by the FDA because it is consistent with recommendations and government experts, who encourage reduced sodium intakes.

Salt and other sodium compounds used in food processing are the largest contributors of sodium to most diets, Brewer said. One teaspoon of salt has about 2,000 mg of sodium. The sodium compounds are used for preserving, flavoring and stabilizing other ingredients, and they turn up with various sodium names on canned, frozen and other processed foods. Kosher beef, lamb and chicken have added salt, and sodium is found naturally in foods such as milk, cheese, meat, fish and some vegetables. For a definition of "salt free," "sodium free," etc., on the new food labels, refer to Table 34.1. Those with high blood pressure may also want similar definitions for calcium and potassium.[3]

It has long been established that a severe reduction in sodium intake will help lower the blood pressure of some individuals with hypertension, stated Louise Fenner in *Sourcebook on Food and Nutrition*. In 1920, one researcher reported successfully treating 20 patients with a low salt (sodium) diet, and many other reports have appeared in medical literature since then. Fenner added:

> A substantial amount of evidence suggesting a relationship between sodium and high blood pressure comes from studies of populations that have different levels of sodium in their diets. Several geographically diverse populations, varying in size from a few hundred to a few thousand persons, do not exhibit essential hypertension—hypertension that cannot be traced to an underlying disorder. A low sodium intake is often cited as a characteristic of these groups, who range from South Sea Islanders to Brazilian Indians to Alaskan Eskimos. In contrast, some populations with a lot of sodium in their diets, such as the northern Japanese, have a very high incidence of hypertension and death from stroke.[4]

Many factors other than sodium are cited as possible contributors to blood pressure patterns, including:

- Stress
- Age
- Body weight
- Genetic factors
- Chronic kidney infection and
- Potassium intake.

As we know, the proper sodium-potassium balance is very important for proper physiological function. Medical experts recognize high blood pressure as a complex disease, including race (blacks seem to be more susceptible than whites), obesity, variations in kidney and endocrine function, congenital kidney abnormalities and others, Fenner said.

"From 10 to 30 percent of all Americans are born with a genetic predisposition to hypertension," Fenner continued. "Evidence suggests that when this genetic factor is present, a diet high in sodium will increase the risk of hypertension. It is not widely accepted that sodium actually causes hypertension. Many experts

TABLE 34.1

NUTRIENT CLAIM GUIDE

SODIUM

Sodium-free: less than 5 milligrams (mg) per serving

Very low sodium: 35 mg or less per serving or, if the serving is 30 grams (g) or less or 2 tablespoons or less, 35 mg or less per 50 g of the food

Low-sodium: 140 mg or less per serving or, if the serving is 30 g or less or 2 tablespoons or less, 140 mg or less per 50 g of the food

Light in sodium: at least 50 percent less sodium per serving than average reference amount for same food with no sodium reduction

Lightly salted: at least 50 percent less sodium per serving than reference amount (If the food is not "low in sodium," the statement "not a low-sodium food" must appear on the same panel as the "Nutrition Facts" panel.)

Reduced or less sodium: at least 25 percent less per serving than reference food

SALT (SODIUM CHLORIDE)

Salt-free: sodium-free (see above definition)

Unsalted, without added salt, no salt added:
• no salt added during processing, and
• the food it resembles and for which it substitutes is normally processed with salt
  (If the food is not "sodium free," the statement "not a sodium-free food" or "not for control of sodium in the diet" must appear on the same panel as the Nutrition Facts panel.)

POTASSIUM

High-potassium: 700 mg or more per serving

Good source of potassium: 350 mg to 665 mg per serving

More or added potassium: at least 350 mg more per serving than reference food

CALCIUM

High-calcium: 200 mg or more per serving

Good source of calcium: 100 mg to 190 mg per serving

More or added calcium: at least 100 mg more per serving than reference food

From *FDA Consumer*, September 1994.

feel that if sodium consumption is high, the effects of other factors that are associated with high blood pressure might be intensified.

"Substantial amounts of sodium are regularly added to processed foods, but not just in the form of salt," Fenner said. Other common ingredients include sodium nitrite (a curing agent and preservative); sodium benzoate (a preservative); monosodium glutamate (MSG, a flavor enhancer); sodium bicarbonate (baking soda, a leavening agent); and sodium phosphate (a wetting agent for quick-cooking cereals).[4]

A 154-lb. male athlete who exercises vigorously for four hours on a hot and humid day can lose nearly two quarts of fluid from sweat each hour, according to Susan M. Kleiner, Ph.D., R.D., in the July 1993 issue of *The Physician and Sportsmedicine*. But water is not the only thing lost in sweat. In addition to water, he will lose electrolytes, which help to regulate fluid balance, nerve conduction and muscle contraction. While sodium, potassium, chloride and magnesium are some of the electrolytes that are lost, sodium is lost in the greatest amounts. Sodium and potassium balance can be disrupted by excessive sweating, she added, and this electrolyte imbalance can lead to muscle cramps.

Most Athletes Don't Need Added Sodium

The better trained an athlete you are, the better your body is able to get rid of excess heat and conserve sodium, Kleiner maintained. Becoming used to a hot, humid environment also enhances this ability. And eating a well-balanced diet that contains sufficient nutrients, such as sodium and water, will help to maintain fluid and electrolyte balance.

"If your workout lasts less than four hours, you don't need to replace sodium during exercise," Kleiner said. "If you are a well-trained athlete participating in a standard endurance marathon, for instance, you may be sweating up a storm, but you will reserve enough sodium to complete the competition. Your post-event meal should contain some sodium to replace what you may have lost."

If you are participating in events that last more than four hours, Kleiner continued, your sodium balance will be affected by the amount you sweat. This usually means that you will need to replace sodium during the event. In one study, for example, 10 to 20 percent of ultra-endurance runners and triathletes and one marathon runner competing in the heat were diagnosed with hyponatremia, which is a depletion of salt in the blood. Symptoms include drowsiness, muscle weakness and cramping, mental confusion and seizures.

To replace lost sodium, Kleiner recommends sports drinks, which contain 50 to 100 mg of sodium per cup. Sodium is added to these drinks to enhance water absorption, stimulate the drive to drink and to replace sodium lost during endurance events as well as for flavor. For reference, table salt is 60 percent chloride and 40 percent sodium.

"Drinking one-half to three-fourths of a cup of a sports drink every 10 to 20 minutes during the event is enough to replenish your fluid needs if you are an endurance athlete, and your sodium needs if you are an ultra-endurance athlete," Kleiner said. "But if you decrease your intensity during an event (if you stop running during a race and slow to a walk, for instance), decrease your fluid intake. Because you won't be perspiring as much, you won't need as much fluid or sodium replenishment."[5]

For a selected list of foods containing sodium (milligrams per 100 grams or one serving) see Table 34.2.

Reducing sodium chloride (salt) in the diet reduces the amount of calcium spilled in the urine, thus reducing the amount of calcium intake needed to maintain calcium balance, reported Ailsa Goulding in the *New Zealand Medical Journal*, March 28, 1990. Sodium competes with calcium for reabsorption in the renal tubules, and the more sodium that is excreted in the urine, the higher the loss of calcium in the urine. For every teaspoon of salt (100 mmol) urinary calcium increases about 1 mmol, Goulding added. And an uncompensated calcium loss of 1 mmol per day can dissolve one percent of the skeleton annually or 10 percent in a decade. Increasing salt intake can increase parathyroid hormone levels, which may cause an increase in blood pressure and result in bone resorption. Sodium is not a panacea for the curtailment of bone loss, but it is a simple, low-risk approach, Goulding added.[6]

Several experts have challenged the low-salt diets in relation to high blood pressure. For example, David A. McCarron, director of the hypertension program at Oregon Health Sciences University, warned that widespread restriction of sodium intake may actually end up harming more people than it helps, reported Philip M. Boffey in the September 14, 1982 issue of *The New York Times*.

"We've got an awful lot of information about sodium, a little about potassium and calcium, and not very much about anything else," McCarron said. "It's dangerous to tell people to change one nutrient (sodium) when we don't know what impact that will have on other nutrients. We're setting the stage for problems down the line."

McCarron admitted that his findings are controversial, but said that there is evidence that a deficiency in calcium may be a factor in high blood pressure. If people try to restrict their sodium intake by cutting back on dairy products,

TABLE 34.2

SODIUM CONTENT OF SELECTED FOODS

POPULAR FRUITS & VEGETABLES	SODIUM (MG PER 100 G)	OTHER FOODS	SODIUM (MG PER 100 G)
More than 50 mg of sodium per 100 g		Beef, ground	48
		Beef liver	136
Beet greens	130	Pork chops	60
Celery	126	Ham, cured	860
Dandelion greens	76	Bacon	1,077
Kale	75	Bacon, Canadian	2,555
Spinach	71	Sausage, link	958
Beets	60	Codfish	70
Watercress	52	Cheese, blue	1,396
		Cheese, brick	557
From 10 to 49 mg of sodium per 100 g	49	Cheese, cream	294
Turnips	49	Cheese, Parmesan	1,848
Carrots	47	Cheese, process	1,421
Artichokes	43	Milk, whole	50
Collards	43	Butter	224
Mustard greens	32	Eggs	122
Chinese cabbage	23	Olives, green	2,400
Cabbage	20	Peanuts	5
Radishes	18	Peanuts, salted	418
Broccoli	15	Soda crackers	1,100
Brussels sprouts	14	Ice cream	83
Garden cress	14	Sherbet	45
Cauliflower	13	Pickle, dill	4-5,000
Green pepper	13	Pretzels	7,800
Cantaloupe	12	Soy sauce (mild)	3,569
Honeydew melon	12	Soy sauce (regular)	6,082
Parsnips	12		
Onions (dry)	10		
Sweet potatoes	10		

From the Institute of Food Technologists, Chicago, January 1980; Watt and Merrill, 1963.

they will also be reducing their calcium intake and thus might actually drive their blood pressure up, McCarron said.

"I don't recommend sodium restriction as a broad public health measure," McCarron continued. "We could turn around 20 years from now and see that it had caused more problems than it prevented."[7]

John H. Laragh, director of the hypertension center at the Cornell University Medical Center in New York City, agreed that the government's efforts to reduce sodium intake were "misguided." His research has found that "calcium has a lot to do with blood pressure and may be more important than sodium—so don't go off the deep end and pick on sodium."[7]

"You can't get hysterical about salt and consider it a poison without considering all the marvelous things it does," Laragh added. "Salt is the number-one natural component of all human tissue. The concept that you don't need much is wrong."

He is convinced that only a minority of the public would benefit from sodium restriction, which, he said, might carry "harmful tradeoffs" for many people.[7]

Diet may determine the development of untoward side effects, according to Seymour L. Halpern, M.D., in *Quick Reference to Clinical Nutrition: A Guide for Physicians*. As an example, he said, sodium depletion enhances lithium toxicity. Therefore, a severe sodium-restricted diet should be prescribed with caution to a patient receiving lithium carbonate therapy for emotional disturbances. If a sodium-restricted diet is a medical necessity, lithium should be discontinued, he added.[8]

Writing in the *Journal of Urology* in June 1990, Richard W. Norman and Wanda A. Manette, of the Stone Clinic, Halifax Infirmary Hospital in Canada, reported that five patients with a history of recurrent kidney stones of cystine origin were placed on a sodium-restricted diet (2 g/day or less). They believe that sodium restriction and a high fluid intake should be prescribed as a therapeutic approach for patients with these stones. They also said that alkalizing the urine should be done with potassium citrate rather than sodium bicarbonate.[9]

ROLE IN CYSTIC FIBROSIS

Between 1989 and 1992, sodium chloride deficiency was observed in the first year of life in 12 of 46 cystic fibrosis patients, according to researchers at Hacettepe University, Faculty of Medicine, in Ankara, Turkey, and reported in the *European Journal of Pediatrics* in 1994. During an attack, the infants were sweating, they had lost their appetite, had a fever, were vomiting, they were also weak and dehydrated. Low urinary sodium and high urinary potassium were observed in four patients. The children were treated with intravenous fluids and electrolyte solutions.[10]

In the same journal, researchers at the Basque University School of Medicine, Bilbao, Spain, found that 13 children with cystic fibrosis had a chloride deficiency. The researchers said that serum electrolytes should be assessed regularly in children with this disorder.[11]

Joel Belmin, M.D., of Hopital Gerontologique in Sevran, France, said in the March 1992 issue of the *Journal of the American Geriatric Society* that a low-sodium diet, often prescribed early in congestive heart failure, is often poorly tolerated in the institutionalized elderly patients, resulting in appetite loss, weakness, low amounts of sodium in the blood or confusion. A reduction in food intake due to a low-sodium diet might worsen the nutritional status of the patient and increase the risk of cardiac cachexia, respiratory infection and decubitus ulcers. The researcher recommends a low sodium diet (0.8 to 1.6 g/day) in the end stages of chronic congestive heart failure, or for only a few days in acute congestive heart failure in order to control the symptoms.[12]

Researchers at the National Institute of Health and Nutrition in Tokyo reported in the *International Journal of Vitamin and Nutrition Research* in 1991 that excess dietary salt increases the loss of calcium in the urine and may be a risk factor in the development of osteoporosis and high blood pressure. The study involved both men and women 60 years of age or older who were healthy.[13]

Jadwiga M. Alexiewicz and colleagues at the University of Southern California Medical Center in Los Angeles, reported in the *American Journal of Hypertension* in 1992, that in salt-sensitive people, a high dietary sodium intake can increase blood pressure by 10 percent. They also reported that there is a link between abnormalities of sodium and calcium metabolism in salt-sensitive people with high blood pressure.[14]

The restriction of dietary salt to levels that are often prescribed for therapeutic purposes might affect both lipid and glucose metabolism, researchers at Medizinische Universitats-Poliklinik on Bonn, Germany, reported in *Klin Wochenschr* in 1991. They found that salt restriction increased serum total and low-density lipoprotein cholesterol (LDL, the harmful kinds) as well as increased serum insulin and uric acid levels.[15]

In a temperate climate, the healthy adult can maintain sodium balance with a very low intake of sodium (Kempner, 1948), according to *Recommended Dietary Allowances*, 10th Edition. Dole, et al. (1950) estimated obligatory urinary and fecal losses by adults to be 23 mg (1 mEq) per day. Loss from sweat normally averages a sodium concentration of 25 mEq/liter (Consolazio, et al. Sanchez-Castillo, et al., 1987) found that sweat and fecal excretion contributed only two to five percent of the sodium lost by British men and women. Obligatory dermal losses have been assumed to range from 46 to 92 mg (2 to 4 mEq) per day (Fregley, 1984). (1 mEq of sodium is 23 mg and 1 mmol of sodium chloride is 58.5 mg.) According to *Recommended Dietary Allowances*:

> Thus a minimum average requirement for adults can be estimated under conditions of maximal adaptation and without active sweating as no more than 5 mEq/day, which corresponds to 115 mg of sodium or about 300 mg of sodium chloride per day. In consideration of the wide variation of patterns of physical activity and climatic exposure, a safe minimum intake might be set at 500 mg/day. Such an intake is substantially exceeded by usual diets in the United States, even in the absence of added sodium chloride. Although no optimal range of salt intake has been established, there is no known advantage in consuming large amounts of sodium, and clear disadvantages for those susceptible to hypertension. From this and other considerations, a Food and Nutrition Board committee recently recommended that daily intakes of sodium chloride be limited to 6 g (2.4 g of sodium) or less (NRC, 1989).[16]

During pregnancy, there is an increased need for sodium because of the increased extracellular fluid volume in the mother, the requirement of the fetus and the level of sodium in the amniotic fluid, the publication added. This need is usually met in part by physiological responses to the renin-angiotensin-aldosterone systems (Pike and Smiciklas, 1972). Assuming a pregnancy weight gain of 11 kg (70 percent of which is extracellular water containing 150 mEq of sodium per liter), the average total sodium requirement for the duration of the pregnancy is 3 mEq (69 mg) per day in addition to the normal requirement. Since the average intake is considerably above that, the sodium requirement for pregnancy is met by usual salt intake.[16]

Breast-feeding increases sodium requirements considerably. Since human milk contains about 7.8 mEq of sodium (180 mg) per liter (AAP, 1985), and the average milk secretion when established is about 750 ml, lactation would add about 6 mEq (135 mg) per day to the usual adult requirement. But this increase is easily met by the usual dietary sodium intake.

The sodium requirement is obviously highest in infants and young children, since their extracellular fluid volume is rapidly increasing. Forbes (1952) calculated that from birth to three months of age, 0.5 mEq/kg (11.5 mg/kg) daily is needed for growth, or about 2 mEq (46 mg) per day for the reference infant. At six months of age, the daily requirement for growth is about 0.2 mEq (4.6 mg/kg).[16]

In addition to the sodium in foods, we often fail to realize that there is considerable sodium in over-the-counter and prescription drugs. These are typical sodium compounds found in drugs and medicines: sodium cloxacillin and sodium ampicillin (antibiotics); sodium pentobarbitol (sedative); sodium sulfo-succinate (laxative); sodium sulfacetamide (ophthalmic (eye) drug); sodium bicarbonate (antacid); sodium salicylate (pain reliever); sodium citrate (cough medicine); sodium saccharin (various medications).[17]

Here is the sodium content for a few nonprescription drugs (mg of sodium per dose):[18]

- Aspirin: 49
- Bromo-Seltzer (antacid): 717
- Alka-Seltzer (sodium citrate): 521
- Sal Hepatica (laxative), sodium bicarbonate, sodium citrate, etc.: 1,000
- Rolaids (antacid), dihydroxy aluminum and sodium carbonate: 53
- Brioschi (antacid), sodium bicarbonate, etc.: 710
- Fleet Enema (laxative), sodium biphosphate and sodium phosphate (absorbed): 250 to 300
- Miles Nervine (effervescent, sleep aid): 544.

For a complete list of sodium in foods and beverages, write for "The Sodium Content of Your Food," Home and Garden Bulletin No. 233, published by the U.S. Department of Agriculture.[19]

REFERENCES

1. Guinness, Alma E., editor. "The Paradox of Salt," *ABC's of the Human Body*. Pleasantville, N.Y.: The Reader's Digest Association, Inc., 1987, p. 243.
2. Mitchell, Helen S., Ph.D., Sc.D., et al. *Nutrition in Health and Disease*, 16th Edition. Philadelphia: J. B. Lippincott Co., 1968, pp. 57–58.
3. Kurtzweil, Paula. "Scouting for Sodium and Other Nutrients Important to Blood Pressure," *FDA Consumer*, September 1994, p. 18ff.
4. Fenner, Louise. "Salt Shakes Up Some of Us," *Sourcebook on Food and Nutrition*. Chicago: Marquis Academic Media, 1982, p. 128ff.

5. Kleiner, Susan M., Ph.D., R.D. "Workouts Worth Their Salt," *The Physician and Sportsmedicine* 21(7):25–26, July 1993.

6. Goulding, Ailsa. "Osteoporosis: Why Consuming Less Sodium Chloride Helps to Conserve Bone," *New Zealand Medical Journal*, March 28, 1990, pp. 120–122.

7. Boffey, Philip M. "Experts Challenge Low-Sodium Diet," *The New York Times*, September 14, 1982, pp. C1, C6.

8. Halpern, Seymour, L., M.D., editor. *Quick Reference to Clinical Nutrition: A Guide for Physicians.* Philadelphia: J. B. Lippincott Co., 1979, p. 106.

9. Norman, Richard W., and Manette, Wanda A. "Dietary Restriction of Sodium as a Means of Reducing Urinary Cystine," *Journal of Urology* 143: 1193–1194, June 1990.

10. Oxcelik, Ugur, et al. "Sodium Chloride Deficiency in Cystic Fibrosis Patients," *European Journal of Pediatrics* 153:829–831, 1994. ·

11. Sojo, A., et al. "Chloride Deficiency as a Presentation or Complication of Cystic Fibrosis," *European Journal of Pediatrics* 153:825–828, 1994.

12. Belmin, Joel, M.D. "Low Sodium Diet and Congestive Heart Failure in the Elderly," *Journal of the American Geriatric Society* 40(3):298–299, March 1992.

13. Itch, R., et al. "The Interrelation of Urinary Calcium and Sodium Intake in Healthy Elderly Japanese," *International Journal of Vitamin and Nutrition Research* 61:159–165, 1991.

14. Alexiewicz, Jadwiga M., et al. "Effect of Dietary Sodium Intake on Intracellular Calcium in Lymphocytes of Salt-Sensitive Hypertensive Patients," *American Journal of Hypertension* 5:536–541, 1992.

15. Ruppert, M., et al. "Short-Term Sodium Restriction Increases Serum Lipids and Insulin in Salt-Sensitive and Salt-Resistant Normotensive Adults," *Klin Wochenschr* 69:51–57, Supplement XXV, 1991.

16. *Recommended Dietary Allowances*, 10th Edition. Washington D.C.: National Academy Press, 1989, p. 250ff.

17. "Straight Talk About Salt," Salt Institute, Alexandria, Virginia, 1983.

18. Bennett, D. R. "Sodium and Potassium in Foods and Drugs," American Medical Association, 1979.

19. "The Sodium Content of Food," *Home and Garden Bulletin No. 233.* Washington, D.C.: U.S. Government Printing Office, 1980.

35

Sulfur: There's Plenty to Go Around

SULFUR, which is essential to life, is a nonmetallic element that occurs widely in nature. It is found in every cell of animals and plants, with one-fourth of one percent of the body consisting of sulfur. Approximately one-half of the total body sulfur is concentrated in the muscles, skin and bones. An estimated four to six percent of the body sulfur is in the hair. The blood contains 1.2 mg of inorganic sulfate per 100 milliliters.

According to *The Complete Book of Minerals for Health*, "Our chief concern with sulfur in human dietetics is the fact that proteins contain sulfur," the authors said. "Carbohydrates and fats do not. This means that proteins contain two substances—nitrogen and sulfur—whose waste products must be excreted by the kidneys rather than the lungs, as is the carbon dioxide produced when carbohydrates and fats are burned in the body furnace. Nitrogen and sulfur are closely related in foods, occurring in approximately the ratio of 16 parts of nitrogen to one part of sulfur."[1]

Nitrogen and sulfur are acid-forming, therefore, the waste products resulting after the body has used the two elements give an acid rather than an alkaline reaction in the urine. By contrast, calcium, sodium, potassium and magnesium have an alkaline reaction in the body.

One of the most important angles of metabolism (e.g., the process of burning and using food) is keeping a proper balance between acidity and alkalinity. Some experts conclude that the healthy body is equipped to maintain this balance and that, regardless of what you eat, the ratio between acid and alkaline will always be correct. Another view is that one must exercise a wise choice of food to help the body preserve this balance. The latter seems to be the prevailing view in that, although protein is rich in sulfur and nitrogen, and is essential to life since all body cells are made of it, one must eat the right amount of foods containing alkaline elements for good health.[1]

Sulfur, which is derived from the Latin word *sulphurum*, is sometimes referred to as nature's "beauty mineral," because it is reputed to keep the hair glossy and the complexion clear and youthful. Sulfur is also a necessary component of the sulfur-containing amino acids methionine, cystine and cysteine. It is present in keratin, the tough protein substance in the skin, nails and hair, and it is apparently necessary for the synthesis of collagen. As a component of biotin, the B vitamin, sulfur is important in fat metabolism, and as a constituent of thiamine (vitamin B1) and insulin, it is necessary for carbohydrate metabolism. As a component of coenzyme A, sulfur is important in energy metabolism, and as part of certain complex carbohydrates, it is important for various connective tissues. Insulin and glutathione, an amino acid, which are regulators of energy metabolism, also contain sulfur. Also, sulfur compounds link with toxic substances (phenols and cresols) and convert them to a nontoxic form so that they can be excreted in the urine.[2]

Since inorganic sulfur is poorly utilized by humans, the body's sulfur needs are largely met from organic complexes, notably the amino acids, rather than from inorganic sources. The average mixed diet contains about one-percent sulfur.[2]

As previously mentioned, sulfur is obtained primarily from foods containing methionine and cysteine, according to Eric R. Braverman, M.D., and Carl C. Pfeiffer, M.D., Ph.D., in *The Healing Nutrients Within*. The other two sulfur-amino acids, taurine and cystine, are synthesized from cysteine. If the diet contains enough methionine or cysteine, glutathione levels are likely to be adequate. The exception is in infants: Since their bodies cannot yet manufacture cysteine or taurine from methionine, their cysteine needs are supplied by breast milk. Cow's milk is not suitable in this instance.[3]

Abram Hoffer, M.D., Ph.D., said that one of the products manufactured by the body of the alcoholic, acetaldehyde, is more toxic than the alcohol itself. H. Sprince, M.D., of Thomas Jefferson University in Philadelphia, and colleagues, found that vitamin B1 and L-cysteine protected alcoholic rats against damage from acetaldehyde. The two substances together were more effective than either one taken by itself.[4]

Besides giving other related proteins rich in sulfur, the Pennsylvania scientists added vitamin C and found they got very good protection against alcohol's toxicity. L-cysteine, plus thiamine, plus vitamin C gave 100-percent protection against the toxicity which developed in other animals who were not thus protected. Sprince said that a combination of cysteine, vitamin B1, plus vitamin C, might be useful for protecting alcoholics and also smokers from the harmful effects of acetaldehyde.[4]

Carl C. Pfeiffer, M.D., Ph.D., pointed out that the only two foods which contain enough sulfur to darken a silver spoon are egg yolk and red-hot peppers. He added that vegetarians may become deficient in sulfur, especially if they don't eat eggs. And, he said, many adults may be deficient in sulfur because of the warnings not to eat too many eggs, because of their cholesterol. Two eggs a day raise blood cholesterol by only two percent, which is not sufficient to cause hardening of the arteries, Pfeiffer said. Onions and garlic also contain appreciable amounts of sulfur, he added.[4]

The Goodies in Garlic and Onions

"Our ancestors downed sulfur and molasses every spring for their tonic effect and Pfeiffer tells us that homeopathic physicians still give small amounts of sulfur for many ailments," Ruth Adams reported in Today's Living. "The evil-smelling water of many health spas smells that way because of its sulfur content. Pfeiffer also tells us that sulfur has been used, along with zinc, for treating psoriasis. Pfeiffer said that arthritics are notably apt to avoid eggs in their diets, and perhaps one reason for their condition may have something to do with lack of sulfur. He advises patients with rheumatoid arthritis to eat at least two eggs per day to provide adequate sulfur for their needs."[4]

Garlic is rich in sulfur compounds and may be important in several detoxification pathways, reported Judith G. Dausch, Ph.D., R.D., and Daniel W. Nixon, M.D., in Preventive Medicine in May 1990. They added that garlic has anti-tumor and cancer-inhibition properties. Other documented effects of garlic include antibiotic and anti-fungal activity, fibrinolysis and platelet-aggregation inhibition. And, they added, selenium and germanium, antioxidants in their own right, are constituents of Japanese garlic.[5]

Researchers have recently put a new spin on what killed off the dinosaurs and other creatures some 65 million years ago, reported the January 3, 1995 issue of The New York Times. The new hypothesis originates from geological studies of a buried crater in the Yucatan Peninsula of Mexico, a huge scar as much as 180 miles wide that is thought to be the site where a giant asteroid collided with Earth just before the time of the dinosaur extinctions. Geologists found the rock in the crater, named Chicxulub, to be especially rich in sulfur. If it had not been, the researchers said, the dinosaurs might well have survived the impact and changed the course of evolution.

"In a detailed analysis, geologists and atmospheric physicists determined that the asteroid, estimated to be six to 12 miles wide, would have vaporized much of the sulfur and spewed more than 100 billion tons of it into the air," the *Times* said. "This would have filled the air with sulfur dioxide in the lower altitudes, casting a pall reeking of the Devil's own brimstone, and also a sulfuric acid haze in the upper atmosphere, the result of interactions between solar ultraviolet radiation and sulfur dioxide."

The researchers said that the dust and soot from most of the debris would have drifted back to Earth within six months, presumably too short a time for any global darkness to have caused the mass extinctions. But in a report in *Earth and Planetary Science Letters*, scientists said that the lighter sulfur particles would have stayed aloft and created a dense haze covering the entire planet for at least a decade, perhaps 20 or 30 years, the *Times* reported.[6]

What was bad for the dinosaurs turned out to be good for us human beings, since sulfur is so essential to our lives.

REFERENCES

1. Rodale, J. I., and Staff. *The Complete Book of Minerals for Health*. Emmaus, Pa.: Rodale Books, Inc., 1972, p. 237ff.
2. Ensminger, Audrey H., et al. *Foods and Nutrition Encyclopedia*. Clovis, Calif.: Pegus Press, 1983, pp. 2071–2072.
3. Braverman, Eric R., M.D., and Pfeiffer, Carl C., M.D., Ph.D. *The Healing Nutrients Within*. New Canaan, Conn.: Keats Publishing, Inc., 1987, p. 111.
4. Adams, Ruth. "Diet-Supplements Protect Against Alcohol Toxicity," *Today's Living*, July 1977, pp. 14–15, 54.
5. Dausch, Judith G., Ph.D., R.D., and Nixon, Daniel W., M.D. "Garlic: A Review of Its Relationship to Malignant Disease," *Preventive Medicine* 19(3):346–361, May 1990.
6. Wilford, John Noble. "Dinosaur Theory: Sulfur Was Villain (But Hero for Humans)," *The New York Times*, January 3, 1995, p. B21.

36

Vanadium May Help You Lose Weight

PROBLEMS in carbohydrate metabolism play a large causative role in the American tendency to put on excess weight, reported Dallas Clouatre, Ph.D., in his book *Anti-Fat Nutrients*. Some of the discussion centers on an anti-fat nutrient, hydroxycitric acid (hydroxycitrate or HCA), which is extracted from the rind of the fruit, *Garcinia cambogia*, a plant that is native to South Asia, chromium and vanadium (vanadyl sulfate).

One of the primary substances involved in fat storage is the hormone insulin, therefore, it is reasonable to presume that foods and nutrients which make insulin more effective and which mimic insulin's actions in the body might aid in controlling appetite and weight gain, Clouatre said.

"An enormous amount of scientific attention is now being directed toward a number of micronutrients which appear to perform just these functions," he continued. "Among them are the trace minerals chromium and vanadium, the Ayurvedic herb *Gymnema sylvestra* and some cooking herbs and spices, including bay leaves, allspice, cinnamon, cloves and turmeric. The mechanisms by which these work vary."[1]

Interest in vanadium dates to 1985 when an article in *Science* indicated that the mineral controlled diabetes in laboratory animals, Clouatre said. This data created excitement because it showed that vanadium is effective when taken by mouth, whereas insulin must be injected to be effective, he added. Other studies confirmed these results and it is now known that vanadium plays a significant role not only in controlling blood sugar levels, but also, as is the case with chromium, prevents the development of excessive levels of low-density lipoprotein cholesterol (LDL, the so-called bad kind) and triglycerides. Other evidence shows that vanadium assists in the development of the bones and teeth, he said.[1]

"These impressive recent findings actually constitute a rediscovery of the uses of vanadium," Clouatre continued. "In France vanadium was already a medically recommended treatment for diabetes and some forms of fatigue in the late 19th century. In the English-speaking world, the 1932 edition of *Dorland's Medical Dictionary* listed vanadium as a treatment for diabetes and neurasthenia [nervous exhaustion]; with the addition of selenium, it was also suggested as a treatment for cancer. In the 1958 edition of *Dorland's*, hardening of the arteries was added to the illnesses for which vanadium was recommended. Vanadium, therefore, has a track record of usage with human beings, not just with laboratory animals."[1]

USEFUL FOR ATHLETES AND THE OBESE

Although not as successful as injected insulin for the treatment of extreme cases of diabetes, which is the reason it originally disappeared from medical usage, vanadium in the form of vanadyl sulfate (its biologically active form) can mimic many of the activities of insulin. Vanadyl sulfate is even more impressive than chromium in this instance, he said. Chromium potentiates the body's insulin, but the vanadyl form of vanadium is biologically active even in the absence of insulin. For example, it significantly increases liver glycogen (stored glucose) and improves the uptake of glucose by muscle tissues.

"These actions help to spare lean tissue during dieting and to improve athletic performance by lessening fatigue and by reducing the breakdown of muscle protein for energy," Clouatre added. "Vanadyl sulfate thus possesses anti-catabolic properties. It also acts to inhibit the storage of excess calories from carbohydrates as fat, apparently stabilizing the body's production of insulin. These properties are useful for controlling weight gain and for improving athletic performance."[1]

Although it is recognized that a deficiency of vanadium is detrimental to the health of both animals and humans, there is currently no Recommended Dietary Allowance for the mineral. The average diet provides about 2 mg/day, mostly from fats and vegetable oils. Absorption is only about five to 10 percent of the amount ingested; unused amounts are readily excreted.

"The recommended supplemental dosage of vanadyl sulfate is 1 to 2 mg/day, and more for special purposes," Clouatre said. "Some studies have used 22.5 mg of vanadyl sulfate per day for 16 months without toxic effects, but others report that this amount is actually in excess of what can be absorbed, and that no further benefits can be expected in dosages over 15 mg of vanadyl sulfate per day, with the exception of diabetics under medical supervision. In other words, there is no consensus on effective dosage levels. The vanadate forms of vanadium should not be taken as supplements. A new form of vanadium, bis(maltolato)oxo-vanadium(IV), has recently been developed, which is both more potent and even safer than is vanadyl sulfate."[1]

Vanadium is a possible essential trace element with significance in disease conditions as disparate as herpes and mania, reported Eric B. Braverman, M.D., and Carl C. Pfeiffer, M.D., Ph.D., in *The Healing Nutrients Within*. Glutathione, the amino acid, is essential for normal vanadium metabolism, maintaining the mineral in a reduced state and increasing its physiologic availability (Macara, et al., 1980), they said. In turn, vanadium may enhance the effects of glutathione under certain conditions.[2]

Vanadium was initially identified in 1931 by Sefstrom, a Swedish scientist, who named it after the Norse goddess of beauty Vanadis, because of the beautiful color of its compounds, reported *Foods and Nutrition Encyclopedia*. It was not obtained in pure form until 1927. In 1970, Dr. Klaus Schwarz indicated that the mineral is needed by higher animals. As an example, vanadium-deficient diets resulted in retarded growth, impaired reproduction, increased packed blood cell volume, and iron in the blood and bone of rats, as well as increased hematocrit in chicks.

William H. Strain, M.D., D.D.S., of the University of Rochester in New York, speaking at a symposium of the American Public Health Association in 1964, said that we might try lowering our cholesterol levels with gelatin, which has a rather high content of vanadium. In a test, giving 7 grams of gelatin before each meal lowered blood cholesterol, but he admitted that large-scale trials are needed to prove this point. However, he admitted that gelatin from Argentina contains up to 2 ppm of vanadium, whereas gelatin made from animal bones in the United States contains only 0.1 ppm.

"The low vanadium content of gelatin prepared from domestic bones is consistent with the high cholesterol level that is characteristic of civilization," Strain said. "The extensive use of calcium fertilizers without compensating addition of vanadium may inadvertently be the cause of this decrease in the dietary supply of vanadium throughout the food chain. Our analyses have shown that the vanadium content of hair ranges to 450 parts per billion (ppb). High blood cholesterol levels are associated with hair vanadium levels of 50 ppb or less."[4]

Vanadium has been found to be related to goiter incidence and tooth decay. Two German scientists reported that there are remarkable geographical differences in the vanadium content of drinking water or mineral water, therefore, food cooked in different waters might have widely varying amounts of vanadium.[4]

LINKED TO CHOLESTEROL LEVELS?

Scientists aren't sure whether vanadium keeps excessive cholesterol from forming, or breaks it down when it has formed, or perhaps both, reported *The Complete Book of Minerals for Health*. The question came to the fore when researchers discovered that vanadium is abundant in the hard drinking waters of certain areas of the southwest, where death rates from degenerative heart disease are lowest in the United States. The mineral is barely present in the soft water of the Coastal and Great Lakes states, where heart disease rates are the highest.[5]

Speaking at a meeting of the American Association for the Advancement of Science, December 29, 1961, William H. Strain said that there are very significant geographical variations in death rates for all causes and for cardiovascular diseases that may be due to a variable intake of trace elements, especially vanadium and zinc.[5]

In 1956, a study of the Scandinavian countries found that the death rates from heart disease in these countries is exceptionally low. Scientists evaluated the consumption of fat, meat and milk in each country but this showed no relationship to the death rates. They theorized that the low rates might be due to the intake of trace minerals.[5]

"In seaside Scandinavian countries, ocean fish are eaten in large quantities and sea salt (rich in trace minerals) is used for preserving fish, for cattle and for household consumption. To add credibility to the importance of the water-surrounded situation of these countries, Prof. Niels Dungal reported in 1953 on 2,200 autopsies in Iceland. The arteries of the Icelanders, at age 60, compared well with the arteries of Austrians at age 40. Strain suggested that their lack of cholesterol accumulation might be credited to the ingestion of vanadium and other trace minerals," according to *The Complete Book of Minerals for Health*.[5]

J. T. Mountain and associates, reporting in *Federal Proceedings* (1959), described an elaborate study with rabbits that showed that vanadium added to the standard diet at premeasured levels lowered free cholesterol and fat content of the liver of the animals. When vanadium was added to a one-percent cholesterol diet, it held down the elevation of free and total cholesterol in the plasma. When the rabbits were fed cholesterol to raise the plasma level, and then the cholesterol was omitted from the diet, the presence of vanadium in the diet was given credit for a faster return to normal cholesterol readings than occurred when no vanadium was furnished. The researchers concluded that vanadium both inhibits the formation of cholesterol and speeds the destruction of it.[5]

G. L. Curran and R. L. Costello reported in the *Journal of Experimental Medicine* (1956) that six weeks of administering vanadium resulted in statistically significant lowering of the serum total and free cholesterol levels, the publication said. The vanadium lowered tissue cholesterol stores in four of the five men studied. A small group of vanadium workers were observed (vanadium has industrial uses, such as in vanadium steel), and, compared with a control group, the workers had a significantly lower cholesterol value.[5]

Writing in the *Archives of Environmental Health* in 1968, W. H. Allaway and colleagues studied the vanadium content in the blood of men who visited blood banks across the U.S. They found that the highest concentration of vanadium was 2/mcg per 100 ml of whole blood. But 90 percent of the samples examined contained less than 1/mcg per 100 ml.[6]

"Nutritional aspects of vanadium have been reviewed by Underwood, Schroeder, et al., and Soremark," the researchers said. "The distribution of vanadium in plants in different parts of the United States has been reported by Cannon. Although vanadium at high concentrations (above 5 ppm) in diets is detrimental to some animals, there is evidence that lower amounts of vanadium may reduce serum cholesterol levels. If the levels of vanadium in blood reflect the level of vanadium intake, the results of our study may indicate that the blood donors involved were subject to suboptimal vanadium intake."[6]

Food sources of vanadium include buckwheat, herring, sardines, soybeans, parsley, oats, eggs, safflower oil, sunflower oil and olive oil.

As fat-burning nutrients, which cut sugar cravings and reduce fat storage, Dallas Clouatre, Ph.D., recommends 5 to 15 mg/day of vanadyl sulfate and 200 to 600 mcg/day of chromium.[7]

REFERENCES

1. Clouatre, Dallas, Ph.D. *Anti-Fat Nutrients*. San Francisco: Pax Publishing, 1993, p. 20ff.
2. Braverman, Eric R., M.D., and Pfeiffer, Carl C., M.D., Ph.D. *The Healing Nutrients Within*. New Canaan, Conn.: Keats Publishing, Inc., 1987, p. 114.
3. Ensminger, Audrey H., et al. *Foods and Nutrition Encyclopedia*. Clovis, Calif.: Pegus Press, 1983, p. 2145.

4. Adams, Ruth, and Murray, Frank. *Minerals: Kill or Cure?* New York: Larchmont Books, 1974, p. 231ff.

5. Rodale, J. I., and Staff. *The Complete Book of Minerals for Health.* Emmaus, Pa.: Rodale Books, Inc., 1972, p. 249ff.

6. Allaway, W. H., et al. "Selenium, Molybdenum and Vanadium in Human Blood," *Archives of Environmental Health* 16:342–348, March 1968.

7. Clouatre, Dallas, Ph.D. op. cited.

PART IV

Minerals You Can Do Without

37

Aluminum

ONE of the most recent metal discoveries, aluminum was initially produced in 1825 by Hans Christian Oersted (1777-1851), a Danish physician, and introduced to the public at the Paris Exposition. In industry, the United States utilizes more aluminum than any other product except iron and steel. Aluminum is a food additive that is found in baking powder, pickles, processed cheeses, aluminum-containing antacids and aluminum cooking utensils.

"Abnormally large intakes of aluminum irritate the digestive tract," the *Foods and Nutrition Encyclopedia* reported. "Also, unusual conditions have sometimes resulted in the absorption of sufficient aluminum from antacids to cause brain damage. Aluminum may form non-absorbable complexes with essential trace elements, thereby creating deficiencies of the trace elements. Aluminum toxicity has been reported in patients receiving renal dialysis."[1]

Although aluminum is naturally present in air, soil, water and plants, it has no known biological function in humans, reported Scott A. Rogers, D.C., in the February 1988 issue of *The American Chiropractor*. Circumstantial evidence implicates aluminum in human toxicology, but most mechanisms of pathology remain unknown, he said. While conclusive proof that aluminum is a causative factor in senility is lacking, some authorities are recommending that the intake of the element be reduced. The role of aluminum in Alzheimer's disease remains controversial, he added.[2]

MANY SOURCES, SOME UNEXPECTED

"Those seeking to reduce their aluminum intake will find that alternatives are readily available to commodities that contain the metal," Rogers said. "For example, some baking powders use monocalcium phosphate for leavening agents, and most pickles are prepared in calcium oxide. At least 25 brands of aluminum-free antacids are sold over-the-counter, and some aspirins are buffered by calcium carbonate. Many health food stores carry non-aluminum makeup and deodorants. Aluminum cookware can be replaced by porcelain, glass or stainless steel. Foods and beverages packaged in aluminum may usually be purchased fresh, frozen or bottled in glass. If the local water supply is contaminated, most cities have companies that will deliver purified water to businesses and residences."[2]

In a British government study, researchers reported high levels of aluminum in drinking water which substantially increases a person's risk for developing Alzheimer's disease, stated Elizabeth Somer, M.A., R.D., in *The Nutrition Report*, March 1989. Their conclusions were based on findings involving 4,000 volunteers, ranging in age from 40 to 69, who lived in 88 counties in England and Wales. During the 10-year study, the researchers compared the incidence of Alzheimer's disease with the levels of aluminum in the local water supply.[3]

"The results showed adults who consume water containing large amounts of the mineral have a 50-percent greater risk of developing Alzheimer's than those whose water does not contain aluminum," Somer said. "In addition, people who are younger than 65 are at even greater risk if exposed to water containing excessive levels of aluminum. And they are 70 percent more likely to develop Alzheimer's if they live in areas with high average concentrations of the mineral. High levels of aluminum were defined as more than 0.11 mg per liter of water."[3]

If you often take aluminum-containing antacids, such as Maalox or Amphojel, you should avoid eating or drinking citrus fruit or citrus juice at the same time, according to the October 1994 issue of *Environmental Nutrition*. To avoid possible aluminum buildup, wait two or three hours after taking aluminum-containing antacids before ingesting citrus products.[4]

Although the small amount of aluminum in most antacids is considered safe, the acidity of the citrus (a small glass of orange juice) can increase absorption of the aluminum as much as ten-fold. But small amounts of aluminum absorbed on a regular basis can accumulate in the tissues and reach levels that might affect your health, the publication said.[4]

CUMULATIVE ACTION

Aluminum is a strong cross-linking agent found in foods which can accumulate in tissues, stated Johan Bjorksten, Ph.D., and colleagues at the Bjorksten Research Foundation in Houston, Texas. They reported in the *International Journal of Vitamin and Nutrition Research* in 1988, that tissue concentrations of aluminum increase approximately 50 percent in an individual between one year and 60 years of age. And the rate of accumulation increases from age 60 to 99.[5]

In studying the aluminum content of various foods, they found wide variations between samples of the same foods. For example, milk contained as little as 4 parts per billion (ppb) to as much as 5,706 ppb; orange juice ranged from 80 ppb to 49,618 ppb; fish ranged from 6 ppb to 8,760 ppb; cereals ranged from 40 ppb to 29,330 ppb; beef ranged from 132 ppb to 20,448 ppb. The researchers suggest that the accumulation of aluminum in tissues might contribute to progressive organ dysfunction, which could eventually lead to death.[5]

Between 1944 and 1979, miners were given aluminum powder as a prophylaxis against silicotic lung disease, reported S. L. Rifat, et al., of the Clarke Institute of Psychiatry, in the November 10, 1990 issue of *Lancet*. When researchers studied these miners between 1988 and 1989, they found that the volunteers performed less well on cognitive state examinations when compared to nonexposed miners. And their impaired range continued to increase with the duration of the exposure, prompting the researchers to conclude that chronic aluminum exposure can result in neurotoxicity.[6]

A research team from the University of Alberta in Canada and the University of Cincinnati in Ohio reported in the *Journal of the American College of Nutrition* in 1988 that highly processed infant formulas containing many additives, such as soy formulas, preterm infant formulas and formulas for various disorders, are heavily contaminated with aluminum, which might result in aluminum toxicity in the infants. The risk is apparently greater in children with chronic kidney insufficiency, those on long-term parenteral nutrition and preterm infants with low aluminum-binding capacity. Side effects of aluminum toxicity include impairment of bone matrix formation. But mineralization may be reconciled by aluminum's direct effect on bone cells or indirectly by its effect on parathyroid hormone and calcium metabolism. To minimize tissue burden, the researchers suggest that the aluminum content of infant formulas should be similar to that of whole milk.[7]

Jose L. Domingo, M.D., et al., of the University of Barcelona in Spain, reported that when 13 healthy volunteers were given three daily oral courses of aluminum hydroxide, 900 mg three times a day alone, or with 2 g/day of ascorbic acid (vitamin C), it was found that ascorbic acid together with aluminum hydroxide caused a significant increase in aluminum excretion in the urine, which the researchers believed was due to enhanced gastrointestinal absorption. In animal models, the authors reported in the December 7, 1991 issue of *Lancet*, increased concentrations of aluminum in the liver, brain and bone were caused by giving vitamin C with aluminum hydroxide. They recommend caution when giving vitamin C to patients with kidney failure who are taking aluminum-containing compounds, since this may accelerate uptake of the mineral.[8]

In *The Medical Journal of Australia*, May 4, 1992, John M. Duggan, et al., at John Hunter Hospital, New Lambton Heights, Australia, said that when they evaluated the aluminum content of 106 cans and bottles, representing 52 different beverages, they found that all had a higher aluminum content than the water in that area. If there is a confirmation between the link of aluminum and Alzheimer's disease, they said, then beverages from aluminum cans, especially soft drinks, may be a risk factor.[9]

A LINK TO ALZHEIMER'S?

A research team at the Johns Hopkins University School of Medicine, Francis Scott Key Medical Center in Baltimore, evaluated the neurocognitive effects of aluminum on 35 patients undergoing hemodialysis. They reported in the October 1992 issue of *Archives of Neurology* that higher aluminum levels were associated with a reduction in visual memory. As the aluminum levels increased, said Karen L. Bolla, Ph.D., the lead researcher, there were reduced vocabulary scores as shown by a decline in the tension-concentration, frontal lobe function and neurocognitive measures. Those who had higher vocabulary scores exhibited no aluminum-related decline. In animal models, they added, reductions in glucose utilization involving the striatal, cortical and hypothalamic areas have been noted. A reduction in glucose metabolism may inhibit the appropriate synthesis of the neurotransmitter acetylcholine, which is involved in neurocognitive function. They noted that Alzheimer's patients have reduced levels of acetylcholine.[10]

Twenty-five workers at an aluminum smelting plant were studied by David H. White, Ph.D., et al., of the University of Washington Medical Center in Seattle. They reported in the July 1992 issue of *Archives of Internal Medicine* that 88 percent of the workers reported frequent loss of balance; 84 percent had memory loss; 84 percent reported signs of incoordination; 70 to 75 percent revealed mild to greater impairment on memory tests; 89 percent exhibited depression on the Minnesota Multiphasic Personality Inventory.[11]

At a conference on Alzheimer's disease and the environment, sponsored by the Royal Society of Medicine, June, 1991, and reported in the February 1992 issue of the *Journal of the Royal Society of Medicine*, Lord Walton of Detchant said that aluminum's role in Alzheimer's disease is questioned because chronic renal failure patients exposed to years of high blood aluminum levels have an absence of neurofibrillary tangles associated with Alzheimer's disease. A transferrin defect, a binding release of free aluminum available for deposition in the brain cells, might release the free aluminum available for deposition in brain cells and possibly be a factor. Reduction of aluminum in food, fluids and medicines might be warranted for the elderly, the conference was told. This includes patients with Alzheimer's disease, Parkinson's disease and those with chronic kidney failure.[12]

The June 1, 1992 issue of *Family Practice News* reported on a study of 30 women who were taking calcium citrate to prevent osteoporosis. It was found that they had significant aluminum levels on days 19 and 38 in the blood and urine. Aluminum, which is available in baking powder, nondairy creamers, antacids, etc., binds to phosphorus, where it is insoluble. When citrate is present, the phosphorus binds to it and aluminum remains insoluble. Researchers have found that, in animal models, supplementation with citric acid causes an accumulation of aluminum in the brain and bone. It is not known whether this is a risk for patients using citric acid, but there is concern for females who have 20- to 30-percent kidney dysfunction, the publication added. These patients should switch to other forms of calcium. If calcium citrate is used, antacids or other aluminum-containing products should be avoided. If this study confirms aluminum accumulation in women with normal kidney function, then calcium citrate use is a significant problem. Aluminum has been implicated in encephalopathy and osteomalacia in uremic patients, the publication added.[13]

Miklos L. Boczko, M.D., was quoted in *Clinical Pearls* in 1992 as saying that dementia is the fourth leading cause of death for those over the age of 60, and that Alzheimer's disease kills an estimated 100,000 people annually in the United States. At least $50 billion a year is spent on caring for these demented patients.

It is believed that multiple concurrent effects, rather than a single agent, may explain the development of Alzheimer's, Boczko said. Neuronal accumulation of aluminum, along with a nutritional deficit of dysmetabolism of calcium, magnesium and zinc, seems to be a toxic agent. He added that the disruption of the blood brain barrier appears to be involved in the effect of many agents. Therapies such as removing the accumulated aluminum, improving zinc nutrition and decreasing peroxidative chain reactions—and possibly using calcium channel blockers—may be useful.[14]

Dialysis Danger

The Food and Drug Administration reported in the September 1992 issue of its *FDA Medical Bulletin* that hemodialysis personnel and dialysis patients may be exposed to dangerously high levels of aluminum and other trace elements from components in the dialysate delivery systems. The Centers for Disease Control and Prevention in Atlanta identified a significant number of patients with elevated blood aluminum levels at large dialysis facilities. And three patients have died from aluminum toxicity.[15]

The CDC stated that 72 percent in a survey of dialysis facilities reported using a bicarbonate-based dialysate, which can result in a corrosive action due to the low pH of the solutions. This increases the leaching of metals used in the components of the delivery system. Additional information is available from the Center for Devices and Radiological Health, FDA, HFZ-240, 5600 Fishers Lane, Rockville, Maryland 20857.[15]

REFERENCES

1. Ensminger, Audrey H., et al. *Foods and Nutrition Encyclopedia*. Clovis, Calif.: Pegus Press, 1983, pp. 1790–1791.
2. Rogers, Scott A., D.C. "The Aluminum Controversy," *The American Chiropractor*, February 1988, pp. 28–39.
3. Somer, Elizabeth, M.A., R.D. "Alzheimer's Disease and Aluminum: New Findings," *The Nutrition Report*, March 1989.
4. "Antacids and Orange Juice May Not Mix," *Environmental Nutrition* 17(10):6, October 1994.
5. Bjorksten, J., et al. "Control of Aluminum Ingestion and Its Relation to Longevity," *International Journal of Vitamin and Nutrition Research* 48:462–465, 1988.
6. Rifat, S. L., et al. "Effect of Exposure of Miners to Aluminum Powder," *Lancet* 336:1162–1165, November 10, 1990.
7. Koo, W., and Kaplan, L. "Aluminum and Bone Disorders—With Specific Reference to Aluminum Contamination of Infant Nutrients," *Journal of the American College of Nutrition* 7:199–214, 1988.
8. Domingo, Jose L., et al. "Effect of Ascorbic Acid on Gastrointestinal Aluminum Absorption," *Lancet* 338:1467, December 7, 1991.

9. Duggan, John M., et al. "Aluminum Beverage Cans as a Dietary Source of Aluminum," *The Medical Journal of Australia* 156:604–605, May 4, 1992.

10. Bolla, Karen L., Ph.D., et al. "Neurocognitive Effects of Aluminum," *Archives of Neurology* 49:1021–1026, October 1992.

11. White, David M., Ph.D., et al. "Neurologic Syndrome in 25 Workers from an Aluminum Smelting Plant," *Archives of Internal Medicine* 152:1443–1448, July 1992.

12. Walton, Lord. "Alzheimer's Disease and the Environment," *Journal of the Royal Society of Medicine* 85:69-70, February 1992.

13. "Preliminary Findings Suggest Calcium Citrate Supplements May Raise Aluminum Levels in the Blood," *Family Practice News*, June 1, 1992, pp. 74–75.

14. Boczko, Miklos, M.D. "Dementia: A Review of Current Environmental Issues," *Clinical Pearls*, 1992, p. 44, 3301 Alta, Sacramento, CA 95825.

15. "Dialysis Patients Face Danger from Aluminum and Other Trace Elements," *FDA Medical Bulletin*, September 1992, p. 8.

38

Arsenic

THE thoughts of arsenic conjure up the Broadway play, "Arsenic and Old Lace," in which the Brewster sisters dispatch lonely, old men with their special mixture of elderberry wine and arsenic. Arsenic migrates into the food chain through arsenic-containing insecticides and weed killers, the smelting of metals and the burning of coal.

A beneficial use of arsenic is Arsenicum album, a homeopathic substance, used by homeopathic physicians to treat asthma, hay fever, dry eczema, psoriasis, anxiety, minor depression, gastroduodenal ulcers, diarrhea resulting from spoiled food and other complaints. In homeopathy, however, generally toxic substances are used only in infinitesimal amounts, and their efficacy has been proven for several hundred years.[1]

"In 1900, Dr. Gautier of Paris found that traces of arsenic are to be found in the epidermis, hair, glands, brain and breast and in a few organs," according to Harvey Day in the *Encyclopedia of Natural Health and Healing*. "It is possible, by taking gradually increasing doses, such as the women of Kashmir do to gain pale complexions, eventually to imbibe enough arsenic to kill a man, with complete immunity to themselves."[2]

The alchemists' symbol of arsenic, a menacing coiled serpent, symbolizes the element's evil reputation through the ages. Arsenic compounds were the preferred homicidal and suicidal agents during the Middle Ages. And arsenic was reportedly used on several occasions to attempt to do away with Napoleon Bonaparte during his exile on St. Helena. Paris green, or copper acetoarsenite, was the first pesticide to be used in modern agriculture.

Symptoms of arsenic poisoning include burning pains in the throat or stomach, cardiac abnormalities and the odor of garlic on the breath. Other symptoms include diarrhea, extreme thirst and a choking sensation. Small amounts of arsenic taken over an extended period may produce hyperkeratosis (irregularities in pigmentation), arterial insufficiency and cancer. And inorganic arsenic is thought to be a skin and lung carcinogen in man.

"Cases of arsenic toxicity in man are rather infrequent," the *Foods and Nutrition Encyclopedia* said. "Two noteworthy episodes occurred in Japan in 1955. One involved tainted powdered milk; the other, contaminated soy sauce. The toxic milk caused 12,131 cases of infant poisoning, with 130 deaths. The soy sauce poisoned 220 people. To treat arsenic poisoning, induce vomiting, followed by an antidote of egg whites in water or milk. Afterward, give strong coffee or tea, followed by epsom salts in water or castor oil."[3]

Children with a history of headaches and reactive airway disease should be studied for possible environmental contaminants at home, school, etc., reported the December 15-31, 1991 issue of *Family Practice News*. For example, wooden playground equipment should be assessed for arsenic-containing compounds and creosote; tobacco smoke; wood and gas stoves; formaldehyde; insulation; radon and asbestos; chemicals from insect repellants and home products; paint contamination, especially from older homes; play sand not from the ocean may contain tremolite, which is a carcinogen; arts and crafts materials may contain lead and other toxic metals.[4]

A CANCEROUS COMBINATION

W. J. Blot and J. F. Fraumeni, Jr., reported in *Lancet* in 1975 that there was a significant increase in lung cancer near refineries and smelters where arsenic concentrations were abnormal.[5]

Irva Hertz-Picciotto, et al., of the University of North Carolina in Chapel Hill, found a synergistic effect between smoking and arsenic exposure on lung cancer, they reported in the January 1992 issue of *Epidemiology*. They insisted that there is compelling evidence that arsenic and smoking act in a synergistic manner to produce lung cancer.[6]

In the October 19, 1994 issue of the *Journal of the American Medical Association*, the magazine discussed an article in JAMA in 1894 (their "JAMA 100 Years Ago" regular feature), in which it was reported that the use of arsenic by women to improve their complexion and personal appearance has become so common throughout the country as to lead to an official investigation by Dr. Cyrus Edson, Health Commissioner for the city of New York, and others.

These gentlemen have been "filled with alarm" by the disclosures of their investigation, and "are moving to have heroic measures adopted to put an end to the pernicious use of the drug." It is further stated that, as a result of their efforts "the health authorities of 30 of the largest cities and of nine states have combined to crush out the growing evil," and that a bill has been drafted, to be introduced in State Legislatures, designed to impose restrictions, under heavy penalties, upon the sale of the drug, except on a physician's prescription; and that the investigation was undertaken none too soon, and no measures too severe can be adopted to stamp out a habit in which "has been discovered the secret of many a mysterious death and of many an untimely-filled grave."[7]

Arsenic contamination of subsoil water used for drinking, has produced some cases of portal high blood pressure in areas of southern Bengal, India, according to D. N. Mazumdar, et al., in *The Journal of Hepatology* in 1991. High levels of arsenic were found in the hair, nails and liver tissue of five of 13 patients studied. The patients had drunk well water containing from 0.22 to 2 mg/liter for from one to 10 years. In addition to abnormal liver pathology, some of the patients exhibited chronic arsenicosis—raindrop pigmentation of the skin and buccal mucosa, keratosis of the palms and soles, and peripheral neuropathy.[8]

F. Nevens, et al., reported in the *Journal of Hepatology* in 1990, that eight of 47 patients with noncirrhotic portal high blood pressure had taken arsenic-containing Fowler's solution for psoriasis. All of the patients had enlarged esophageal veins and enlargement of the spleen with signs of other abnormalities in the spleen. Half of the patients had malignant skin lesions. One patient developed lung carcinoma, while another had abnormal ovarian growth which resulted in death. The authors suggest that chronic arsenic intake should be observed in patients with psoriasis and noncirrhotic portal hypertension, with a thorough history of the patient encouraged. And, they added, these patients should be followed for years to see if malignant lesions in the skin, lung and liver develop.[9]

There are thousands of toxic substances in factory-made cigarettes (from tobacco, paper and filters), including arsenic, cyanide, DDT and asbestos, reported Timothy R. Stockwell, M.Sc., Ph.D., in the July 6, 1992 issue of *The Medical Journal of Australia*. Government experts have said that the amounts of these substances and risks are small when compared to the tar, nicotine and carbon monoxide from cigarettes. But in a survey of 510 smokers, few of them were aware of carbon monoxide and other toxic chemicals in cigarettes. Eighty-five percent of the responders felt that tobacco companies should inform smokers about these toxic elements, and two-thirds told Stockwell that the pesticide/chemical warnings, especially mentioning arsenic, DDT, lead and asbestos, would induce them to cut down or quit smoking.[10]

REFERENCES

1. Horvilleur, Alain, M.D. *The Family Guide to Homeopathy*. Alexandria, Virginia: Health and Homeopathy Publishing, Inc., 1986, p. 32.
2. Day, Harvey. *Encyclopedia of Natural Health and Healing*. Santa Barbara, Calif.: Woodbridge Press Publishing Co., 1979, p. 10.
3. Ensminger, Audrey H., et al. *Foods and Nutrition Encyclopedia*. Clovis, Calif.: Pegus Press, 1983, pp. 1790–1791.
4. "Taking Child's Environmental History Advocated," *Family Practice News* 20(24):34, December 15-31, 1991.
5. Blot, W. J., and Fraumeni, Jr. "Arsenical Air Pollution and Lung Cancer," *Lancet* 2(7926):142-144, July 26, 1975.
6. Hertz-Picciotto, Irva, et al. "Synergism Between Occupational Arsenic Exposure and Smoking in the Induction of Lung Cancer," Epidemiology 3(1):23–30, January 1992.
7. "Why Arsenic Only?" *Journal of the American Medical Association* 23:620–621, 1894. (In JAMA 272(15):1170ff, October 19, 1994).
8. Mazumdar, D. N., et al. "Arsenic and Non-Cirrhotic Portal Hypertension," *The Journal of Hepatology*, 1991, p. 376.
9. Nevens, F., et al. "Arsenic and Non-Cirrhotic Portal Hypertension: A Report of Eight Cases," *Journal of Hepatology* 11:80–85, 1990.
10. Stockwell, Timothy R., M.Sc., Ph.D. "Pesticides and Other Chemicals in Cigarette Smoke," *The Medical Journal of Australia* 157:68, July 6, 1992.

39

Cadmium

In the early 1970s, there were many cases of cadmium toxicity in the Jinzu River basin near Toyama, Japan, which is located about 160 miles from Tokyo. The disease caused by this pollution is called *Itai-Itai* ("ouch-ouch"), because of the pain its victims suffer. The poisonings were traced to consumption of rice and soybeans containing about 3 parts per million (ppm) of cadmium which came from the wastes of nearby mines and smelters. Cadmium levels of about 1 ppm have been found in soybeans grown in soil fertilized by sewage sludge, and oysters taken from water contaminated with industrial wastes contained about 3 ppm of the metal.

Cadmium contamination has also been traced to cigarette smoke, electroplating processes, paint pigments (cadmium red and orange are two popular oil colors), the cadmium-nickel type of automobile storage battery, certain phosphate fertilizers and some of the older types of galvanized water tanks.

"While severe cadmium toxicity like that which occurred near Toyama has not been found elsewhere, it is suspected that mild to moderate types of chronic cadmium toxicity may cause disorders of the kidneys leading to high blood pressure," the *Foods and Nutrition Encyclopedia* said. "However, the milder forms of cadmium poisoning may be counteracted by such essential minerals as calcium, copper, iron, manganese, selenium and zinc. Therefore, a few scientists believe that high ratios of cadmium to zinc in the diet and in the various tissues of the body are better indicators of potential cadmium toxicities than the dietary and tissue levels of this toxicant alone."[1]

ENVIRONMENTAL HAZARD

Dr. James D. Ebert of the Carnegie Institution of Washington, spoke at the 4th International Conference on Birth Defects on September 3, 1973, in Vienna. He said that the American baby has only one microgram of cadmium in his body at birth. But, by the time he is 50, he may have 30 milligrams or 30,000 times more. He added that the hazards of environmental agents which cause birth defects are so great that the development of new screening techniques is essential.[2]

Dr. Russell N. Hirst, Jr., of Washington University, was quoted as saying that, in autopsy studies, he and his associates have found high amounts of cadmium in lung tissue of emphysema patients, and that the severity of disease is correlated with the amount of cadmium and a history of cigarette smoking. Dr. Gordon L. Snider and associates at Boston University said that one cigarette contains about 1 mcg of cadmium, and that one pack deposits between 2 and 4 mcg of cadmium into a smoker's lungs.[2]

Seventy percent of the cadmium in tobacco passes into the smoke, which is inhaled or goes out into the room to be inhaled by all, smokers and nonsmokers alike. Studies of the livers of people dying from emphysema and bronchitis show three times more cadmium than those of people dying of other diseases. Dr. Harold Petering of the University of Cincinnati has shown that the tobacco smoke from one pack of cigarettes, smoked over an 8-hour period in a 10- by 12-foot room, releases over 100 times the amount of cadmium in the outside air.[2]

Cadmium in the air is absorbed from the lungs and deposited in the kidney, liver and arteries, added Henry Schroeder, M.D. This can produce destructive kidney changes and liver damage has been caused by chronic exposure to large amounts. Cadmium is released into the air as a result of incineration or disposal of cadmium-containing products (rubber tires, plastic containers, etc.) and as a byproduct in the refining of other metals, primarily zinc.[2]

In one survey, cadmium was detected in 42 percent of some 720 samples of drinking water from rivers and reservoirs in the United States. In addition, the mineral accumulates in water stored in galvanized or plastic water pipes. Phosphate detergents may carry cadmium, along with arsenic, as a pollutant of the phosphates. Refining grains eliminates the zinc, which, to some extent, protects from possible harm from cadmium.

Science reported that when foods were grown in soil heavily fertilized with phosphate they absorbed cadmium. Vegetables normally containing cadmium picked up more of the mineral when the phosphate fertilizer was used—and none in its absence. Therefore, phosphate fertilizers may be the source of the cadmium in some vegetable foods.[2]

Cadmium can accumulate to toxic levels over a lifetime because the mineral is not well excreted by the body, reported Robert H. Garrison, Jr., M.A., R.Ph., and Elizabeth Somer, M.A., R.D., in *The Nutrition Desk Reference*. It is also poorly absorbed. Workers exposed to copper-cadmium alloys have a high incidence of pulmonary emphysema, and anemia, protein in the urine and amino aciduria are associated with high concentrations of cadmium (10 to 100 times normal) in the liver and kidneys, they added. Since cadmium excretion is slow, high concentrations can remain in the body for years after cessation of exposure. The estimated daily intake of the cadmium is 13 to 24 mcg, with urinary excretion at about 10 mcg/liter.[3]

A study reported in the *British Journal of Urology* in 1982 concerned copper-smiths who had been chronically exposed to cadmium. The researchers said that the prevalence of urinary tract stones was almost 40 percent, compared to about 3.5 percent in the general population.[4]

Researchers at Teikyo University in Japan reported in *Toxicology Letters* in 1990 that cadmium exposure altered the fatty acid metabolism in the liver of laboratory rats. The research team added that there is an increase in saturated and omega-6 fatty acids in the liver phospholipids and a decrease in omega-9 fatty acids, and that these changes are similar to what occurs with dietary zinc deficiency. Cadmium appears to be a zinc antagonist, which inhibits various zinc enzymes and, therefore, alters the metabolism of fatty acids, they said.[5]

In the *American Journal of Epidemiology*, May 1992, Leslie Stayner, Ph.D., and colleagues at the Robert A. Taft Laboratories in Cincinnati discussed their evaluations of workers exposed at a cadmium smelter. There was a large number of deaths due to lung cancer, with mortality the greatest among non-Hispanic workers, workers in the highest cadmium exposure group and workers with 20 or more years since their initial exposure. According to the current Occupational Safety and Health Administration standard, between 50 and 111 lung cancer deaths per 1,000 can be expected among those exposed to cadmium for 45 years. The researchers added that the relationship between cadmium and lung cancer might also be related to arsenic exposure.[6]

A review of available data and a follow-up as to the causes of deaths among cadmium workers in six different cohorts found that long-term, high-level exposure to cadmium is related to an increased risk for prostate and lung cancer, reported the *British Journal of Industrial Medicine* in 1985.[7]

Twenty-four-hour urine cadmium levels were studied in 1,523 volunteers, who were not exposed to the metal occupationally, and who lived in various areas of Belgium, reported Francis Sartor, et al., in the September-October 1992 issue of *Archives of Environmental Health*. The research team reported that the highest 24-hour cadmium levels in the urine were found in those who lived in areas with cadmium-polluted soils. Elevated cadmium levels were associated with locally grown vegetables and contaminated well water used for cooking and drinking.[8]

Edmund Lui, Ph.D., et al., of Victoria Hospital in London, Ontario, Canada, assessed the storage of metals in the livers of 17 Alzheimer's disease patients and 17 controls. They found that hepatic cadmium and zinc were greatly elevated in the Alzheimer's patients. In other words, the metabolism of cadmium and zinc are apparently altered in these patients.[9]

Alginic acid and its salts are seaweed derivatives that maintain the "heads" on beer, provide creamy bodies to milk shakes, are used to make dental impressions and are beneficial for the treatment of heartburn caused by acid reflux from the stomach, according to Sheldon Saul Hendler, M.D., Ph.D., in *The Purification Prescription*.[10]

Alginates have been found to strongly bind strontium. Radioactive strontium-90 is one of the more common radioactive pollutants. Strontium-90 gets deposited in the bones and has been associated with increased incidence of bone cancer and other forms of cancer. Sodium and calcium alginate both bind to radioactive strontium in the gastrointestinal tract, preventing its absorption into the body. In addition, the alginates have been shown to reduce the amount of radioactive strontium that has already accumulated in the bones. The alginates can thus be used as both preventives and as treatments. Alginates can also bind to cadmium, barium, radium and, to a lesser extent, to lead.

In addition to the alginates, selenium, zinc, copper, iron, calcium and vitamin C protect against cadmium toxicity, Hendler added.

K. Borowiak, et al., of the Pomeranian Academy of Medicine in Szczecin, Poland, stated in *Z Rechtsmed* in 1990, that a 52-year-old woman developed a progressive illness for which no cause could be found. Symptoms developed about two years after she had a gold dental prosthesis inserted. Symptoms intensified during the next three years. Since the prosthesis had been in place for five years, the researchers decided to do a toxicological examination, which revealed an elevation of cadmium in the blood and urine. Since the cadmium content of the prosthesis was excessive, the researchers removed it, and the cadmium content in the blood and urine returned to normal levels within 12 weeks. The patient's health improved and her symptoms were restored to normal, the researchers added.[11]

In *Archives of Environmental Health* in 1967, H. A. Schroeder, et al., reported that, in an experimental study involving animals, a zinc chelate supplement reversed the cadmium-induced high blood pressure in the animals.[12]

REFERENCES

1. Ensminger, Audrey H., et al., *Foods and Nutrition Encyclopedia*. Clovis, Calif.: Pegus Press, 1983, p. 1523.
2. Adams, Ruth, and Murray, Frank. *Minerals: Kill or Cure?* New York: Larchmont Books, 1974, p. 222ff.
3. Garrison, Robert H., Jr., M.A., R.Ph., and Somer, Elizabeth, M.A., R.D. *The Nutrition Desk Reference*. New Canaan, Conn.: Keats Publishing, Inc., 1990, p. 79.
4. Scott, R., et al. "The Importance of Cadmium as a Factor in Calcified Upper Urinary Tract Stone Disease—A Prospective 7-Year Study," *British Journal of Urology* 54:584, 1982.
5. Kudo, Naomi, et al. "The Effect of Cadmium on the Composition and Metabolism of Hepatic Fatty Acids and Zinc-Adequate and Zinc-Deficient Rats," *Toxicology Letters* 50:203–212, 1990.
6. Stayner, Leslie, Ph.D., et al. "A Dose Response Analysis and Quantitative Assessment of Lung Cancer Risk and Occupation Cadmium Exposure," *American Journal of Epidemiology* 2(3):177–194, May 1992.
7. Elinder, C. G., et al. "Cancer Mortality in Cadmium Workers," *British Journal of Industrial Medicine* 42(10):651–655, 1985.
8. Sartor, Francis, et al. "Impact of Environmental Cadmium Pollution on Cadmium Exposure and Body Burden," *Archives of Environmental Health* 47(5):347–353, October 1992.
9. Lui, Edmund, Ph.D., et al. "Metals and the Liver in Alzheimer's Disease: An Investigation of Hepatic Zinc, Copper, Cadmium and Metallothionein," *Journal of the American Geriatric Society* 38(6):633–639, June 1990.
10. Hendler, Sheldon Saul, M.D., Ph.D. *The Purification Prescription*. New York: William Morrow and Co., Inc., 1991, pp. 67, 228.
11. Borowiak, K., et al. "Chronic Cadmium Intoxication Caused by Dental Prosthesis," *Z Rechtsmed* 103:537–539, 1990.
12. Schroeder, H. A., et al. "Cadmium Hypertension: Its Reversal in Rats by a Zinc Chelate," *Archives of Environmental Health* 14:693, 1967.

40

Lead

ANYONE who has read Gibbon's *Decline and Fall of the Roman Empire*—or seen the "I Claudius" series on TV—must have been impressed with what a bunch of monsters most of the Roman emperors were. It has been suggested that they were driven crazy by the lead in the vessels from which they drank so much wine, reported the December 10, 1988 issue of *Lancet*.[1]

In more recent years, other sources of lead have been the targets of those charged with protecting the public welfare, the magazine said. In the U.S., for example, in the 1970s, federal agencies made strenuous efforts to reduce population exposure by banning lead-based interior house paints, reducing the lead content of tinned foods, and phasing out leaded gasoline for cars. These efforts succeeded because, between 1976 and 1980, blood-lead levels in the U.S. population fell by one-third.

Lead, which has been mined and used for centuries, was considered by the alchemists to be the oldest metal, according to *Foods and Nutrition Encyclopedia*. The mining and processing of lead dates back to pre-Christian times. The Roman Empire declined and finally fell, according to authoritative speculation, not because of the barbarian hordes, overextended colonization or because of moral decadence, the encyclopedia added, but mainly because of lead poisoning. The upper-class Romans unwittingly poisoned themselves by eating and drinking from vessels containing lead and dabbing themselves with lead-laden cosmetics, which sapped their vitality and that of their society. A study of early Roman tombstone inscriptions revealed a life expectancy of 22 to 25 years among upper-class Romans, and their birth rate was one-fourth of what was needed to replace themselves. The poor people ate out of cheap earthenware utensils and didn't use cosmetics, so they were generally spared lead intoxication.[2]

"Today, there is great concern over acute lead poisoning in young children—ages 1 to 6—who live in urban slums where they may eat chips of lead-containing paints, peeled from painted wood," the encyclopedia added. "The effects of such poisoning may be anemia, hyperactivity, learning disabilities, mental retardation or even death. There is also concern for older children and adults who might develop chronic lead poisoning from exposure to sources such as automobile exhaust fumes, cigarette smoke, fumes from lead smelters or smoke from coal fires; consumption of beer held in lead-containing pewter mugs; produce from orchards sprayed with lead arsenate; or fruits and vegetables grown near heavily traveled highways."[2]

GREATEST RISK

Children and pregnant women appear to be the most susceptible to lead poisoning, because they are likely to have deficiencies of calcium and iron, which protect against lead toxicity; rapidly growing children absorb more lead and excrete less of the metal than other people; and there is a rapid transfer of lead from the blood of pregnant women, through the placenta to the fetus.[2]

The Centers for Disease Control and Prevention (CDC) in Atlanta estimates that lead poisoning kills 200 children annually, and that between 400,000 to 600,000 children have elevated levels of lead in their blood. Most of the lead exposure comes from homes built before 1945. Since then, lead-free paint has reduced this exposure.[2] Children can also get lead poisoning by eating dirt near the house where lead from an old house remains in the soil, or where lead is deposited there by automobile exhausts.

Acute lead poisoning causes colic, cramps, diarrhea or constipation, leg cramps and drowsiness. In children exposed to large amounts of lead, or heavy drinkers of illicitly distilled whiskey, there may be disturbances of the central nervous system; permanent damage to the brain; kidney damage; and shortened life span, of the erythrocytes or red blood cells. Chronic lead poisoning results in colic, constipation, palsy in the forearm and fingers, mental depression, chronic nephritis, convulsions and a blue line at the edge of the gums.[2]

A number of recent studies have shown that lead poisoning of children can affect their rate of growth and intelligence and school performance. The effects of lead in the blood and growth were explored by Carol A. Huseman and co-workers at the University of Nebraska Medical Center in Omaha, and reported the August 29, 1992 issue of *Science News*. Their study involved 12 children and measured growth rates and levels of hormones that play a significant role in regulating growth.

At the beginning of the year-long study, the researchers studied six of the children before and after they were administered chelation therapy to reduce their toxic levels of lead. The other six children did not have abnormal amounts of the metal. In the full study, which appeared in *Pediatrics*, the team reported diminished levels of growth hormone and insulin-like growth factor-1 (IGF-1) among the children in the higher-lead group. In contrast with the low-lead group, children requiring chelation grew far more slowly than normal, the publication added. After receiving chelation therapy, however, the children experienced a growth spurt. In one case, the bone-growth rate almost tripled.[3]

"The researchers also assayed several growth-hormone characteristics every 20 minutes throughout one 24-hour period prior to chelation therapy in two children with extremely high blood-lead levels," the magazine continued. "Nearly all of the features . . . such as average and peak nighttime growth-hormone concentrations, and the number of hormone pulses released into the blood, compared unfavorably with values seen in normal short children and even in children suffering from growth-hormone neurosecretory dysfunction."[3]

In an earlier study, the Nebraska researchers found that high levels of lead inhibited thyroid-stimulating hormone, a pituitary-gland secretion that also helps to regulate growth.[3]

When David Bellinger, Ph.D., of the Harvard Medical School in Boston studied 150 children, he found that the higher the children's lead concentrations at the age of two years, the lower their IQ scores on mathematics and other tests at the age of 10, according to the January 7, 1993 issue of *Medical Tribune*. The children had lead levels that ranged from 0 to 15 mcg/dl of blood. The Centers for Disease Control and Prevention has suggested the upper limit of safe lead concentrations is 10 mcg/dl, but they do not actually know if levels below 10 mcg are without effect or even safe.

Bellinger determined that, for every 10-mcg increase in lead concentrations, there was a 6-point decrease in IQ scores and a 9-point decrease in scores achieved in tests measuring performance in mathematics, spelling and other academic areas, the publication continued. He added that, "while most previous studies have demonstrated the effects of lead in disadvantaged children, the new study involved only children from middle- and upper-middle-class homes."[4]

Although the major sources of lead contamination were previously thought to be lead-based paints in deteriorating homes and dust, a new study suggests an equally ominous source: water from the faucet. The Environmental Protection Agency said that 20 percent of the lead intake in this country comes from drinking water.[5]

As previously mentioned, another source of lead contamination is dirt that children play in. Children can get lead poisoning from playing in lead-contaminated soil and putting their fingers in their mouths, reported Rufus Chaney of the USDA's Agricultural Research Service in Beltsville, Maryland. In a report in 1991, Chaney found lead levels as high as 5,000 or more parts per million (ppm) in tests of some gardens in Baltimore. Soil with more than 500 ppm of lead is considered hazardous waste by the EPA.

Generally, lead contamination ranges between 15 and 40 ppm in most soils, Chaney said. But soils in older cities accumulate much higher lead levels from airborne paint chip dust and dust contaminated by auto exhausts. A number of Cooperative Extension Service offices, such as in Maryland, Minnesota, Texas, Wisconsin and other states will test soil for a charge of $10.[6]

Although experts do not recommend that all children be tested for lead contamination, they do recommend it for those who have a high risk. The CDC has called for an annual screening of high-risk children under the age of six, and that perhaps all children in that age group should be screened during the first years of their life, according to the November 17, 1992 issue of *Medical Tribune*. Although lead was banned from paint in the 1970s, it is still found in schools and homes that used lead-based paints.[7]

"Some studies have shown that 55 percent of urban African-American children under the age of six, and 7 percent of suburban middle-class children in that age group, have moderately elevated levels of lead in their blood," the publication added. "But Mary Ellen Mortensen, M.D., of Ohio State University, warned that chelation for lead poisoning carries risks of its own, and doctors should be selective in administering the treatment to children with moderate lead levels."[7]

Originally tested on adults with occupational plumbism, the drug, DMSA (2,3-dimercaptosuccinic acid), significantly reduces blood levels of lead with no apparent side effects, reported Marguerite Holloway in the January 19, 1989 issue of *Medical Tribune*. She quoted Joseph Graziano, M.D., professor of pharmacology at Columbia University's College of Physicians and Surgeons in New York City, as saying that similar results in children suggest that DMSA may find its greatest application in the treatment of pediatric lead poisoning.[8]

LURKING IN DRINKING WATER

Research suggests that water from self-contained systems, such as water coolers and fountains, is prone to lead contamination, stated Heda Lugo de Slosser in the March 1989 issue of *Consumer News*, a publication of Cornell University

Cooperative Extension, New York City. Linda Wagenet added that, "In water coolers and fountains, water can sit undisturbed for many hours each day and night, when the school is closed." Wagenet, who is home water-quality specialist with Cornell Cooperative Extension, added that the longer water sits, the more lead is liable to leach out from lead-soldered pipes. The solution, she said, is to let the water run for several minutes before drinking it. And ask your school to thoroughly flush fountains each morning, she added.[9]

The EPA and the Office of Drinking Water have published a 58-page report, "Lead in School's Drinking Water," which school administrators can purchase from the Office of Drinking Water at 202 783-3238 for $3.25. The publication provides general information on the significance of lead in school drinking water; how it affects children; how to pinpoint the source of contamination; how to reduce or eliminate lead in the water system; etc. The booklet can also be purchased for $3.25 from the Superintendent of Documents, Dept. 36-ES, Washington, D.C. 20402.[10]

By lowering the levels of lead in the blood of moderately lead-poisoned children, it is possible to reverse any possible damage as well as to raise intelligence scores, according to Roger Field in the April 29, 1993 issue of Medical Tribune.[11,12]

The study, initially reported by Holly Ruff, M.D., John Rosen, M.D., and colleagues at the Albert Einstein College of Medicine, Bronx, New York, in the April 7, 1993 issue of The Journal of the American Medical Association, involved 154 children, ranging in age from one to seven, with blood-lead levels between 25 and 55 mcg/dl. On average, Field quoted Rosen as saying, the treated children experienced an 8 mcg/dl decrease in lead levels in their blood. Six months later, the children had a 2.7 percent increase in cognitive index and IQ. He noted that, although this is a modest improvement in intelligence score, it "may turn out to be the difference between graduation from high school and future productivity in the workplace."[11,12]

The New York researchers used a number of procedures to lower the lead levels in the children, including inspection of the children's homes for possible lead toxicity. Therapies included the chelating agent edetate calcium disodium and an iron supplement.[11,12]

Ten percent of all American children have been exposed to unsafe levels of lead at one time or another, reported The Journal of the American College of Nutrition in October 1992. Abnormal amounts of lead in the blood are related to high blood pressure, lower class standing, absenteeism from school, kidney dysfunction, lower verbal scores, poor coordination and other health problems. Lead levels can sometimes be reduced with iron, calcium, zinc and calcium EDTA, the publication added.[13]

In an article in the August 18, 1993 issue of *The Journal of the American Medical Association*, based on data from the CDC, it was found that exposure to lead-based paint is the leading cause of high-dose lead exposure among children in the United States. Sources of lead contamination in the study group included paint; bean pots or other large holloware, which leach lead; lead-contaminated soil; azarcon and greta, two Hispanic remedies; paylooah, a Southeast Asia remedy; surma, an Asian Indian remedy; and others.[14]

An adequate dietary intake of calcium may reduce lead absorption and toxicity, reported K. Kostial and colleagues from the University of Zagreb in former Yugoslavia in *Biological Trace Element Research* in 1991. Blood levels of lead were lower in a region where women had a dietary intake of 940 mg/day of calcium.[15]

NUTRIENTS CAN PREVENT ILL EFFECTS

Adequate calcium nutrition can protect against the toxicity of such environmental toxins as lead and cadmium, stated Sheldon Saul Hendler, M.D., Ph.D., in *The Purification Prescription*. He added that this may, in part, explain why calcium is beneficial in the control of high blood pressure, which is sometimes related to heavy-metal toxicity. He said that lead can enter our bodies from air, water and food, and that lead sources include leaded gasoline, old plumbing, newer plumbing containing lead solder, certain imported ceramics, batteries and paint pigments. This can contribute to depression, memory problems, fatigue and other related problems, he said.

"Some nutrients are known to protect against lead toxicity," Hendler continued. "These include calcium, magnesium, copper and iron. Also, vitamin B6, vitamin B12, vitamin C, vitamin E and selenium offer protection. A vitamin and mineral supplement is recommended for those at risk for lead exposure," he added.

"Milk protects against lead toxicity because of calcium," he continued. "Fats increase the absorption of lead into the body. A low-fat diet is, therefore, protective. Alginates, which are found in brown seaweed (hijiki, kombu, wakame and arame), and polysaccharides found in red seaweed (nori, agar and dulse) decrease the absorption of lead. Liberal intake of edible seaweed is recommended."[16]

Occasionally, the development of lead poisoning in household pets leads to the identification of children with lead intoxication, according to Robert Dowsett, B.M., B.S., of the University of Massachusetts Medical Center, in Worcester, and Michael Shannon, M.D., M.P.H., of Children's Hospital in Boston, in the December 15, 1994 issue of *The New England Journal of Medicine*. They found three such children in two families.[17]

In the first family, a pet dog had persistent vomiting and weight loss, which surfaced one month after the exterior of the house was painted. A veterinarian diagnosed lead poisoning, and the animal recovered after receiving chelation therapy. But the dog was readmitted nine months later with blood lead levels of 120 mcg/dl, the researchers continued. This prompted the family to have their one- and three-year-old children tested for lead poisoning. They were found to have blood levels of 48 and 37 mcg/dl, respectively. Lead exposure was traced to lead-paint chips found in the yard. The one-year-old child recovered after receiving edetate calcium disodium and penicillamine. Blood levels in the older child subsided when the family moved to deleaded housing, the researchers said.

In the second family, their pet cat exhibited vomiting, somnolence and lack of coordination one month after the exterior of a neighbor's house was renovated. The cat was determined to have lead poisoning and was given chelation therapy. Their two-year-old child was found to have a blood lead level of 24 mcg/dl. The child is being monitored without undergoing chelation therapy.

"Family pets, including dogs, cats, birds, rabbits and iguanas, can show severe signs of lead poisoning with common signs being vomiting, somnolence and seizures," the researchers added. "Pets may thus serve to identify lead-contaminated environments. These cases suggest that screening of young children for lead intoxication should be considered in families with pets who have lead poisoning."[17]

Writing in the May/June 1994 issue of *Women's Health Access*, a newsletter published by Women's Health America, Madison, Wisconsin (608-833-9102), the authors reported that lead paint in older homes is a leading source of lead poisoning. But there are other sources, they said, including:[18]

1. Some crayons can be sources of lead poisoning, such as : 12 Jumbo Crayons by Concord Enterprises; Safe 48 Non-Toxic by Toys 'R' Us; 12 Crayons Glory by Glory Stationery Manufacturing; 18 Crayons That Paint by Glory Stationery Manufacturing; and crayons not carrying the label "Conforms to ASTM-D-4236" should be thrown out according to the Consumer Product Safety Commission.
2. Air, soil and clothing can carry lead used in heavy industry. Industry workers then bring it home on their clothing.
3. Other sources include hobbies, some ceramic dishes, lead-soldered cans, lead pipes, dolomite calcium supplements and the bright red and yellow paints on bread bags.

The organization offers the "Lead Test" kit, which can determine the presence of lead in paint, toys, water pipes, dishes, soil, pottery and cooking utensils without using hazardous materials. The kit, which contains enough materials for eight tests, costs $9.95, plus shipping and handling.[18]

Another kit, "Water Lead Test Kit," can determine the presence of lead in home drinking water. The kit, including a sample vial, cardboard mailer and prepaid mailing label, requires filling the sample vial with tap water and mailing it. Within three weeks a complete analysis report is returned by mail. This kit costs $29.95, including lab fees, but does not include shipping and handling.[18]

"A 1986 EPA draft report cites lead as a significant contributor to high blood pressure and risk of pregnancy complications," stated Robert A. Anderson, M.D., in *Wellness Medicine*. "The positive correlation between blood lead levels and systolic (beating) and diastolic (resting) blood pressures has been shown to be statistically significant. Lead bonds to bone from which it may later be released with prolonged or violent exercise in sufficiently large amounts to bring on acute attacks of lead poisoning. Excretion of lead from the body takes twice as long as its accumulation."[19]

He added that the bones of present-day Americans contain 500 times as much lead as the bones of ancient Peruvians. And it is estimated that worldwide industry spews 400,000 tons of lead into the atmosphere each year. Hippocrates wrote about the lead poisoning, including its treatments, nearly 1,500 years ago, he said.

"Von Hilsheimer reports that many of his long-term adolescent patients with intractable mental problems had high lead values," Anderson continued. "A Mexico Ministry of Health study demonstrated lead poisoning in significant numbers of children in Ciudad Juarez, a city downwind from an El Paso smelter. Lead poisoning is a problem for women of childbearing age who work in the manufacture of batteries.

Lead, mercury and cadmium react with sulfur-containing glutathione, cysteine and methionine, reducing their availability to oppose free-radical formation, Anderson continued. Lead reacts with selenium, which inactivates the selenium-containing antioxidant glutathione peroxidase. Lead and heavy metal intoxication are, therefore, associated with increased risk of cancer, probably through the interference with antioxidant mechanisms, he said.

"Nearly 20 percent of Americans consume levels of lead in drinking water from public systems exceeding federal standards of safety," Anderson added. "Dietary lead comes chiefly from food stored in soldered tin cans. The solder used to seal the vertical seams on standard three-piece tin cans contains 97 percent lead. The varnish used to seal the inner surface of cans may be totally inadequate; one investigator found a concentration of lead in canned tuna which was 10,000 times that of fresh tuna. Soldered tin cans may be recognized by peeling the paper label from the outside and observing the rough patch of silvery-gray metal over the seam, which differs in color and texture from the smooth, shiny surface of the can."[19]

Lead has no known functions or health benefits for humans, reported Alexandra Greeley in the July-August 1991 issue of *FDA Consumer*. It is considered a metabolic poison, meaning that it inhibits some of the basic enzyme functions, causing humanity untold ills.[20]

She quoted Joseph LaDou, M.D., chief of the division of occupational and environmental medicine at the University of California at San Francisco, as saying that, "Once lead enters the body, it is treated like calcium because the body can't tell the difference between the two." After several weeks, he added, lead leaves the bloodstream and is absorbed by bone, where it can continue to accumulate over a lifetime.[20]

"Probably the first published link between lead ingestion or inhalation and illness or death was made in the second century B.C. by the Greek physician Nicander, who wrote graphically about the tortures of lead poisoning—foaming lips, bloated belly, drooping limbs and an inflamed mouth," Greeley continued. "Without intervention, Nicander observed, 'the sick man descends to the Stygian shades.' "[20] (Characteristic of the river Styx, the river encircling Hades over which Charon ferried the souls of the dead.)

Since that time, Greeley continued, scientists and physicians have catalogued a lengthy list of health effects that they attributed to lead, such as: damage to the kidney and liver, and to the nervous, reproductive, cardiovascular, immune and gastrointestinal systems. In addition, lead interferes with the manufacture of heme, the oxygen-carrying part of hemoglobin in red blood cells. Very high levels of lead in the body cause encephalopathy, or degenerative brain disease, which, if untreated, results in death, she said.[20]

HYPERACTIVITY OR LEAD POISONING?

Greeley quoted LaDou as saying that damage to a child's nervous system is permanent, and some experts are now suggesting that low doses of lead may be responsible for some behavioral problems that most people call hyperactivity, such as the Puerto Rican child (discussed in the article) who could not sit still in the doctor's office. Even the subtle effects may be permanent, said Sue Binder, M.D., chief of the Lead Poisoning Prevention Branch of the CDC. Added Herbert Needleman, M.D., professor of psychiatry and pediatrics at the University of Pittsburgh, "It is a reasonable assumption that 20 percent of delinquency is associated with lead intake."[20]

Since lead accumulates over a lifetime, added Kathryn Mahaffey, Ph.D., science advisor in the office of the director, National Institute of Environmental Sciences in North Carolina, people may be harboring in their bones deposits of a toxic chemical. And, she added, lead may reenter the bloodstream at any time as a result of severe biologic stress—such as renal failure, pregnancy and even meno-pause. Richard Wedeen, M.D., associate chief of staff, research and development, V.A. Medical Center, East Orange, New Jersey, and author of *Poison in the Pot: The Legacy of Lead*, added that lead may also reappear during prolonged immobi-lization and a very severe disease.[20]

It is reasonable to assume that lead contaminates every biochemical function, Wedeen continued. And, he said, there may be racial implications as well. As an example, black males are six times overrepresented in end-stage renal disease programs in our society, and these figures may well be related to lead exposure, he said. It is a well-known fact that black male children have the highest lead exposure and blood lead levels of any group in the United States, he added.

"Symptoms of lead exposure may not be identified unless the doctor does specific kinds of testing," Wedeen said. "Many adults with mental symptoms due to lead encephalopathy may be misdiagnosed as alcoholics. Conversely, adults who suffer from acute lead poisoning may become alcoholics and end up in mental institutions.

Measuring the level of lead in blood is the most common way to estimate how much lead is circulating in the body, Greeley continued. But, since lead migrates to bones several weeks after entering the bloodstream, a number of scientists are in favor of using a more precise technique, such as measuring the amount of lead in bones and teeth, she said. In the 1970s, scientists set the maximum safe blood lead level for adults at 45 mcg/dl, and in 1985 for children at 25 mcg/dl. Since then, however, research has shown that adverse effects can occur at lower levels. For adults, according to Mike Bolger, M.D., toxicologist at FDA's Center for Food Safety and Applied Nutrition, lead toxicity is associated with blood lead levels as low as 30 mcg/dl. For children, toxicity occurs at 10 mcg/dl, he said.[20]

According to Gregory D. Miller, Ph.D., senior research scientist and chairman of the International Life Sciences Institute, Nutrition Foundation Committee on Diet and Behavior:

An interaction between lead and essential elements might be a mechanism involved in the neurobehavioral sequelae of low level lead exposure during development. Developing animals exposed to lead slowly accumulate lead in the brain and only to low levels, with a concomitant reduction of brain levels of zinc and iron. Additionally, animals exposed to low levels of lead exhibit behavioral abnormalities, such as impaired learning performance, increased behavioral excitability and altered motor activity patterns that are behavioral perturbations similar to those observed with dietary deficiencies of zinc and iron. Thus, alterations in the central nervous system's functioning might result from lead-induced alterations in the absorption or metabolism of zinc and/or iron.[21]

Increased body concentrations of lead or decreased tissue levels of essential elements can have detrimental effects on many different biochemical systems in many different cell types, Miller added. And the normal development of the brain can be adversely affected by undernutrition and/or toxic agents. Understanding the role of nutritional status and dietary intake of essential elements on lead intoxication in developing animals might help in developing public health policy directed toward the prevention and treatment of this health hazard, he said.[21]

In the *Journal of Learning Disabilities*, in 1985, C. Moon, et al., studied the relationship between cognitive functioning and hair-metal concentrations of lead, arsenic, mercury, cadmium and aluminum in 69 randomly selected elementary children. Their data showed that increases in arsenic and the interaction of arsenic and lead resulted in decreased reading and spelling achievement. And increases in aluminum and the interaction between aluminum and lead were significantly related to decreased visual-motor performance.[22]

STILL ON THE JOB

Phillip J. Landrigan, M.D., M.Sc., of Mt. Sinai Medical Center in New York City, reported in the *American Journal of Public Health* in 1990 that overexposure of American workers to lead is a "national scandal," and that nonessential uses of lead can no longer be tolerated. He added that there is a subclinical toxicity involved with lead exposure, which can cause inhibition of enzymes, kidney damage, high blood pressure, sperm malformation, slowing of nerve conduction and central nervous system dysfunction. These conditions have apparently occurred in healthy workers at levels of exposure to airborne lead below OSHA's permissible limit, he added.[23]

Thiamine (vitamin B1) appears to decrease lead deposition in blood, liver and kidney, and the combination treatment with calcium ethylenediamine tetraacetic acid or other chelating agents may enhance the treatment of lead intoxication, according to a rat experiment reported by Barry R. Blakley, et al., in the *Journal of Applied Toxicology* in 1990.[24]

High exposures to lead have been linked to a range of neurological problems, including reduced IQ, impaired hearing and trouble maintaining motor control and balance, reported the January 14, 1995 issue of *Science News*. Science does not yet understand how lead affects the brain, but it seems that it may eventually enlist the body's immune system in its attacks.[25]

During the past two years, Hassan A. N. El-Fawal at New York University's Institute of Environmental Medicine in Tuxedo, New York, has correlated brain proteins circulating in the blood of lead-exposed rodents with bloodborne antibodies to them, the publication reported. If he and his colleagues could link lead exposure to these antibodies, they would have a simple blood test to pick up early effects of lead on the brain.[25]

"Though preliminary, the NYU group's research 'is very suggestive' that antibodies to brain proteins might be 'setting up an immunological attack on the brain,' noted David A. Lawrence of New York State's Wadsworth Center in Albany," the publication continued. "His own work indicates that exposure to lead and various other heavy metals can upset the balance between two classes of the immune system's helper T-cells in favor of cells less able to ward off certain viral infections."[25]

Exposure to lead can cause miscarriages, developmental retardation, hearing loss and impaired vitamin D metabolism, according to Joel Schwartz at the Harvard School of Public Health in Boston, reported the September 3, 1988 issue of *Science News*. He found "a robust relationship between low-level lead exposure and blood pressure," even though the mean blood lead level in the group tested was 17 mcg/dl, well below the 25 mcg/dl considered excessive for children.[26]

Schwartz went on to say that although a 10 mcg/dl increase in blood lead levels may correspond to no more than a 2 ml mercury increase in average systolic blood pressure, this small change could have important consequences, *Science News* continued. Herman A. Tyroler, an epidemiologist at the University of North Carolina in Chapel Hill, concurred, noting that data from the national Hypertension and Detection Follow-Up Program indicates that a 2 ml mercury decrease in blood pressure might be associated with as much as an eight to 10 percent decrease in premature death.[26]

DEADLY DRINKS

The Bureau of Alcohol, Tobacco and Firearms completed a study in June, 1991, which found that three to four percent of table wine tested contained more than 300 ppb of lead, reported the December 1991 issue of *The FDA Medical Bulletin*. The Agency advised health professionals to warn pregnant and nursing mothers that wine can contain low levels of lead that may be hazardous to the mother and her fetus. At the time the FDA was considering legislation to tighten existing standards for lead-glazed ceramic products and to prohibit the use of lead-soldered food cans.[27]

"Scientists from Columbia University in New York recently reported that tiny amounts of lead began to migrate within a few minutes after wine was poured into many lead crystal decanters and wine glasses," reported Lawrence K. Altman in the February 19, 1991 issue of *The New York Times*. "Large amounts of lead were found in wine that had been stored for a long time in a decanter but the amounts varied widely among the crystal containers tested."[28]

Altman quoted Joseph H. Graziano, M.D., of Columbia University, as saying that apple juice and infant formula leached lead from crystal baby bottles about as fast as alcohol does. Since the developing nervous system of an infant is so sensitive to lead, Graziano and his colleagues, including Conrad Blum, M.D., recommended a ban on the sale of crystal baby bottles. At least one company, Waterford Wedgwood P.L.C., has discontinued production of the bottles.[28]

The Columbia University researchers said that, after port was poured into one decanter, periodic tests showed that the amount of lead in the liquid rose steadily over four months to 5,331 mcg/liter from 89, Altman reported.[28]

Members of a Westchester County, New York family were falling ill and they couldn't figure out why, reported Dale Blumenthal in "Food Risk: Perception vs. Reality," an *FDA Consumer* special report in 1990. Marco Tulio Rey, 67, went to see his doctor about his stomach pains. The doctor initially thought that Rey might have stomach cancer, but other symptoms troubled him, such as severe anemia. After tests showed that Rey had an abnormally high level of lead in his blood, he was treated for lead poisoning. He recovered after two weeks of hospitalization, Blumenthal reported. Other members of the family began complaining of fatigue and dizziness. Tests showed that six members of the Rey family had seriously high blood lead levels, but, fortunately, only one required hospitalization.

While the family was recovering, a Westchester County public health worker visited the Rey home and found the culprit: a brown jug that a friend had purchased in Mexico and given them as a gift. It was used to store a fermented sugar and bean drink. The worker noticed the glaze inside the jug was corroded and the jug was lined with a powder residue that may have contained a high lead content.[29]

"Most glazes for ceramic products contain lead but are safe because they have been properly formulated and fired to prevent the release of toxic amounts of metal into foods," Blumenthal continued. "However, some pottery, especially earthenware made by individuals and in small cottage industries abroad, have not been treated properly. In these pieces, acid substances may interact chemically with the glaze and accelerate the lead release. Therefore, acidic foods—orange, tomato or other fruit juices, tomato sauces, wines and vinegar—stored in improperly glazed containers are potentially the most dangerous. In the 1987 case of the brown jug from Mexico, says Frederick Morrisey, a program coordinator at the Westchester County Department of Health, the acidic nature of the bean drink gradually ate away at the glaze."[29]

Edward A. Steele of the FDA was quoted as saying that many ceramic products he found at roadside stands and local shops in various countries would dangerously violate the American standard. When he tested a small fruit dish he purchased at a shop in Spain, he found that it leached 25.5 ppm of lead. The U.S. legal limit for a small dish is 5 ppm.[29]

Military personnel and others stationed abroad are at high risk for lead poisoning, Steele was quoted as saying. U.S. citizens who move to foreign countries often purchase an entire set of dinnerware for use. But often this dinnerware does not meet U.S. standards for lead, he said.

"Such was the case with Donald and Frances Wallace," Blumenthal continued. "While stationed in Italy, they bought new household items, including a pair of terra cotta coffee mugs. They each drank eight to 10 cups of coffee a day from their mugs, and after three years it nearly killed them. The symptoms of lead poisoning are insidious and often misdiagnosed. Wallace underwent two operations for carpal tunnel syndrome, a painful wrist disorder that he didn't have. Mrs. Wallace's doctors thought she was suffering from porphyria, a rare, incurable metabolic disorder. Her body ached; she was dehydrated and anemic. To regain strength, she drank bouillon and juice daily from her terra cotta mug.

On his own, Wallace began researching their conditions and learned that lead poisoning caused many of the symptoms that continued to weaken them. A doctor measured their blood for lead levels, and found that both of the Wallaces were victims of acute lead poisoning.

"Although ceramic products purchased from vendors in foreign countries remain the chief concern, FDA is looking to a quick color test developed by FDA chemists John Gould and Stephen Capar to set up inspection of imports," Blumenthal said. "This test can determine—within 30 minutes—whether a ceramic product leaches excessive amounts of lead. As this article goes to press, the patent is pending for the FDA quick-color test."[29]

The Food and Drug Administration recommends that ceramic tableware, especially when purchased in Mexico, the People's Republic of China, Hong Kong and India, be tested for lead release by a commercial laboratory on your return or be used for decorative purposes only.[29]

Writing in *The Journal of the American Medical Association*, November 16, 1994, Howard Hu, et al., said that their study provides new clues in understanding the full toxicological implications of lead exposure and accumulation. Since bone lead may be a better biological marker than blood level of lead for chronic toxicity, they suggested that further research should be directed at the relationship of bone lead to the outcomes explored in their study, as well as others, such as cognitive functioning, peripheral nerve conduction and reproductive outcomes.[30]

They had previously reported a case study in which bone lead was found to be the source of recurrent lead toxicity long after environmental lead exposure had ceased in a 37-year-old woman who had developed increased bone turnover during an excessive production of thyroid hormone. Their new study involved construction trade union members, who engage in carpentry, demolition and other construction activities, and is believed to be the first such study to determine if the concentration of lead in bone constitutes a biological marker that is more sensitive to chronic toxicity than blood lead levels.[30]

In spite of the extent of lead exposure in industrialized societies, great gaps exist in our knowledge of the chronic toxicity of lead, reported Phillip J. Landrigan, M.D., M.Sc., and Andrew C. Todd, Ph.D., in an editorial in the January 19, 1994 issue of *The Journal of the American Medical Association*.[31]

"Lack of a sensitive and specific biologic marker of cumulative exposure has long been an impediment to research in this field," the authors said. "The fundamental problem is that the blood lead level, the traditional index of absorption, reflects only relatively recent exposure because the half-life of lead in blood is only about 36 days. In persons with chronic exposure, there is little correlation between a single, randomly obtained blood lead level and either a cumulative index of absorption or the body lead burden."[31]

A new technology—X-ray fluorescence (XRF) analysis of lead in bone—appears to hold substantial promise for overcoming those limitations. The XRF technique, which was detailed in the same issue of *JAMA* by Kosnett, et al., takes advantage of the fact that absorbed lead is stored in bone and has a half-life in dense cortical bone of at least 25 years. Thus, they added, it is hypothesized that direct measurement of lead in bone will provide data on cumulative past exposure and these data will be useful for epidemiologic analysis as well as for clinical assessment. The new technique involves less than 2.5 percent of the radiation of a chest X-ray examination, they said.[31]

REFERENCES

1. "Lead Poisoning from Ceramics," *Lancet*, December 10, 1988, p. 1358.
2. Ensminger, Audrey H., et al. *Foods and Nutrition Encyclopedia*. Clovis, Calif.: Pegus Press, 1983, pp. 1524, 1794.
3. "Why Lead May Leave Kids Short," *Science News*, August 29, 1992, p. 143.
4. "Lead/Learning Link Strengthened," *Medical Tribune*, January 7, 1993, p. 25.
5. Burros, Marian. "A Report Concludes Lead Can Be in Any Home's Water," *The New York Times*, January 27, 1993, p. C4.
6. Comis, Don. "Soil Test Identifies Potential Lead Poisoning," *USDA Scientific Research News*, April 1992.
7. "Panel Rejects Routine Lead Testing of Children," *Medical Tribune*, November 12, 1992, p. 10.
8. Holloway, Marguerite. "Oral Chelator Clears Lead from Blood Without Any Side Effects," *Medical Tribune*, January 19, 1989, p. 1.
9. de Slosser, Hada Lugo. "Lead in Water Fountains: Hazard to Children," *Consumer News*, Cornell University Cooperative Extension, March 1989.
10. Cameron, Jim. "Report Analyzes the Content of Lead in School Drinking Water," *Government Publications Outlook*, undated.
11. Field, Roger. "Removing Lead from Blood May Raise IQ," *Medical Tribune*, April 29, 1993, p. 4.
12. Ruff, Holly, M.D., et al. "Declining Blood Levels and Cognitive Changes in Moderately Lead-Poisoned Children," *The Journal of the American Medical Association* 269:1641–1646, April 7, 1993.
13. "Overview of Lead Toxicity Early in Life, Effects on Intellect Loss and Hypertension," *Journal of the American College of Nutrition* 11(5):608, October 1992.
14. "Lead Poisoning Associated with Use of Traditional Ethnic Remedies—California, 1991-1992," *The Journal of the American Medical Association* 270(7):808, August 18, 1993. For readers' comments concerning the Ruff, et al. study see Reference 12, pp. 827–830.

15. Kostial, K., et al. "Dietary Calcium and Blood Levels in Women," *Biological Trace Element Research* 28:181–185, 1991.
16. Hendler, Sheldon Saul, M.D., Ph.D., *The Purified Prescription*. New York: William Morrow and Co., Inc., 1991, pp. 45, 228.
17. Dowsett, Robert, B.M., B.S., and Shannon, Michael, M.D., M.P.H. "Childhood Plumbism Identified After Lead Poisoning in Household Pets," *The New England Journal of Medicine* 331(24):1661–1662, December 15, 1994.
18. "Lead Poisoning: The Silent Killer in Older Homes." *Women's Health Access*, May/June 1994.
19. Anderson, Robert A., M.D., *Wellness Medicine*. New Canaan, Conn.: Keats Publishing, Inc., 1987, pp. 45–46.
20. Greeley, Alexandra. "Getting the Lead Out of Just About Everything," *FDA Consumer*, July/August 1991, pp. 26–31.
21. Miller, Gregory D., Ph.D. "Interactions Between Lead and Essential Elements: Behavioral Consequences," *The Nutrition Report*, February 1991, pp. 9, 16.
22. Moon, C., et al. "Main and Interaction Effects of Metallic Pollutants on Cognitive Functioning," *Journal of Learning Disabilities* 18(4):217–221, 1985.
23. Landrigan, Phillip J., M.D., M.Sc. "Lead in the Modern Workplace," *American Journal of Public Health* 80(8):907–908, 1990.
24. Blakley, Barry R., et al. "The Effects of Thiamine on Tissue Distribution of Lead," *Journal of Applied Toxicology* 10(2):93–97, 1990.
25. Raloff, J. "Lead May Foster Immune Attack on Brain," *Science News*, January 14, 1995, p. 23.
26. "Has Lead Got Your Blood Pressure Up?" *Science News*, September 3, 1988, p. 158.
27. "Lead and Table Wines Could Pose Hazards for Pregnant and Nursing Women," *The FDA Medical Bulletin* 21(3):6–7, December 1991.
28. Altman, Lawrence K. "Storing Wine in Crystal Decanters May Pose Lead Hazard," *The New York Times*, February 19, 1991, p. C3.
29. Blumenthal, Dale. "An Unwanted Souvenir: Lead in Ceramic Ware," an *FDA Consumer* Special Report, "Food Risk: Perception vs Reality," 1990, pp. 39–42.
30. Howard, Hu, et al. "The Relationship Between Bone Lead and Hemoglobin," *The Journal of the American Medical Association* 272(19):1512–1517, November 16, 1994.
31. Landrigan, Phillip J., M.D., M.Sc., and Todd, Andrew C., Ph.D. "Direct Measurement of Lead in Bone: A Promising Biomarker," *The Journal of the American Medical Association* 271(3):239–240, January 19, 1994.

41

Mercury

IN our book, *Minerals: Kill or Cure?* Ruth Adams and I reported on the plight of W. Eugene Smith, a world-famous photographer, and his Japanese-American wife, Aileen, who, while living in the Japanese village of Minamata, observed the death and anguish that local residents suffered after eating mercury-tainted fish from polluted waters. As explained by Deidre Carmody in the January 27, 1971 issue of *The New York Times*, the Smiths began collecting evidence to be put in a book about the horrible conditions in the small fishing village.

> On July 7, 1972, during the course of a protest against the Chisso Corporation, a chemical company in Minamata that had been dumping industrial waste into the water, Mr. Smith was severely beaten by six men. As a result of his injuries, he is now almost entirely blind. Two weeks ago his condition worsened considerably. His failing vision disappeared and he was suffused with such violent pain that he kept blacking out. The beating occurred when Mr. Smith, his wife and some of the victims of the poisoning were waiting to see a union leader at the Chisso Company. According to Mr. Smith, he was suddenly surrounded, kicked in the stomach and then slammed across a chair. The six men grabbed his legs and swung him—like a cat, he said, onto the cement courtyard. He landed on his neck as his assailants jumped on him.[1]

He eventually died as a result of his injuries.

Although chemical companies usually do not resort to such extreme measures, they often practice more subtle forms of pollution, often dumping their wastes into rivers and streams at night when nobody is watching.

We reported an item from *Chemical Week*, which said that there are 7,000 hospitals in the United States, and that even a small one may dump as much as 150 pounds of mercury a year. And *Chemical and Engineering News* told the story of a dental assistant who, after her death, was found to have relatively enormous amounts of mercury in her kidneys, presumably because she had handled mercury (amalgam) fillings during her 20 years of work. Another source of mercury, which is not now so widespread, is the use of calomel or mercurous chloride in medicine.[1]

In ancient times, mercury was known as quicksilver, because of its slimy appearance and slippery form. Mercury is discharged into air and water from industrial operations and is used in herbicide and fungicide treatments. Mercury poisoning has occurred where mercury from industrial plants has been discharged into water and then accumulated as methyl mercury in fish and shellfish. Accidental consumption of seed grains treated with fungicides that contain mercury, used for the control of fungus diseases of oats, wheat, barley and flax, has also been reported.[2]

About 1,200 cases of mercury poisoning identified in Japan in the 1950s were traced to the consumption of fish and shellfish from Minamata Bay contaminated with methyl mercury. Children of exposed mothers were born with birth defects, and many victims suffered central nervous system damage. Another outbreak of mercury toxicity occurred in Iraq. More than 6,000 people were hospitalized after eating bread made from wheat that had been treated with methyl mercury.[2]

The organic compounds of mercury, such as the various fungicides, affect the central nervous system but are not corrosive. The inorganic compounds of mercury include mercuric chloride, a disinfectant; mercurous chloride (calomel), a cathartic; and elemental mercury. The toxic symptoms include corrosive gastrointestinal effects, such as vomiting, bloody diarrhea and necrosis of the alimentary mucosa.[2]

DANGEROUS EFFECTS

Robert A. Anderson, M.D. said in *Wellness Medicine*:

Mercury, one of the heavy metals, leads to toxic effects in man and is now ubiquitous in the environment as a result of the leaking of mercury from cinnabar (mercury sulfide in the earth's crust), industrial contamination, coal burning and use in fungicides. It adheres to the lipid tissues and is difficult to displace from the body. Among its effects is renal damage. Chronic mercury intoxication or poisoning gives symptoms of apathy, insomnia, anorexia, tachycardia, loss of hair and nails, restlessness, irritability and muscle weakness and pain. Other symptoms of chronic mercury toxicity may include dizziness, drowsiness, fatigue, depression, tremors, memory loss, shyness, headache, incoordination, dermatitis, numbness and paresthesias of the lips and feet, some loss of vision and hearing and emotional instability.[3]

Dental amalgams may contain mercury, silver, tin, zinc and copper, Anderson added. Gold and amalgam placed side by side in the mouth may act as a voltaic cell, generating potentials of 1,000 millivolts or more. These currents may electrolytically dissolve the amalgam, causing toxic or allergic reactions because of the dispersed metal ions which may include mercury.[3]

Almost 300 dentists were studied, using an X-ray fluorescent technique to assess their tissue levels of mercury. Twenty-three were found to have tissue levels over 20 mcg/g of tissue; 30 percent of this group had peripheral nerve damage. The low-mercury concentration group had no polyneuropathy.[3]

In 1973, the American Conference of Industrial Hygienists set the top limit of safety at 0.05 mg of mercury per cubic meter of air, according to *NIH News & Features*, September 25, 1976. Somewhat higher levels would not harm patients who are in dental offices only occasionally and for brief intervals, but could cause chronic fatigue and neurological damage to dentists and their assistants if they were constantly exposed, the NIH said. Wilmer B. Eames, D.D.S., et al., reported in the June 1976 issue of the *Journal of the American Dental Association* that there are three methods of decontaminating an office with unacceptable levels of mercury. A type of vacuum cleaner with special filters works best on hard surfaces and provides some help with close-woven carpets. But it is not recommended by the manufacturer for rugs with long naps.[4]

"A water-soluble powder applied to carpets quickly reduced the mercury which appears in the air after spills on carpets," NIH continued. "However, when such a rug was disturbed by foot-scuffing for several days, vapor levels increased to unacceptable levels again. The most satisfactory results, Eames found, came from a device that quickly filtered the air, provided the filters were changed frequently. Good outside ventilation, or air conditioning, helped reduce the burden from accidentally spilled mercury."

The best protection, Eames maintained, is prevention that comes from proper work habits. The main recommendation is to abstain from expressing mercury when mixing amalgam by using a ratio of no more than 1:1, mercury to alloy, NIH added. Avoidance of spilling is important, and so is consistent maintenance of ventilation without recirculating the air. The use of screw-cap capsules to prevent leakage while mixing amalgam, and the employment of water spray when removing old amalgam fillings at high speeds are also important, Eames said. NIH continued:

Carpets are not usually a factor in contamination, but mercury should be removed at once if a spill occurs, because ordinary vacuuming tends to disperse the metal in fine droplets and increases the chances of toxicity. Dentists who have practiced for many years in the same location may want to check their premises, and should ask their state or nearest federal agency in charge of occupational safety for information and help. The larger instruments used to detect mercury in the air are expensive and might best be purchased by dental societies for loan or rent by those who would like to be sure their offices and laboratories are safe. Badges and discs are more economical for individual use. The survey found that most laboratories have lower mercury levels than operatories, while waiting rooms are entirely safe.[4]

In their book, *Toxic Metal Syndrome*, H. Richard Casdorph, M.D., and Morton Walker, D.P.M., wondered whether or not silver-mercury amalgams might be related to Alzheimer's disease. Germany and Sweden have acknowledged that fact and have banned the use of mercury as dental filling material, they added. The Swedish Health and Welfare system demanded in July 1993 that the Swedish government submit a five-year plan for discontinuing the use of amalgam permanently because of environmental pollution and disease development in dental patients, they said.[5]

The authors added that John Miller, D.D.S., a New York dentist, has not filled a tooth with amalgams for nearly 15 years. Throughout his practice, Iowa family dentist, Carl W. Svare, D.D.S., was steadily replacing his patients' amalgam fillings with gold. New York allergy specialist, Alfred V. Zamm, M.D., has had all silver fillings removed from his own mouth. And, they continued, Colorado dental researcher Dr. Hal A. Huggins, author of *It's All in Your Head*, an expose on the dangers of mercury amalgams—is traveling across the North American continent to lecture about the dangers amalgam fillings present.[5]

They also reported that Massachusetts dentist and physician, Dr. Victor Penzer, has lost his license to practice dentistry because he has gone public with warnings about mercury amalgams. The Massachusetts Dental Association, which brought the charges against Dr. Penzer, fears that it, along with the American Dental Association, will be in jeopardy of class-action suits for malpractice if dental amalgams are shown to cause dementia and/or other degenerative diseases.[5]

MS, AD AND OTHER CONDITIONS

"These courageous health professionals are taking actions against mercury in our mouths," the authors said. "The toxic metal content in fillings of silver-mercury amalgam could possibly cause conditions ranging from diarrhea and insomnia to multiple sclerosis and Alzheimer's disease. Informed dentists and physicians advise that they are detecting mercury toxicity in their patients, and they urge those who test positive for the metal to have their dental amalgams replaced with some other material as soon as possible."[5]

Reporting in *Lancet* in 1990, F. L. Lorscheider and M. J. Vimy, of the University of Calgary in Canada, said their primate studies show that dental amalgams release more mercury vapor and more mercury is absorbed in other tissues than was previously thought. For that reason, they said that dental silver-mercury amalgams should not be put in pregnant females.[6]

Writing in the *Townsend Letter for Doctors*, July 1990, Sandra Denton, M.D., of Anchorage, Alaska, said that over 100 million people have mercury fillings in their mouth. She added that mercury is more toxic than lead, cadmium or arsenic, and that mercury vapor is released from fillings, especially after chewing, bruxism (clenching of teeth), hot and/or acidic food and tooth brushing. She added that the release of mercury from dental amalgams is probably the most significant cause of human exposure to inorganic mercury. Multiple sclerosis patients have been found to have up to eight times higher levels of mercury in their cerebrospinal fluid than neurologically healthy controls. And scrap metal amalgam was declared a hazardous waste in 1988 by the EPA.[7]

Strength vs Safety

Denton pointed out that, outside of your mouth, mercury has to be stored in unbreakable, tightly sealed containers away from heat; it cannot be touched; it should be stored under liquid glycerine or photographic fixer solution. So, she added, the paradox is once it is taken out of the mouth it is toxic, but when it is placed in the teeth it is "nontoxic." And, she said, the American Dental Association has not produced studies showing the safety of amalgam fillings; they have been tested for their strength but never their safety.[7]

She went on to say that dentists have the highest rates of suicide and divorce among professionals. She quoted Gerald Butler, Ph.D., of the University of North Texas at Denton, as saying that he found neuropsychological dysfunction in 90 percent of the dentists tested. And, she said, female dental personnel have higher rates of spontaneous abortion, raised incidence of premature labor and elevated perinatal mortality. In a Polish study of 81 females, 45 dentists and 35 dental assistants, hair mercury levels were much greater than in 34 nonexposed controls. There was a positive correlation between total mercury levels and reproductive failures as well as a prevalence of menstrual cycle disorders. There were five cases of spina bifida out of 117 pregnancies. Denton noted that folic acid deficiency has been associated with spina bifida (a deformed brain or spinal cord), and that mercury is a known inhibitor of folate metabolism in the body.[7]

Although there has been an awareness of mercury toxicity since the 1500s, occupational and residential exposure remains a source of poisoning, according to *Clinical Toxicology* in 1992. Death is an infrequent outcome, and is generally due to acute exposure to mercury. The patient is usually asymptomatic during the first one to four hours after acute exposure to high concentrations of mercury vapor; then symptoms begin abruptly, including fevers, chills, nausea, general malaise and respiratory difficulties. In some cases pulmonary edema can bring death in a few days. After inhalation, elemental mercury is absorbed through alveolar membranes and transported by the blood to the brain and other tissues of the nervous system. Mercury is rapidly converted by the blood to mercuric ions and is excreted in urine and feces, the publication said.[8]

The potential for indoor mercury exposure is increased when indoor air exchange is reduced, the publication added, such as when windows and doors are closed. Warm air from heating ducts and vents can increase volatilization when circulated over spilled mercury. Potential sources of elemental mercury in the home include mercury switches and mercury-containing devices—thermostats, thermometers and barometers. Family members can bring home elemental mercury from laboratories, dental offices or other industrial sources.[8]

In the same issue of *Clinical Toxicology*, Yiu K. Fung, Ph.D., and Michael P. Molvar, D.D.S., M.S., give an in-depth analysis of the possible hazards of amalgam restorations. They conclude that there is a need for further research to clarify the short- and long-term effects of mercury that is released from dental amalgam restorations into the dental environment.[9]

CATCH OF THE DAY

Fish is an important source of high-quality proteins, vitamins and minerals, and FDA seafood specialists say that eating a variety of types of fish, the normal pattern of consumption, does not put anyone in danger of mercury poisoning, according to Judith E. Foulke in the September 1994 issue of *FDA Consumer*. It is when people frequently eat only one type of food or a particular species of fish that they put themselves at risk, Foulke said.[10]

Fish absorb methyl mercury from water as it passes over their gills and as they feed on aquatic organisms, she continued. Larger predator fish are exposed to higher levels of methyl mercury from their prey. Methyl mercury binds tightly to the proteins in fish tissue, including muscle. Cooking does not appreciably reduce the methyl mercury content of the fish. For the amounts of mercury in various fish, see Table 41.1.

"Nearly all fish contain trace amounts of methyl mercury, some more than others," Foulke added. "In areas where there is industrial mercury pollution, the levels in the fish can be quite elevated. In general, however, methyl mercury levels for most fish range from less than 0.01 ppm to 0.5 ppm. It's only in a few species of fish that methyl mercury levels reach the FDA limit for human consumption of 1 ppm. This most frequently occurs in some large predator fish, such as shark and swordfish. Certain species of very large tuna, typically sold as fresh steaks or sushi, can have levels over 1 ppm."

She said that canned tuna, composed of smaller species of tuna such as skipjack and albacore, has much lower levels of methyl mercury, averaging only about 0.17 ppm. The average concentration of methyl mercury for commercially important species (mostly marine in origin) is less than 0.3 ppm.

Nevertheless, FDA scientists responsible for seafood safety agree that swordfish and shark are safe, providing they are eaten no more than once a week as part of a balanced diet. This is especially true for pregnant women.[10]

REFERENCES

1. Adams, Ruth, and Murray, Frank. *Minerals: Kill or Cure?* New York: Larchmont Books, 1974, pp. 235ff.
2. Ensminger, Audrey H., et al. *Foods and Nutrition Encyclopedia.* Clovis, Calif.: Pegus Press, 1983, pp. 1796–1797.
3. Anderson, Robert A., M.D. *Wellness Medicine.* New Canaan, Conn.: Keats Publishing, Inc., 1987, pp. 44–45.
4. "Mercury Vapor in Dental Offices Is Investigated," *NIH News and Features*, September 25, 1976.
5. Casdorph, H. Richard, M.D., and Walker, Morton, D.P.M. *Toxic Metal Syndrome.* Garden City Park, N.Y.: Avery Publishing Group, 1995, pp. 131ff.
6. Lorscheider, F. L., and Vimy, N. J. "Mercury from Dental Amalgams," *Lancet*, December 22-29, 1990, pp. 1578–1579.
7. Denton, Sandra, M.D. "The Mercury Cover-Up: Controversies in Dentistry," *Townsend Letter for Doctors*, July 1990, pp. 488–491.

TABLE 41.1

METHYL MERCURY LEVELS IN FISH

Results of FDA sampling for methyl mercury by species for October 1990 to October 1991 (the action level is 1 ppm).

FISH SPECIES	RANGE (PPM)
Bass, fresh water	0.15-0.34
Catfish, fresh and salt water	<0.10-0.31
Cod	Trace
Crabs	0.10-0.15
Croaker	0.13-0.32
Flounder	ND-0.08
Grouper	0.35-0.48
Haddock	Trace
Lobster	0.10-0.14
Mackerel	0.10-0.23
Mahi mahi (dolphin)	0.11-0.21
Marlin	0.10-0.92
Orange roughy	0.42-0.71
Oysters	<0.10
Perch, fresh water	ND-0.31
Perch, ocean (rosefish, red rockfish)	Trace-0.03
Pike	Trace-0.16
Pollock	ND-0.10
Salmon	ND-0.11
Shrimp	<0.10
Shark	0.23-2.95
Snapper, red	0.07-0.26
Swordfish	0.26-3.22
Trout	Trace-0.13
Tuna, canned	ND-0.75

ND means none detected

From *FDA Consumer*, September 1994.

8. "Acute and Chronic Poisoning from Residential Exposure to Elemental Mercury—Michigan, 1989-1990," *Clinical Toxicology* 30(1):63–67, 1992.

9. Fung, Yin K., Ph.D., and Molvar, Michael P., D.D.S., M.S. "Toxicity of Mercury from Dental Environment and from Amalgam Restorations," ibid, pp. 49–61.

10. Foulke, Judith E. "Mercury in Fish. Cause for Concern?" *FDA Consumer*, September 1994, pp. 5–8.

Index

A